P9-CBT-637

The Complete
MIND&

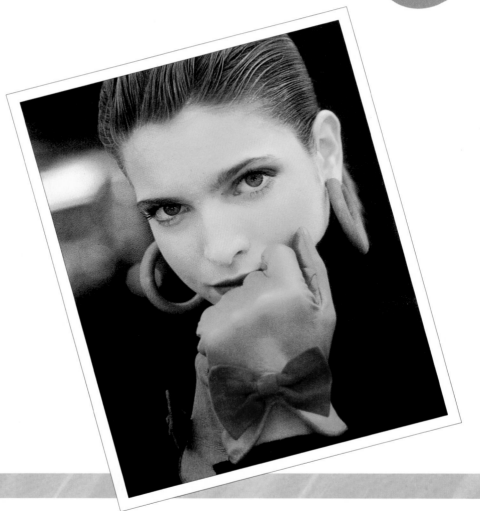

BODY BOOK

Total Bodycare

Edited by
Dr. Jean Ann Graham
—— *and* ——
Dr. Louise M. Wallace

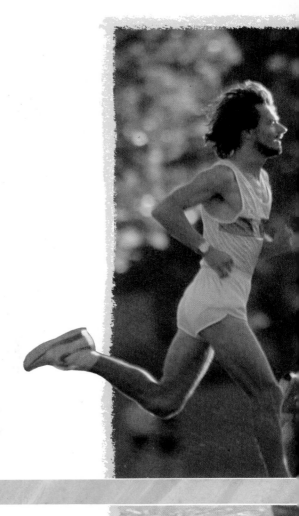

SIMON & SCHUSTER

New York   London   Toronto   Sydney   Tokyo   Singapore

CONTRIBUTORS

First published in the USA in 1990 by
Academic Reference Division
Simon & Schuster
15 Columbus Circle
New York, NY 10023

Devised and produced by
Andromeda Oxford Ltd
Dorchester-on-Thames
Oxford OX10 7JU, UK

Copyright © 1990
Andromeda Oxford Ltd

All rights reserved. No part of
this book may be reprinted or
reproduced or utilized in any form
or by any electronic, mechanical,
or other means, now known or
hereafter invented, including
photocopying and recording, or
in any information storage or
retrieval system, without
permission in writing from
the publishers.

Originated by Scantrans, Singapore

Printed and bound in Spain by
Graficas Velasco Torerias SA, Madrid

**Library of Congress
Cataloging-in-Publication data**

The Complete mind and body book:
total bodycare / [edited by] Jean Ann
Graham, Louise Wallace.
     p.   cm.
ISBN 0-13-924911-7
1. Health. 2. Beauty, Personal. 3. Mind
and body. I. Graham, Jean Ann.
II. Wallace, Louise
RA776.C753 1990
613–dc20
                         90-9795
                              CIP

Andromeda Oxford Ltd has
produced this publication with the
intention of making generally
available the result of serious
academic research and it would be
wholly inappropriate for the
editors and publisher to make any
substantive change to a contributor's
work. For this reason the editors
and publishers do not accept any
responsibility for the advice or
suggestions contained in this book.
As with all matters concerning
personal health, the application
of any techniques by any individual
should be taken with medical
advice.

VOLUME EDITORS

Dr Jean Ann Graham
International Psychological
Consultant, Cosmetics and
Appearance, North Wales, UK

Dr Louise M Wallace
Top-Grade Clinical Psychologist
(Physical Health), South Birmingham
Health Authority, UK

AUTHENTICATORS

Marie Johnston PhD
Reader in Health Psychology,
Royal Free Hospital School of
Medicine, University of London, UK

Dr J M Argyle
Department of Experimental
Psychology, Oxford University, UK

KEY TO AUTHORS

ACK   Dr Abby C King,
Stanford Center for Research in
Disease Prevention, Stanford
University School of Medicine, USA

AER   Anthony E Reading PhD,
Director, Psychological Studies,
Center for Reproductive Medicine,
Associate Clinical Professor, UCLA
School of Medicine, USA

CE   Dr Christine Eiser,
Senior Research Fellow in
Psychology, University of Exeter,
Devon, UK

CM   Dr Charles Morin,
Department of Psychiatry, Virginia
Commonwealth University, USA

CT   Dr Charles Twining,
Psychology Department, Whitchurch
Hospital, Cardiff, UK

DC   Dr Dan Cavanaugh,
Instructor, Department of Speech
Communication, University of
Texas at Austin, USA

DGS   David G Schlundt PhD,
Assistant Professor of Psychology and
Medicine, Vanderbilt University, USA

DJC   Dr David J Cooke,
Top-Grade Psychologist, Douglas
Inch Centre, Glasgow, UK

EH   Professor Elaine Hatfield,
Professor of Psychology, University
of Hawaii, USA

JAB   James A Blumenthal PhD,
Associate Professor of Medical
Psychology, Assistant Professor of
Medicine, Department of Psychiatry,
Duke University Medical Center, North
Carolina, USA

JAG   Dr Jean Ann Graham,
International Psychological Consultant,
Cosmetics and Appearance, North
Wales, UK

JMGW   Dr John Mark G Williams,
Research Scientist, Medical Research
Council, Applied Psychology Unit,
Cambridge, UK

JP-C   Jamie Pope-Cordle MS RD,
Director of Nutrition, Vanderbilt
Weight Management Program,
Vanderbilt University, USA

KB   Kevin Browne PhD,
Lecturer in Health Psychology,
School of Medicine, Department
of Psychology, University of
Leicester, UK

KW   Dr Keith Williams,
Department of Social Medicine,
University of Birmingham, UK

LE   Louise Earll,
Department of Neurology, Gloucester
Royal Infirmary, UK

LMW   Dr Louise M Wallace,
Top-Grade Clinical Psychologist
(Physical Health), South Birmingham
Health Authority, UK

MG   Professor Martin Gipson PhD,
Psychology Department, University of
the Pacific, Stockton, California, USA

MA   Dr J M Argyle,
Department of Experimental
Psychology, Oxford University, UK

MK   Dr Mark L Knapp,
Professor and Chair of the Department
of Speech Communication, University of
Texas at Austin, USA

MW-R   Margaret Walsh-Riddle MS,
Department of Psychiatry, Duke
University Medical Center, North
Carolina, USA

NEA   Nancy E Adler PhD,
Professor of Medical Psychology,
University of California, San Francisco,
USA

OWW   Dr O Wayne Wooley,
Department of Psychology, University of
Cincinnati Medical Center, Ohio, USA

PH   Dr Patrick Hill,
Department of Neurology, Gloucester
Health Authority, UK

RR   Rita Roberts,
International Cosmetic Consultant,
London, UK

SL   Susan Ledwith BSc MSc,
Principal Clinical Psychologist, South
Derbyshire Health Authority, UK

SLP   Dr Stephanie L Pinder,
Department of Psychiatry, Duke
University Medical Center, North
Carolina, USA

SW   Dr Stephen J Wright,
Lecturer in Health Psychology,
Department of Social Studies, Leeds
Polytechnic, UK

TWS   Dr Timothy W Smith,
Associate Professor of Psychology,
University of Utah, USA

PROJECT EDITOR
Fiona Mullan

TEXT

Editors
Kate Mertes and
Paul Barnett, Stephanie Boxall
Lauren Bourque, Paul Burns
Carol Busia, Nancy Duin
Justin Pearce, Della Thompson

Indexer
Kate Mertes

Compositor
Reina Foster-de Wit

Typesetting
Pauline Moroney, Lin Thomas

PICTURES

Research coordinator
Thérèse Maitland

Research assistant
Nicola Whale

Researchers
Celia Dearing, Jenny Speller
Suzanne Williams

ART

Senior art editor
Chris Munday

Designer
Martin Anderson

Additional layout designer
Kevin Hinton

Artists
Martin Cox, Simon Driver
Mary Ann Le May, Trevor Mason
Taurus Graphics, Alison Toft

SERIES EDITOR
Stuart McCready

CONTENTS

1

2

THINK OF ALL THE WAYS that your mind and body interact. One of the most important for everyday well-being – one which you may not even have thought about – is the mental image you form of your physical self. This is your body image, closely linked to your self-esteem. Are you healthy enough and do you look good enough for the life you want to live? Being able to answer yes boosts your confidence and happiness.

Very few of us can answer yes unequivocally, and most are at least vaguely aware of some change that would make our bodies more acceptable to our minds. This is the book that explains how to deal with these vague dissatisfactions constructively. The strategies include psychological ones – practicing greater self-acceptance when your ambitions for your body go beyond what is possible; and physical ones – eating a healthy diet and becoming fitter.

You may feel bombarded from all sides with information about what is good or not good for your health. Advice from medical experts and media personalities, family and friends, and even from your own doctor may seem contradictory and ultimately pointless. With so few healthy options left that are also enjoyable, good health might seem unattainable. Yet most of us are basically healthy and can choose whether or not to stay that way.

Part One – YOUR HEALTH – explores the myths that surround fitness and health care and helps you to make practical, informed choices. The health psychologists and medical experts who have contributed are carefully selected from their fields of study and have wide experience of helping people make healthy decisions for themselves.

Researchers have found that people are more concerned about what they can do to improve their health now than ever before. YOUR HEALTH explores why, and takes a look at how patterns of illness are changing. In previous centuries poor hygiene and public health meant that people were likely to die from infectious diseases such as tuberculosis or pneumonia. Now we tend to live longer but are more susceptible to chronic illness like heart disease and diabetes. Ill health is a risk – it is costly, inconvenient and it can disrupt our lives. Good health is largely a matter of lifestyle, and there is a great deal we can do to prolong it into old age.

What is health? Is it only expressed in the body, or does it involve the mind as well? How do body and mind interact? How is your health affected by your gender, age, lifestyle, behavior and body rhythms? Good health is more than a matter of avoiding illness and obtaining good medical care – it is our most valuable asset and is vitally important to the quality of our lives. In good health, we feel alert, fit and confident, are more likely to see our problems as challenges, and to seize life's opportunities instead of letting them go by.

Adopting a healthy lifestyle means taking responsibility for your mind and body and possibly making changes. Knowing what affects your health clarifies what you can and cannot change – it is easier to alter lifestyle if you understand the benefits and costs. It will also help you to assess for yourself your capacity for fitness. Knowing how to monitor your health, when to seek professional advice and how to get the best out of expert diagnosis and treatment will help you to feel in charge of your own body.

YOUR HEALTH gives you the information you need to make healthy choices in your life. It offers practical advice on how to evaluate your present state of fitness, how to get to know your own body, follow a healthy diet, take sufficient exercise, find time for relaxation, have a healthy sex life, get a good night's sleep and control your dependency on artificial stimulants and other drugs. Together with your knowledge of your own medical history and your commitment to a way of living that will benefit mind and body, it will put you in control of the way you look and the way you feel.

Louise M Wallace

INTRODUCTION
Your Appearance

RADIANT GOOD LOOKS depend partly on a healthy lifestyle. In addition, research has shown that lavishing cosmetic care and attention on your appearance can have a dramatic effect on the way you feel inside, and that there are social and psychological benefits to be gained from making yourself look more attractive. The combination of good health and good looks can, in turn, substantially improve the quality of your life.

Part two – YOUR APPEARANCE – discusses these psychological benefits and looks at the resources that are available to all of us to make the most of the way we look. How can we increase the likelihood of success at a job interview? What are the most up-to-date techniques in makeup and haircare, and why do they make a difference? These and many other questions are answered, together with information about how your appearance influences your self-esteem, the significance of being thought attractive by others, and the social and material advantages of looking good in different areas of our lives. More specifically, topics include the psychology of dress and what your clothes say about you, body language, developing a personal style and the techniques of good grooming for men and women alike.

Rapid social changes mean that trends and values in fashion and good looks evolve very quickly: attitudes toward the use of cosmetics by men, for example, have changed significantly. At the beginning of the last decade, it might have been considered odd for a man to visit a manicurist; today it is becoming more acceptable.

Whether you are a man or a woman, whether you think of yourself as an attractive person or not, YOUR APPEARANCE will guide you through the maze of different cosmetic treatments available for the face and body. It will provide insights into why the way we look affects how we feel and explain why self-image and self-esteem affect *the kind of opportunities that come your way in life, influence your chances of success at work control the way people behave toward you and affect your general well-being.* YOUR APPEARANCE *brings you the latest research into the psychology of dress, behavior and general cosmetic care. It shows that however attractive or unattractive you may feel at the moment, you can both improve your appearance and learn to feel better about the way you look.*

The information contained in YOUR APPEARANCE *has been carefully researched by psychologists and other experts in the fields related to professional beautycare. They have drawn from findings in the areas of medicine, the social sciences and cosmetology, particularly when the research has been closely linked with cosmetic care and its psychological impact. The information and advice that they present is offered in a readable and easily digestible form with practical guidance, tips and answers to common queries.*

Your potential for making cosmetic changes to your outward appearance is enormous. Here, at your fingertips, are techniques that can help you to make real changes in the way you look and the way you feel about yourself, especially in areas that you have considered a problem in the past. Good looks are for everyone who is prepared to look after them, and, built on the firm foundation of good health, they can have a dramatic effect on the way in which you live your life.

Jean Ann Graham

SUBJECT GUIDE
Your Health

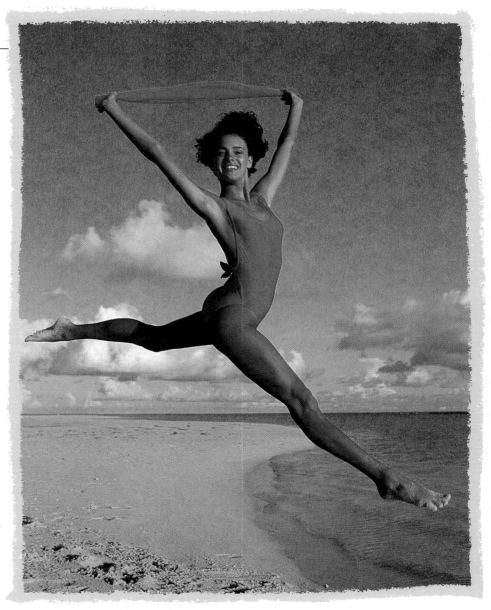

SUBJECT GUIDE
Your Appearance

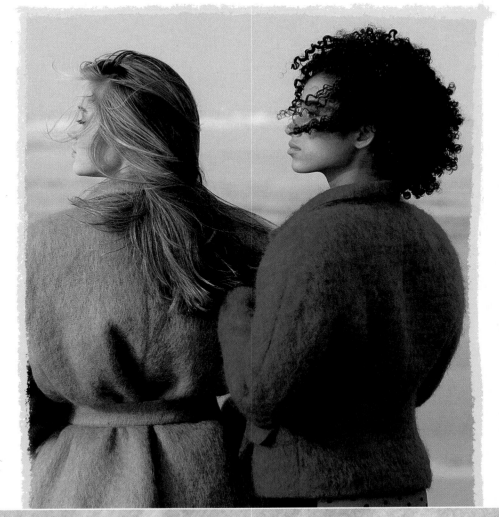

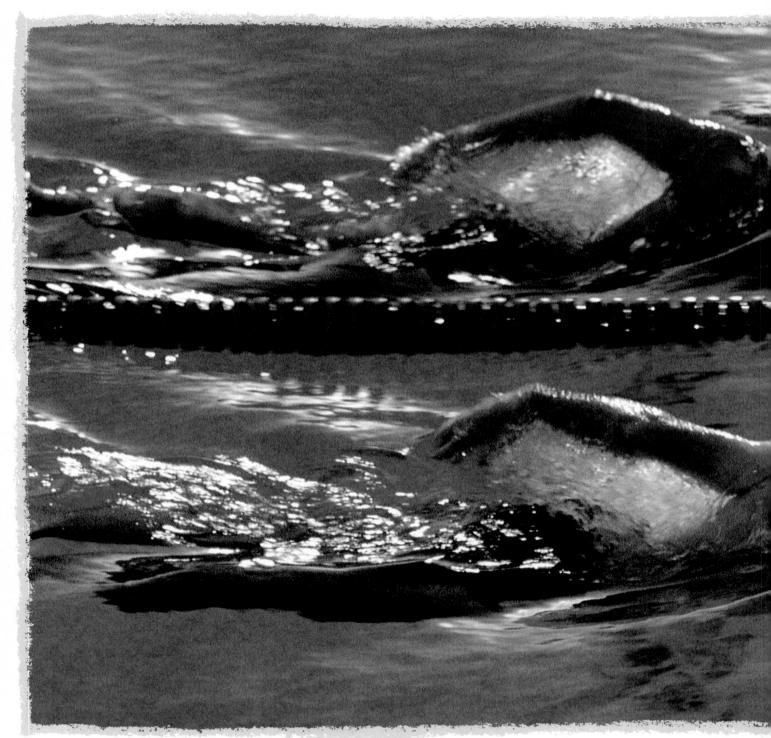

Your Health

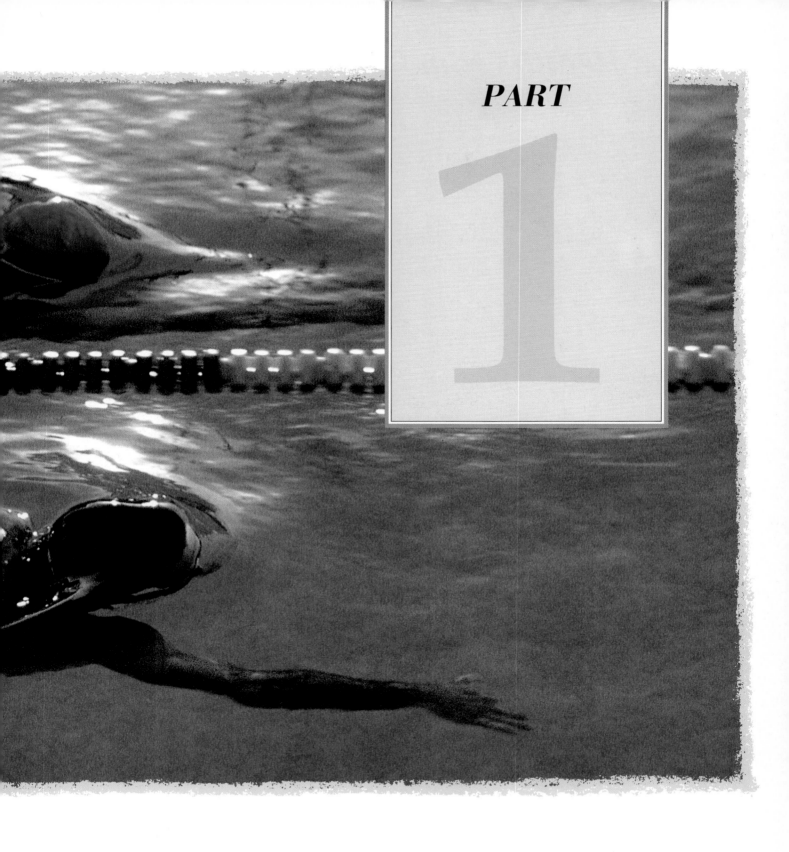

PART

1

Good Health From Birth

How healthy are you? ● *Good health is a balanced relationship between you and your physical, social and spiritual environments* ● *You can vastly improve your own health through making changes in your lifestyle.*

EACH OF US has only one body, and we must make it last a lifetime. How long and how enjoyable that lifetime will be depends on many factors – the society we live in, our wealth or poverty, our natural abilities, the way our career develops – but the most important one of all is ourselves, our own behavior and attitudes. Through attention to our health and well-being we can ensure that our lives are greatly enriched in whatever course we choose to follow.

All too often caring for health and appearance is considered to be a purely physical matter, but the state of our bodies is closely bound up with our mental outlook and our perceptions of ourselves. Just as good physical health encourages greater emotional and psychological strength, so an understand-ing of the way our own minds work and of how to change our negative attitudes can contribute to our bodily well-being and help us improve it.

Children's awareness of health

Even very small children will be curious about why they are ill, and they should be encouraged to take an interest in their bodies. This can be the beginning of a healthy sense of responsibility for their own well-being. Whether a child suffers from a severe illness or is only temporarily incapacitated, medical treatment can be distressing, often because children find it difficult to understand the purpose of what is being done to them. They may have a stomach pain, yet the doctor gives them an injection in the arm. It is very natural for children to resist such puzzling treatment by crying, shouting and struggling.

Try to ensure that the sick child understands both illness and treatment. Remember that children have very different

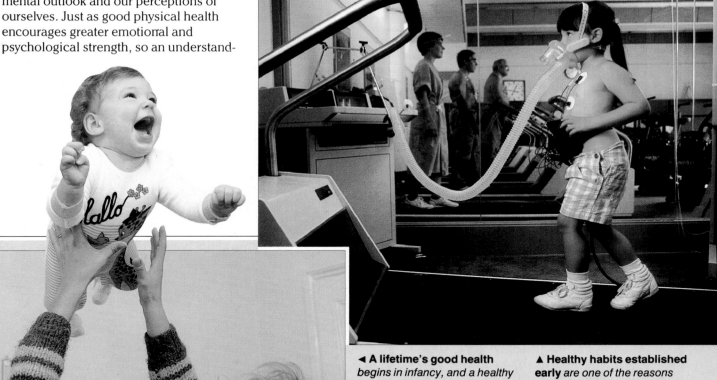

◄ **A lifetime's good health** begins in infancy, and a healthy childhood increases the chances of a healthy adult life. Every phase of our lives from babyhood through old age creates new priorities for how we look after our health. Taking health priorities seriously – including those affecting our social and mental well-being – pays long-term dividends.

▲ **Healthy habits established early** are one of the reasons why the United States Census Bureau predicts that it will count one million centenarians in 2050. Here an American who will probably live long into the second half of the 21st century uses health club equipment to gauge her aerobic capacity (the efficiency with which her body takes up oxygen from the air she breathes).

ideas about why people become ill and about how the body works. Children under 5 years commonly think that illness is caused by magic, or that it is a form of punishment. This is not so surprising – parents often tell children things like "come down from that tree, or you will fall and break your leg." Children can infer from this that accidents and illness are always a kind of punishment for not doing what they are told.

At school age, children learn about contagious diseases such as chickenpox, and then tend to assume that all illnesses are something you "catch." At about 11 years, children understand that the breakdown of a body part can cause an illness. On the verge of adolescence, children are beginning to comprehend the role of stress and anxiety: for example, that heart attacks can be the result of both damage to the organ and a combination of tension, overwork, tiredness and unhappiness.

If you explain to your child about why people get sick,

and what they can do to help themselves get better, your child will have a head start in taking responsibility for their personal health: for instance, try to be clear about why a balanced diet is important. Children will be interested (and more cooperative) if they know why certain kinds of food are good for them. Developing a sound attitude toward health can start now.

Stress and teenage health

The teenage years are turbulent times for both parents and children. Due to hormonal changes and the challenges of greater independence, adolescents are often moody, anxious and withdrawn. Natural curiosity or rebelliousness may lead to health- or life-threatening behavior, while the more common and relatively minor teenage health problems are aggravated by the stresses of becoming an adult.

Teenagers are largely past the stage of common infectious diseases like measles. Acne and spots, migraines,

Children's beliefs about internal anatomy

■ Children under five years have very simple ideas about what is inside them. Little children often draw delightful pictures of chicken, fries, or rice

pudding, mixed up with their bones and blood.

As they get older, they begin to include the heart (often heartshaped), brain and stomach. Later they draw in the

lungs, liver and kidneys, though they may not understand that these parts have a purpose. Anatomical notions may continue to be heavily influenced by cartoon images.

By the time children reach 11 or 12 years old, they have a more biologically sound view of the human body and understand that individual parts work together.

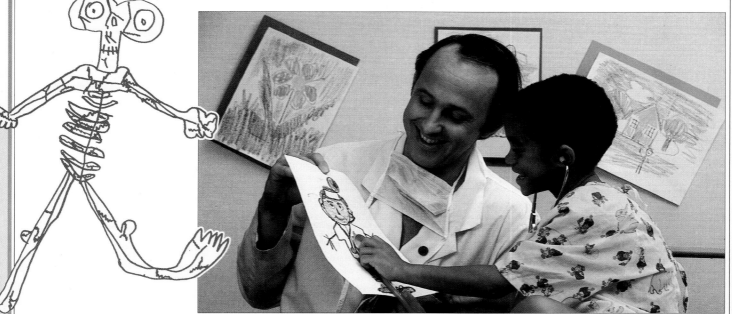

▲ A child's understanding of what we look like inside is influenced as much by fiction as by anatomical fact. In this drawing by a five-year-old the skull is a parody of a pirate flag from a storybook. The bones most clearly represented are those

which are most easily discernible in real life: the ribs and kneecaps.

▲ A trusting relationship with doctors and nurses provides children with a foundation for thorough health care. The unease which children might feel in the unfamiliar environment of the hospital or doctor's office needs to be overcome if

they are to talk freely about their symptoms. Children who see their doctor as a friendly figure are far more likely to let their parents know when they feel something is wrong with them.

17

mononucleosis (glandular fever), hay fever, asthma, period pains and menstrual irregularities are common health problems for adolescents. All of these are exacerbated by stress. Treatment involves not only medical attention, but personal guidance. Now is the time to make young people aware that their behavior and emotions can affect their bodily health. Learning self-control, developing methods of relaxation and learning to "talk things out" with you can help them to feel better.

Adolescents can be very resentful of adult interference, but relating your advice to a health problem that concerns them will make guidance easier, especially if you put your counsel in terms of their own growing responsibility and control. This may also be a basis from which you can begin to discuss more serious issues relating to health and fitness.

Teenagers are generally careless of their health and safety. They are preoccupied with their appearance and often insecure about themselves, which makes them extremely sensitive to peer pressure. As a result, adolescents are prone to experimentation with substances and activities that can be dangerous, such as smoking, alcohol, drugs, sexual experience, excessive dieting (sometimes leading to eating disorders like bulimia or anorexia) or overfast driving. It is important for adolescents to "try out" things in the process of becoming adults, but this natural need to experiment can lead to tragedy. Car and motorbike accidents account for many cases of teenage hospitalization. The teenage mother faces many difficulties in return for an evening's sexual experimentation.

The destructive lifestyles of many adults began in their adolescence. Even if teenagers do not indulge in highly dangerous behavior, they may be forming habits now which will be difficult to break later – eating too much junk food, smoking, avoiding exercise, or too many late nights.

Adolescents recover quickly from such bodily abuse, but when they are older they will find their bad habits more debilitating and difficult to break. Try to encourage them to consider the consequences of their behavior for health.

Teenagers are resistant to parental lectures because they want to control their own lives. As they get older, you can point out to them that they are becoming responsible for their own health and safety in order to urge them to "think

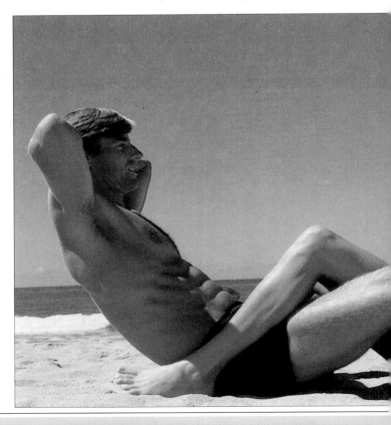

▶ **Carefree living** *for adolescents and young adults includes a much higher level of health-giving exercise than the lifestyle of older age-groups does. Fun, rather than health, is usually the motive and diet is often neglected in very fit-looking young people. The habit of eating excess fat, sugar and salt becomes a health hazard as they grow older and less active. Accidents are the most serious threat to life and health from childhood into the early thirties.*

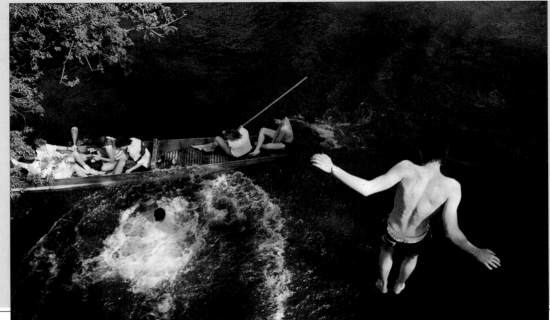

twice" about their actions. Perhaps the best way to encourage adolescents to live well, however, is to develop a healthy lifestyle yourself. **CE**

Young adulthood: enjoying good health

Between the ages of 18 and 35, most people are at their fittest and healthiest. The illnesses of childhood and the troubles of adolescence are left behind. At this stage of life, young people are likely to consolidate the habits that they will follow for the rest of their lives. They often realize for the first time that they are fully responsible for their own health. At this age it is easy to ignore basic fitness and medical care, because the young body can deal with and recover from considerable abuse. However, choices made in this period will affect health in later life.

During young adulthood, the most important healthcare remains the establishment of a healthy lifestyle – proper nutrition, enough sleep, regular exercise, moderation in

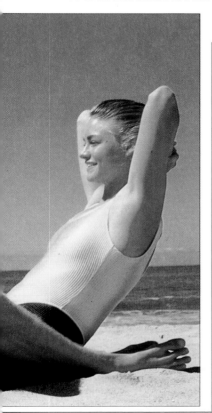

▲ **Exercising for fitness.**
A systematic program, routinely followed and combined with good nutrition, gives greater long-term health benefit than mere youthful activity. A routine that includes exercising in pairs adds a social aspect to your health program, and mutual encouragement will help two people not only to get started on a shared program but to persist with keeping fit.

How well do you understand your doctor?

■ A medical consultation involves two people: yourself and your doctor. Far too often the consultation proves value-less because of poor communication. This can be the fault of the doctor, the patient, or most commonly both.

One important point is that frequently we fail to pass on important information to the doctor. This may be because we are diffident or simply forgetful; it may also be because of poor interviewing on the part of the doctor or anxiety on the part of the patient. You probably know the experience of leaving the consulting room and suddenly remembering that you have forgotten to mention a particular symptom.

Another problem concerns the transmission of information the other way – from the doctor to you. The levels of understanding and remembering among patients are astonishingly low. On average, just over one-half of the information given by doctors in a medical consultation is understood by the patient. About 50-90 percent of the information given verbally is simply forgotten – often because we are so nervous during the interview that we fail to take in what is being said to us, or because we do not fully understand it.

The way to avoid these problems is to approach any consultation methodically. List your symptoms and the questions you want to ask; do not be afraid of coming to the consultation equipped with paper and pen. Write down all relevant information the doctor gives you, and ask about anything that seems unclear. At the end of the interview, give the doctor a summary of what you think you have been told, so that they can correct you if there have been any misunderstandings.

Make sure that your knowledge of the subject of health as a whole is good so that, whenever you are suffering from an ailment, you can apply your knowledge to your own particular case. At the same time, be careful that partial knowledge does not mislead you – listen to what the doctor is saying: do not assume it will merely confirm what you already think.

The best methods for improving your understanding and memory of medical advice can be summarized as follows:
● *improve your knowledge about health in general*
● *use this knowledge to understand the facts of your own case better*
● *ask your doctor, to check that your understanding is correct.*

Finally, if you know you are suffering from a particular complaint, try to get hold of relevant articles, books or leaflets – your doctor may be able to give you one or at least tell you how to get hold of one. Libraries, health-promotion organizations and telephone helplines are all useful. **SW**

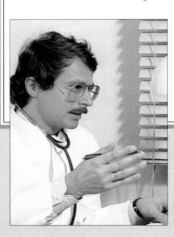

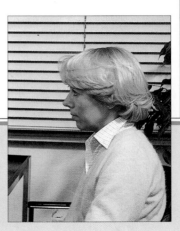

19

When a warning can change your life

■ A change of perspective can prompt life-saving changes in lifestyle. Bill had always prided himself on his good health. At 44, he had rarely had health problems; both his parents were alive and well, and he did not smoke. He felt that, compared to other people, he was unlikely to have heart problems, even though he was under a good deal of stress at work, rarely ate breakfast, and usually grabbed a hamburger or other fast food at lunch. These seemed like normal aspects of life, shared by most of his friends.

Bill intended to start an exercise program, particularly to combat his increasing girth, but there never seemed enough time in the day.

John, a close friend of Bill's with whom he had gone to college, suffered a heart attack. Bill had felt that John, like himself,

was an unlikely candidate for such an event. If it could happen to John, perhaps it could also happen to him. He reanalyzed his risk of heart disease, focusing now on the things that were not favorable.

He soon joined a health club and began to exercise before lunch. He started to eat lunch at the restaurant at the health club, which served low-fat foods, and also had a more substantial breakfast to provide energy for his workout. He found that he felt better on the days that he went to the health club.

In taking the time out to exercise, Bill also discovered that he could still get his work done, and he felt less pressure at the office. Bill talked one of his office friends into joining the club, and they help each other to go on the days that one or the other slips into old routines.

drinking and smoking. Healthy living will influence your body for the good when you are older, and you will feel better now. In addition, all sexually active women should arrange to be screened at least every three years for cervical cancer. Women should also learn to screen themselves for signs of breast cancer. Men should check for testicular cancer (see *Ch3*).

Many couples begin to plan their families now. Attention to well-being before conceiving will make your pregnancy happier and less worried. A pre-pregnancy screening will check the basic health of the potential mother. Both partners will be asked about their lifestyle, and about various hereditary diseases such as cystic fibrosis or hemophilia. Most women in this age group, however, have relatively untroubled pregnancies and a healthy baby at the end of it.

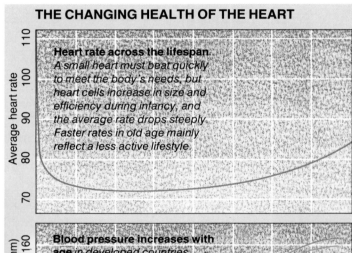
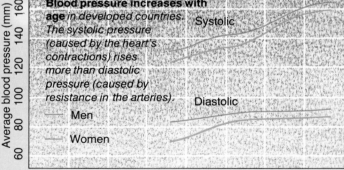
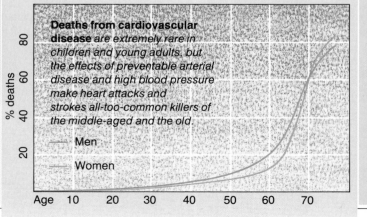

THE CHANGING HEALTH OF THE HEART

Heart rate across the lifespan. A small heart must beat quickly to meet the body's needs, but heart cells increase in size and efficiency during infancy, and the average rate drops steeply. Faster rates in old age mainly reflect a less active lifestyle.

Blood pressure increases with age in developed countries. The systolic pressure (caused by the heart's contractions) rises more than diastolic pressure (caused by resistance in the arteries). — Men — Women

Deaths from cardiovascular disease are extremely rare in children and young adults, but the effects of preventable arterial disease and high blood pressure make heart attacks and strokes all-too-common killers of the middle-aged and the old. — Men — Women

▲ **Middle-age spread** is a risk factor for middle-age heart attacks. Good diet and exercise are now more important than ever before. But it is precisely at this time of life that many people become less active, often finding their jobs involve more stress than physical exertion. This kind of lifestyle is largely responsible for the high incidence of heart disease after 40.

Common problems in middle age

As the human body ages, we expect it to slow down and to be less resilient, so we do not expect as much of ourselves as we grow older. The effects of slowing down to a less active lifestyle, however, add only to the risks you may have taken on by not being careful about your body as a young person. Adopting a healthy, active lifestyle in midlife, even if you have not had one earlier, is still good advice.

It is not until 40 that heart disease, especially sudden heart attacks, becomes a major threat. It is more likely to affect men. The hormones released during menstruation seem to offer some protection to women, but after the menopause women become increasingly vulnerable (see *Ch.3*).

A heart attack occurs when a blood vessel that has been growing more narrow for years suddenly becomes blocked. This starves some part of the heart of oxygen – heart muscle tissue dies and about 50 percent of the victims die. In survivors, the dead tissue is replaced not with new muscle, but with scar tissue: the heart is permanently weakened. High blood pressure, too much fat in the diet and poorly managed stress contribute to arterial wall damage and the build-up of fatty tissues that narrow arteries at sites of damage.

Inadequate exercise increases the risk of heart attack for someone whose heart receives its own oxygen supply through narrowed arteries; an underexercised heart does not always have the power to keep blood flowing through the narrow passages.

High blood pressure is worth avoiding not only because it damages arterial walls but because it places a high demand on the pumping capacity of the heart – and narrowed

arteries feeding the heart may not be able to deliver blood quickly enough when it is working hard.

High blood pressure (hypertension) may have no observable symptoms until the victim has a heart attack. Both men and women can suffer from it, though men seem to develop it more often. Regular testing of blood pressure is therefore a good idea, especially after the age of 40 – earlier if your family has a history of high blood pressure. Doctors are still uncertain about its exact causes, though smoking, alcohol consumption and being overweight all contribute.

Cancer may strike at any age, but becomes more common with increasing age. Partly, this is because the longer you are exposed to cancer-inducing agents – such as the cigarette smoke that has been blamed for lung cancer – the more chances they have of affecting you.

Less serious threats to health faced by the middle-aged include worsening eyesight, gum diseases like gingivitis and arthritis of varying severity. Women between 45 and 58 also experience the menopause, cessation of the menstrual cycle, which can involve mood swings and some physical discomfort as the body adjusts.

Regular medical screening, especially for breast cancer and hypertension, is important as you get older.

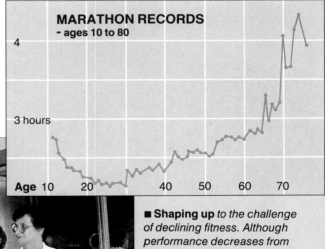

MARATHON RECORDS
- ages 10 to 80

4

3 hours

Age 10   20   40   50   60   70

■ **Shaping up** *to the challenge of declining fitness. Although performance decreases from the early thirties onward, keeping fit enough just to complete the course is as worthy a reward as winning. Marathon runners have finished the race well into their eighties. With or without competitive athletic ambitions, fitness training LEFT is a benefit to any middle-aged person.*

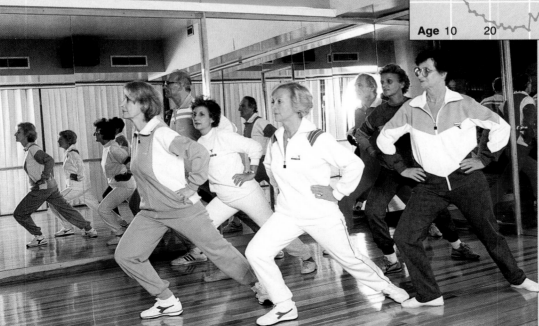

Does aging have to make us ill?

Many people in the industrial world will live into their eighties and beyond. Unfortunately, our images and expectations of late life often include the prospect of returning to a childlike state, where we give up the responsibility for our own well-being. We have even taken age-related words and turned them into terms of abuse. "Senile" does not mean simply "to do with old age." It has come to be a shorthand for feebleness, dependency and, worst of all, the progressive loss of mental faculties.

We can do many things to improve our chances of enjoying a good old age. Growing old is often much more feared by those who have yet to reach it than by those already there. Normal aging does not cause as much physical breakdown as most people fear: it is disease and accidents that make us sick when we are old, just as when we are young.

Normal aging brings changes in the body tissues, but these are not drastic. We all know that tissues such as skin can regenerate, and that torn muscles and broken bones can knit. Healing and replacement processes may take somewhat longer in old age, but they happen whether you are 19 or 90. On the other hand, some tissues such as nerve cells and muscle cells and the structures in the kidneys that filter the blood do not regenerate, and there is a progressive loss. Other cells, which are important because of their products, become less efficient – bone cells produce less osteoid, the material that gives bones their strength and hardness. Women especially are affected (see *Ch3*). However, it is usually not until we are into our seventies that such degeneration has an effect, if ever.

In a sense, aging starts to happen very early in life. It has been estimated that shortly after birth we begin losing an average of 50,000 irreplacable brain cells every day of our lives. An 80-year-old has two-thirds to one half as many purification cells in the kidneys as a 40-year-old. The surviving brain and kidney cells can cope perfectly well in normal circumstances so this aspect of aging is not to be feared.

What is worthy of fear is the catastrophic loss of irreplacable brain tissues during a stroke, when a blockage in a narrowed artery starves part of the brain of oxygen. Arteries feeding the brain become narrow for all of the same reasons as arteries feeding the heart do. Another kind of stroke results when high blood pressure weakens a blood vessel in the brain and eventually it bursts. Doctors do not regard susceptibility to strokes and heart disease as part of the normal aging process – rather they see it in a large measure as a price that older people pay for an avoidable lifestyle

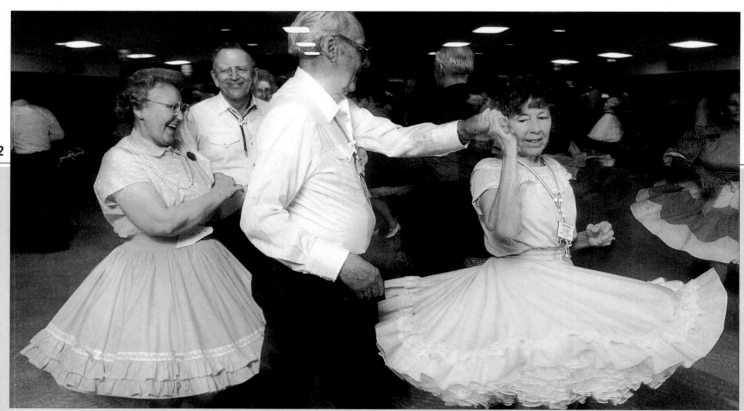

▲ **Staying active** in the later years of your life is part of staying healthy. Physical soundness and active involvement are both essential ingredients of overall health. They are interrelated – social involvement not only boosts self-esteem and other aspects of psychological well-being but encourages physical activity.

they adopted when younger – not enough exercise, poor diet, too much stress.

Respiratory diseases and chronic bronchial infections also cause problems, especially for long-time smokers. Arthritis, rheumatism and some loss of hearing are also more prevalent as we get older.

Older people tire more easily and recover less readily from exertion. These seem to be part of the normal aging process. They have to take life a little more slowly and carefully, but can still be active.

The aging of mental ability

Studies have shown that those who start with the most mental ability tend to show the least decline. Skills which rely on speed and agility, such as mental arithmetic, show more decline from middle age than do those dependent upon acquired experience, such as doing a crossword puzzle. Some forgetfulness is normal as we get older, but serious mental confusion is not due solely to aging and requires medical attention. Alzheimer's disease, for example, is not a disease of normal aging.

Personality also shows gradual changes. Long-standing traits may become more pronounced – we become "more like ourselves" – and there is a tendency to become less extroverted and more emotionally sensitive. However, severe or sudden personality change is abnormal and medical advice should be taken.

Confusion or marked personality change may have a physical cause and will disappear when the cause is treated, but in some cases they may be due to Alzheimer's disease which affects about one in four of the very old, but also some younger people. This is incurable and progressive: the old person becomes less and less capable of looking after themselves, although a certain amount of independence can be maintained if the right kind of support is available. The doctor will advise on this.

Aging is part of the lifespan, and continuity is much more obvious than change. The best way of predicting what sort of person you will be in old age is to take a close look at yourself now. Think positively: it is never too late to cultivate a healthy lifestyle and the effort will be worthwhile. A positive outlook and a sense of purpose and usefulness are crucial in maintaining fitness and well-being, and it makes sense to make the most of your life. **CT**.

It is a mistake to think of health purely in physical terms. Its other two aspects – mental and social health – are much too intimately related to the physical aspect to be treated as separate issues. People with high morale and healthy social relationships tend to be the soundest in body.

It is a mistake to think of health purely in negative terms – as the absence of disease. If you regard it as something more, you are more likely to maintain and improve a good state of health. The World Health organization defines health as "a state of complete physical, mental and social well-being, and not merely the absence of disease or infirmity."

▲ **Continuing mental health** need not be prevented by physical decline. Learning a new skill – for example, the use of a computer – keeps a mind active, involves the learner socially with teachers and provides a sense of personal worth that helps to motivate self-care. Even though confined to a wheelchair, and whatever your age, some form of fitness training may be recommended by your doctor. By working the parts of your body that work best, you may improve circulation, strengthen your heart and increase your respiratory capacity.

It matters to know about health

■ The more you know about health, the greater the improvements you can make to your lifestyle and the more informed the choice you can make about decisions affecting you. Increasingly, people want to make such decisions for themselves rather than accept their doctor's advice without criticism.

Knowledge is also important because of its contribution to the feeling of being in control. Research has consistently shown that feeling more in control tends to be associated with better health. In one study, residents of two old people's nursing homes were observed over a period of several years. No changes were made in the way the residents were treated in one home, while in the other they were given more control and choice about their activities and surroundings – for example, being allowed to choose when to have meals or to choose their own kind of recreation. At a follow-up 18 months later, significantly fewer people had died in the nursing home which encouraged choice and control. **SW**

Why do we take risks with health?

■ Many infectious diseases that were killers in the past have now been brought under control by sanitation, immunization and antibiotics. Today the major causes of illness and premature death are more closely linked to lifestyle. You are at far greater risk, for example, if you smoke, have more than one or two alcoholic drinks each day, miss breakfast, eat large snacks between main meals, are more than 10 percent overweight, take little exercise, sleep less than 7-8 hours each night, drive without a seat belt and ignore safety precautions in the home and workplace. Most of these risk factors can be avoided but we often do not bother. The reasons for our neglect are complex.

The dangers of false optimism

One major reason why people do not change their habits is that they do not view themselves as being at risk of poor health. Neil Weinstein, who has researched this, has called it "unrealistic optimism." He asked people to rate how likely they are, compared to others of their age and sex, to develop health problems like diabetes, cancer and arthritis. Most estimated their risk as a below-average one. Of course, some of them were correct – but clearly not everybody can be less at risk than average. What seems to happen is that people focus on those factors that make them less likely to suffer a particular problem and fail to recognize the other factors that do put them at risk.

One important factor is the common gut-belief that, if a person has yet to experience a problem, they are less likely to experience it in the future; this is totally illogical, of course, but the instinct is part of human nature.

Other factors encouraging unrealistic optimism are the belief that the problem is rare, lack of personal contact with the problem, and knowledge that the problem is theoretically preventable – even though the person is doing nothing at all right now to prevent it ("I am perfectly capable of forestalling heart disease by quitting smoking, and one day I will do it").

Unrealistic optimism may even stop

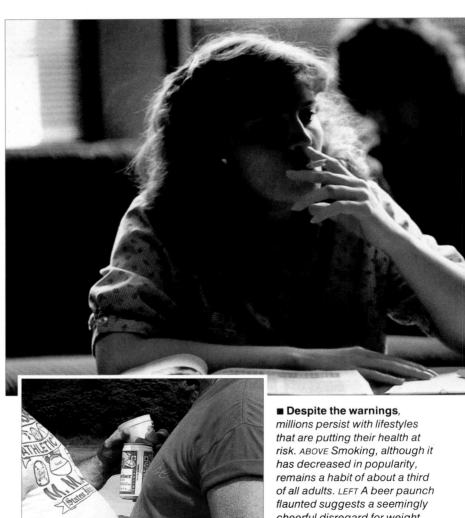

■ **Despite the warnings**, *millions persist with lifestyles that are putting their health at risk. ABOVE Smoking, although it has decreased in popularity, remains a habit of about a third of all adults. LEFT A beer paunch flaunted suggests a seemingly cheerful disregard for weight problems. In fact, most smokers wish that they could quit (see Ch14), and most overweight people, especially overweight women, are discontented at least with their appearance, if not their health (see Ch9). Reasons for not changing include lack of confidence, but many people's motivation is also weakened by confused thinking about the degree of risk they are running.*

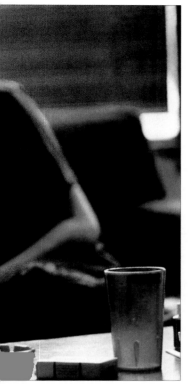

people from engaging in the kind of behavior that actively promotes good health. We all need to be aware of this bias in our outlook and to check our own perceptions of how great a risk we run of developing any specific problem. When you do this yourself, remember your built-in tendency to discount your own risk factors and to assume that you – among all the rest of humanity – are the person who will somehow be spared. None of us is special in that way.

Believing in your own health

Another reason why you may or may not promote your health better concerns your self-image. The more you believe that you are capable of doing something, the more likely you are to achieve it, whatever the obstacles. For example, researchers have shown that smokers who have a greater belief in their own ability to resist a relapse after quitting are able to abstain for longer than others who have less faith in themselves.

The same has been found in people who have suffered heart attacks. Those who believe in their ability to practice regular exercise after they get home from hospital are much more likely to do so. An important result of other surveys has been that such people's faith in themselves can be reinforced if they are put through a treadmill (or similar) test, in which they learn that they can exert themselves without bringing on a new heart attack.

Follow-up studies have revealed an even more significant effect: the influence of the person's partner. When the partner watches the treadmill test, their evaluation of the person's physical abilities rises. At first this might not seem important; however, the surveys showed that people whose partners had watched them undergoing the test developed, on average, significantly better cardiac fitness.

Typically, our commitment to a positive program of self-improvement reflects in some degree our perception of how much the people closest to us want us to succeed, and how strongly they believe in our method. NEA

An upward spiral of self-care

■ Your belief about your own abilities can have a considerable effect on your health-related behavior.

If you focus on the problems involved in changing your habits (lack of time, insufficient physical strength and so on), you are both less likely to try to change and, even after trying, more likely to quit early.

This creates a downward spiral, in which the failure to make the change reinforces your conscious or unconscious belief that you are incapable of doing so.

However, you can use exactly the same effect to create an upward spiral. By making one successful change you learn that you can actually carry it

through. This can raise your faith in your own ability and it can encourage you to try even harder next time.

The best approach is to start off with something that you already know you can do – a half-dozen push-ups maybe – and then use this as a base for your future expectations: 12, 20, 50 or even more push-ups. The important point is that you should show yourself that you are indeed capable of making a change for the better; once you have gained this confidence you will have sufficient belief in yourself to continue changing your habits in ways that are positively beneficial to your health.

Too much information can be bad

■ When we look at why people fail to adopt a more healthy lifestyle we often assume that the failure is one of public education. But never before have people been bombarded with so much health information as they are today. It seems likely that, ironically, the problem is that we receive too much advice.

Faced wherever we turn with news about health risks and recommendations for preventive action, we begin to regard each new warning as an empty threat. We tend to discount each new theory about exercise or diet as it seems to contradict what we were told last week.

People may also focus a great deal of energy on changing one apparently dangerous

habit while paying little attention to another that is far more dangerous.

In 1989, C Everett Koop, the Surgeon General of the United States, highlighted an example of this. Talking about Fresca, a drink that contains artificial sweeteners, he said, "People just have an inappropriate sense of what is dangerous. They get overly upset about minor problems. If you translate the weight and time it takes a laboratory rat to develop bladder cancer to a 200lb (90kg) man drinking Fresca, it comes out to about two bathtubs full each day.

People dropped Fresca in a minute, but they continue to smoke."

2

Your Sex and Your Health

If women really are the weaker sex, why do they live longer than men? ● *Are men and women vulnerable to the same diseases?* ● *How do hormones and lifestyle affect our susceptibility?* ● *What can we do about it?*

WOMEN are generally regarded as the weaker sex, and yet in the industrialized world they tend to outlive men by four to ten years. What are the reasons for this: is it due to biology or behavior? Are women on average healthier because the female body is more resistant to disease than the male body, or is there something about a woman's life-style that promotes better health? Experts have been trying to discover how health is influenced by gender and how the biological causes of disease relate to the way we behave. Their findings show the areas where each sex is particularly vulnerable and suggest ways for both men and women to improve their health and help to combat disease.

Life expectancy and the sexes

Statistics show that as far as health is concerned, women have the advantage over men from the moment they are born. About two boys in every 500 die before they are six weeks old, while the figure for girls is 1.6 in 500. In every age group up to 70, a male's chances of dying are slightly greater than a female's. In the Western world, 84 percent of women are still living at the age of 65, compared with only 70 percent of men for the same year of birth. To compensate,

Why do we go to the doctor?

■ Although women live longer than men, they seem to experience more illness, or at least they use the health services more. There are many reasons for this.

Childbearing itself brings women into contact with the health professions for long periods at a time; women also consult doctors more often on matters of contraception than men do, and they may need help with problems related to menstruation or menopause.

Men tend to make more use of the health services as a result of physical injury, especially during their working life. Such injuries may occur at work (especially in the mining, manufacturing and construction industries) or at leisure, for example when playing sports or driving.

Both men and women may also suffer from long-term chronic conditions resulting from their work: miners and others who work underground, as well as those who are involved in the chemical and metal industries or agriculture, are exposed to toxic substances and various kinds of dangerous dust, leading to respiratory or skin conditions. Those engaged in heavy physical work are especially prone to back problems and joint injuries.

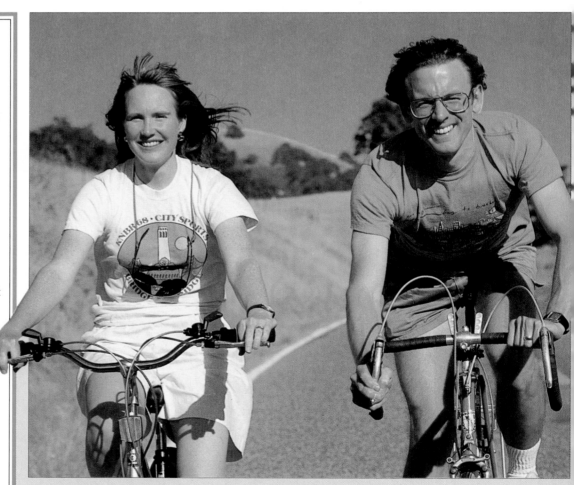

▲ **Different sex,** *different risks. From birth, women have the advantage of being less vulner- able than men – both to disease and to accidents. Throughout the lifespan, sex is a factor in vulnerability to different risks. Whether this is due to biology or* *lifestyle is the subject of on- going research and debate. Women are less likely than men to die of heart disease before the age of 70, and 75 percent of men over 50 will develop an enlarged prostate gland. For a longer, healthier life, men and* *women should take the same approach: no smoking, a proper diet and regular exercise.*

nature allows more boys than girls to be born: the ratio is about 106:100.

It is not known whether more boys than girls are actually conceived – more boys are miscarried after three months of pregnancy, and this led early researchers to calculate that as many as 150 boys are conceived for every 100 girls. It is now known that more girls are miscarried than boys *before* three months.

The causes of premature death in males vary according to age. In infancy and childhood they tend to be related to biology rather than behavior. Girls have a greater chance of survival than boys because they are naturally more robust at a young age. In the second and third decades of life, the behavior of males begins to influence mortality rates. Being more aggressive than females, they are more likely to suffer violent death in the form of homicide, suicide and accidents. This aggression is also biologically triggered in that it is related to the male sex hormone testosterone.

Another notable feature of male behavior which puts men at risk is their tendency to consume more drugs and alcohol than women, making violence, accidents and some types of disease more likely. Until very recently, they have also smoked more, increasing their rate of lung cancer and lung disease. In the industrialized world, young men are also the chief victims of the AIDS virus. As men approach middle age, their risk of cardiovascular disease in the form of heart attacks and strokes increases, while women seem to be protected until after the menopause. This would suggest a link between hormones and heart disease, an area of research that has attracted a great deal of medical attention.

Causes of death among men and women

■ Women not only live longer than men, but are less likely to die of certain causes. A team of researchers at the Alameda County Human Laboratory in northern California made a study of the causes of death according to sex. They took a sample of 5,000 adults and observed them over several decades.

There are four times more male homicide victims than female. Male deaths also led female deaths from lung cancer, accidents, cirrhosis of the liver and heart disease, in that order.

Some of these differences can be explained by behavior. Men generally drink and smoke more than women, accounting for the higher incidence of lung cancer and cirrhosis in men. Men are also more likely to engage in dangerous work RIGHT and leisure activities – such as mining, construction, hang gliding and motor racing and so to have more accidents.

Other disorders, however, are affected by hormones – for example, there is strong evidence to suggest that female hormones may account in part for lower female vulnerability to heart disease.

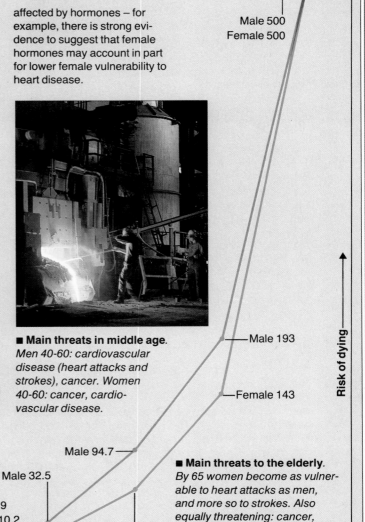

Male 500
Female 500

Male 193

Female 143

■ **Main threats in middle age**. *Men 40-60: cardiovascular disease (heart attacks and strokes), cancer. Women 40-60: cancer, cardiovascular disease.*

Male 94.7

Male 32.5

Male 13.9
Female 10.2

Female 61.1

Female 21.3

■ **Main threats to the elderly**. *By 65 women become as vulnerable to heart attacks as men, and more so to strokes. Also equally threatening: cancer, pneumonia as a complication of bronchitis or emphysema.*

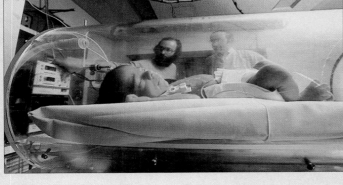

■ **Main threats in early life**: *congenital malformations (especially in the newborn), premature birth, accidents (especially boys), childhood cancers, infection.*

Risk of dying:
Male 4.0 in 1000
Female 3.2 in 1000

Male 2.5
Female 1.0

■ **Main threats for young adults**. *Up to 30: accidents (especially men). Over 30: cancer (especially women), heart disease (especially men), accidents.*

Male 7.0
Female 2.8

Risk of dying

| Age | 10 | 20 | 30 | 40 | 50 | 60 | 70 | 80 |

Major risks for heart disease

■ Eight major risk factors have been identified with heart disease – the leading cause of death in developed countries. Although men are more likely than women to be afflicted, both sexes should be aware of the factors that increase their vulnerability. All of these factors except gender and family history can be modified by regular aerobic exercise.

● Heart disease in family member(s) before age 50
● Being a man
● High blood pressure (over 140/90)
● High cholesterol (cholesterol over 200; LDL more than 130mg%)
● Smoking
● Diabetes
● Physical inactivity
● Stress

■ **The menace of arterial disease.** *Narrowed arteries appear as thin green threads in the upper right of this computer image of a living heart* RIGHT. *The strain on the heart can be so great that it fails. Coronary arteries* BELOW *encrusted with atheroma plaque. A constriction that leaves part of the arterial wall flexible is less dangerous than a "cuff."*

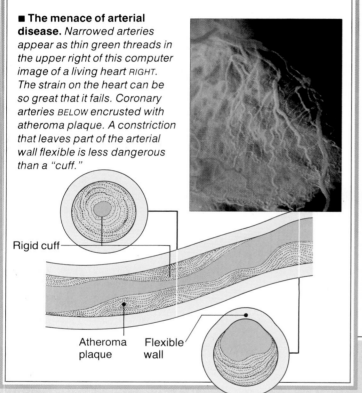

Rigid cuff

Atheroma plaque

Flexible wall

Hormones and heart disease

Because heart disease is the most common cause of death among the people of developed countries, scientists are keen to investigate its causes. The observation that men are particularly vulnerable has led researchers to examine the effect of hormones on the cardiovascular system. Could it be that the male hormone testosterone promotes heart disease, or that the female hormone estrogen is protective? The fact that women become more prone to disease after menopause, when estrogen levels decline, suggests that this may be so. Scientists are still studying how estrogen may be beneficial, but already there seems to be a connection between hormones and the amount of cholesterol in the blood, which is itself an important factor in determining the likelihood of heart disease.

Cholesterol is made up of several components, two of which are low density lipoproteins (LDL) and high density lipoproteins (HDL). It is the low density lipoproteins (sometimes called the "bad" cholesterol) that are dangerous. HDL, on the other hand, seems to be protective. It has been found that estrogen lowers the production of LDL and increases the production of HDL, while testosterone has the opposite effect. This is why women are less likely to develop heart disease than men while their estrogen levels are high

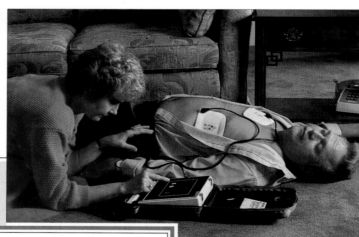

▲ **Wives and daughters** *often provide support for heart attack victims – who, before the age of 60, are mostly men. Here a woman uses a portable defibrillator to apply an electric shock to a heart that has gone into fibrillation – it is twitching rapidly and uselessly instead of pumping blood – following a heart attack. The shock should restore normal beating.*

Preventing heart disease

■ Higher blood cholesterol levels in particular have been found to increase the risk of heart disease, the most serious health problem in the developed world. They can be tackled in the following ways:

1 Eat less fat. It is generally believed that saturated fats, the main component of animal fats, are more dangerous in raising cholesterol levels than polyunsaturated fats. However, the evidence is not conclusive and the best safeguard is to consume less fat of all types (see *Ch 8*). Avoid butter and other high-fat dairy products, fatty meat, lard oils, nuts, chocolate and pastry. Eat more fresh fruits, vegetables, lean meat and fish. Bake, boil, broil, steam or poach your food – do not fry it.

2 Take moderate exercise. Exercise can increase the HDL (high density lipoproteins) in the blood, giving a protective effect. Too much exercise, however, can do the opposite.

3 Drink in moderation. Experiments have shown that not more than 1.5 liters (25 fluid oz) of beer (or the equivalent) daily for men – half this for women – can also increase HDL cholesterol (see *Ch 15*).

4 Avoid stress. High levels of cortisol, produced by stress, can increase cholesterol (see *Ch 4*).

and cholesterol levels relatively low. After menopause, some women undergo hormone replacement therapy or estrogen therapy which means they are given extra doses of estrogen. Again, this seems to reduce their risk of heart disease.

The disadvantages of estrogen

Estrogen offers women protection against fatal heart attacks or strokes but makes other disorders more likely, especially after the menopause when estrogen levels decrease. Rheumatoid arthritis, lupus (any of several skin diseases) and scleroderma (a hardening of the body's connective tissue) and other so-called auto-immune disorders arise when the body's immune system becomes active against its own tissue, setting in motion an inflammatory disease process. Even oral contraceptives containing estrogen can lead to flareups of such disease. In addition, the fluctuations of estrogen and progesterone levels during the menstrual cycle may affect the likelihood of infectious diseases such as herpes, and explain why women are more vulnerable to colds and infections at certain times than others. During pregnancy high levels of progesterone suppress a woman's immune system so that she may accept the fetus rather than reject it as a "foreign body."

Women can avoid brittle bones

■ Brittle bone disease (osteoporosis) affects many elderly women, leading to illness and sometimes to death. It can cause pain, loss of movement and broken bones in elderly women. The hormonal losses caused by the menopause (and sometimes by anorexia and amenorrhea in young women) mean that in later life women lose bone density at a more rapid rate than men, so that the skeleton becomes brittle, frail and easily damaged. Calcium supplements and estrogen replacements help, but exercise is proving to be the best preventative medicine.

It is best if you start the menopause with high bone density, but with proper exercise women in their fifties and sixties can still attain a bone mass greater than they had in their thirties and forties.

Exercise has to be weight-bearing to increase bone mass, but aerobic dance or jogging may be too hard on the joints of an already delicate structure. Swimming (which many women prefer) is not weight-bearing at all and offers no benefits in maintaining bone mass. Weight training with light weights and many repetitions, or cycling, are better alternatives.

Older women can fill two sturdy shopping bags with tin cans and carry them around the house for 15 minutes; even this mild exercise will increase bone mass and prepare the way for more strenuous activity.

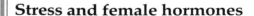

Stress and female hormones

■ Research by health experts has examined whether female hormones make women respond in a different way to stress, and so run a different risk of suffering from heart disease.

In a typical study, people are asked to perform mental arithmetic, compete in challenging video games or talk about an upsetting or stressful experience. Their physical response to the challenge of the task is studied by measuring changes in heart rate, blood pressure, muscle tension and skin conductance (sweating). Blood or urine samples may also be measured in order to assess adrenaline.

If the female hormone estrogen has a dampening effect on arousal, women with low levels of this hormone would be expected to react in ways more resembling men. Studies have indeed confirmed that there is a lower cardiovascular and adrenaline response in women who have not yet reached the menopause, who on average have higher estrogen levels than men and postmenopausal women.

Another way in which gender may affect stress is that women might respond less vigorously to challenge. If this is true, it emphasizes the importance for men to learn ways of dampening their physical response, through relaxation or other means.

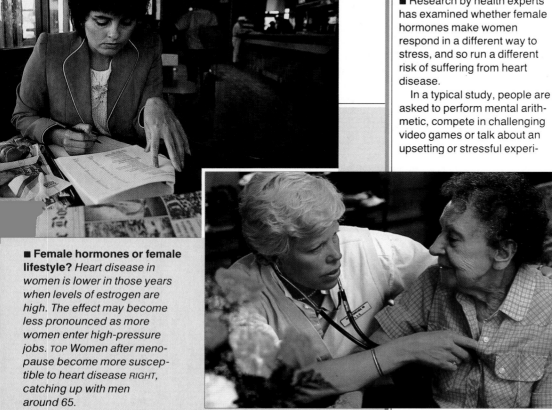

■ **Female hormones or female lifestyle?** *Heart disease in women is lower in those years when levels of estrogen are high. The effect may become less pronounced as more women enter high-pressure jobs.* TOP *Women after menopause become more susceptible to heart disease* RIGHT, *catching up with men around 65.*

Sex differences and cancer

After heart disease, the most serious threat to life in developed countries is cancer. Cancer is not, in fact, just one disease, but about 200 different diseases, all attacking different parts of the body. Some affect both men and women while others are restricted to one sex. Because many cancers seem to be a product of the environment, shown by the fact that incidence changes when people migrate, they should in theory be preventable. Although medicine still has a long way to go in preventing and curing cancer, there are some steps that the individual can take to reduce the chances of developing it.

The most common type is lung cancer, accounting for about 20 percent of all cancers and 27 percent of cancer deaths. It affects both sexes, but especially men, and is caused by hazards in the environment and by smoking. Exposure to dangerous substances in industrial processes, such as asbestos, accounts for some cases of lung cancer, but it has been estimated that about 90 percent of lung-cancer deaths are the result of smoking. It is clear, therefore, that the most effective thing a person can do to guard against this disease is not to smoke.

After lung cancer, men are most prone to cancer of the prostate. More than any other cancer this type is associated with old age, with as many as 30 percent of men over 50 developing it. Like other forms of cancer, it can be cured in its early stages and it is therefore recommended that men over 50 have regular six-monthly examinations to ensure early detection.

Cancer of the bowel and cancer of the rectum occur in both sexes. Both are slow to develop and can be successfully operated on. As with other types of cancer, the important thing is to note and report to the doctor any unusual symptoms.

Breast cancer and cancer of the cervix

The next most widespread form of cancer is breast cancer which affects women almost exclusively and accounts for about 12 percent of all cancers and 20 percent of female cancer deaths. Breast cancer seems to be somehow linked with hormones but its precise causes are not known. It has also been linked with the amount of fat in the diet and the age when a woman has her first child, but again the evidence is inconclusive. The risk of contracting breast cancer increases with age, but if detected at an early stage it can be cured. To this end women are being advised to examine their own breasts every month, especially after the age of about 25, to look for any lumps or changes in shape. Many

Preventing cancer

■ Not all causes of cancer are known, but many are and they are worth avoiding.

● Do not smoke. Do not breathe other people's smoke. Lung cancer is still the most common form of cancer.

● Avoid breathing other irritating fumes and sprays, eg exhaust fumes, pesticides.

● Avoid overexposure to the sun – causing skin cancer.

● Eat more wholegrain cereals and fresh fruit. More fiber in the diet may reduce the risk of colon cancer.

● Avoid heavy consumption of smoked and salt-cured food and food preserved with

nitrites. All are implicated in the production of nitrosamines – a group of chemicals including many that induce cancer.

● Dark green and yellow vegetables contain vitamins A and C, which protect against some cancers.

● Eat lean meat or fish and cut down on use of fat and oils. High levels of fat are suspected of promoting some cancers.

● Limit the number of your sexual partners. Both cervical and rectal cancer can be caused by a herpes virus spread by sexual contact.

Detecting cancer early

■ Cancer cells are out of rhythm with the rest of the body. They may multiply at abnormally fast rates and spread uncontrolled throughout the tissues. Some begin to spread after as long as 10 years, others in less than a year, but in all cases early treatment is vital. Even if your health is good, regular screening for cancer is important.

Each kind of cancer is unique, and even the same kind of cancer may behave differently in different people. It is therefore impossible to predict when a cancer will arise and how it will behave.

Certain early warning signs may – but do not always – indicate cancer. These include lumps in the neck; sores that will not heal; blood in the urine or feces; prolonged constipation or diarrhea; unexplained vaginal bleeding; or changes in any moles on your skin. General symptoms that occur when the cancer is more advanced are constant tiredness, loss of weight or a persistent cough.

If cancer is suspected, a doctor can arrange examinations by X-ray, or biopsy which involves some tissue being removed and analyzed for malignant cells.

■ **Breast and cervix.** Most of the women who are cured of breast cancer discover it themselves, so the importance of self-examination cannot be overestimated. A simple check (see RIGHT) once a month after menstruation will help to detect any problems that may develop. Sexually active women should be tested for cancer of the cervix every three years. This is a "slow" cancer, so any condition discovered during a three-year check can usually be completely cured. Testing may be done more frequently if there is a particular cause for concern.

■ **Testicular cancer** is relatively rare, but it is one of the fastest-growing cancers and it is on the increase. Men between 20 and 40 are most at risk. Check once a month.

1 Hold the scrotum in the palms of your hand. Use the thumbs and fingers of both hands to feel the testicle, using very gentle pressure.

2 Examine the epididymis (where the spermatic cord joins the testicles). It should feel soft and slightly tender.

3 The spermatic cord (a tube that runs behind the testicles from the top of the epididymus) should feel firm and smooth.

4 The testicles themselves should be smooth. Examine each in the same way, checking especially for lumps on the front and sides.

How to look

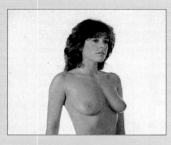

1 *Study appearance of your breasts. Turn from side to side, and hold them up to look underneath.*

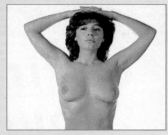

2 *Put your hands on your head and look for anything unusual, especially around the nipples.*

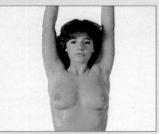

3 *Stretch your arms above your head and have another look, again concentrating on the area around the nipples.*

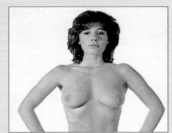

4 *With your hands on your hips, press inward until your chest muscles tighten. Look for any dimpling of the skin.*

How to feel

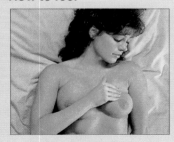

1 *Lie flat, your head and left shoulder slightly raised. Feel left breast with fingers of right hand.*

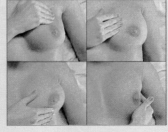

2 *Press in gently and firmly toward your body and feel every part of the breast, circling outward from nipple.*

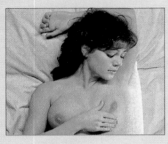

3 *Repeat, with your left arm above your head and the elbow bent. Pay particular attention to outer breast.*

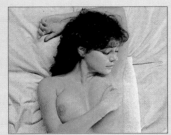

4 *In the same position, feel the part closest to the armpit. Repeat the whole process for the right breast.*

women experience dysplasia, lumpiness in the breasts before periods. With practice, you will learn what is normal for your body – and what to tell the doctor about. Doctors and family-planning clinics also carry out checks if requested, and later in life an annual mammography or X-ray of the breasts may be recommended.

Another form of cancer specific to women is cancer of the cervix – the narrow passage between the vagina and the womb. The occurrence of this disease has been linked to teenage sexual experience and to the number of sexual partners a woman or her partner has had, and therefore seems to be caused by a virus spread by sexual intercourse. Again, this is a slow-growing type of cancer, taking up to 10 years to invade other tissue, that can be treated successfully if diagnosed early. In recent years it has been actively fought by screening programs, and in countries where screening has been widespread there has been a sharp drop in mortality rates compared with countries where no such preventive measures are taken. Women are therefore strongly advised to have a cervical smear test at least every three to five years.

Prostate cancer

■ Cancer of the prostate gland is the most common cancer affecting men. Almost all men over 85 have it; 75 percent of men over 50 will develop an enlarged prostate, and over 30 percent will develop prostate cancer.

The prostate gland is located at the point where the urethra leaves the bladder. Fluids from the prostate help fight urinary tract infections and combine with seminal fluid to transport sperm during ejaculation. Prostate growth in men between 40 and 60 is inevitable and is not a problem in itself.

However, as the gland increases in size, there may be an obstruction of urine flow. Minor symptoms may be a need to urinate more frequently, difficulty starting, and less output. This becomes a problem because the bladder will become infected if it is not emptied completely; pressure in the bladder may also affect the kidneys. Then the obstruction may become dangerous.

Prostate enlargement does not always lead to cancer, and the cancer usually does not spread. Surgery, chemotherapy, radiation and hormonal therapy are some of the options for treatment. An annual rectal examination for men over 40 allows early detection.

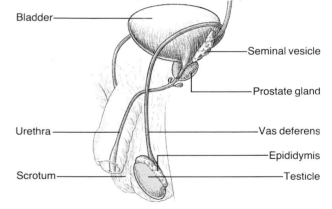

Bladder

Seminal vesicle

Prostate gland

Urethra

Vas deferens

Epididymis

Scrotum

Testicle

31

Hormones and emotional health

While great advances have been made in medical science over the past 100 years, improving people's life expectancy and general health, the incidence of people seeking psychological help has increased enormously, especially since the Second World War. It seems that once people have reached a certain standard of living and physical well-being, they turn their attention to their emotional needs.

Both men and women can become the victims of depression or other mental illness, but women are traditionally portrayed as less emotionally stable than men and more prone to nervous breakdown. Studies have shown that they are two to three times more likely to become depressed than men and that this is true for every age group. Moreover, it is not simply a reflection of their greater willingness to admit to their problems and seek help. In order to try and explain this difference, a possible connection has been suggested between female hormones and women's psychological health.

Everyone has heard of women becoming depressed after childbirth or during menopause. Such depression, like the auto-immune disorders described earlier, is often triggered by times of reproductive change, such as during menstruation, menopause or pregnancy. If depression is caused by hormonal change, then it ought to be treatable by hormones too. For example, doctors know that the level of progesterone drops in a woman's body during the second week of the menstrual cycle. One study showed that women who were given progesterone at that time experienced relief from premenstrual symptoms. This has led to theories linking the female reproductive hormones with neurotransmitters which regulate mood, although no clear-cut picture has yet emerged. In addition to depression, women are more prone to anxiety and ailments brought on by emotional distress, such as headaches or colitis.

In contrast to theories linking emotional health and hormones, it has been suggested that men suffer depression just as frequently as women but are not diagnosed as such because they are less likely to turn to the medical profession for help. Instead they seek refuge in alcohol or drugs or anti-social behavior. Studies of the Amish Society, a self-contained religious sect in Pennsylvania where drugs and alcohol are not available, show no gender difference in the likelihood of depression. This indicates that there may only be a difference in its manifestation rather than in the disease itself. Although more women attempt suicide than men (two to three times as many), men are two to three times as likely to be successful.

Social factors and depression

Apart from hormonal causes, the role of social and cultural conditions and expectations on both sexes has to be taken into consideration when attempting to explain

---

Fertility

■ Between 15 and 20 percent of couples have difficulty conceiving. Half of those who seek help will conceive naturally within five years. In the other half, nearly all will discover a medical problem that has prevented conception. Since 40 percent of infertility is caused by inadequate sperm production, the man is tested first. There may be abnormalities in the testicles due to infection by mumps, radiation or toxic chemicals. Sperm may be blocked from reaching the penis by an infection of the prostate or seminal glands. Hot baths or tight underwear may create an environment that is too warm; the testicles function best at around 32°C/90°F. Drugs and alcohol also affect sperm production.

In women, menstrual irregularity and failure to ovulate are common causes of infertility. There may be blockage of the fallopian tubes following a successful pregnancy, or scarring due to chlamydia or other sexually transmitted disease. Contraception and abortion have also been blamed, but in many cases the reason for infertility remains unidentified.

Women's age is a critical factor in childbearing. A woman of 40 has more fertile menstrual cycles than an 18-year-old based on the occurrence of ovulation, but the possibility of Down's syndrome in a child increases with both the mother's and father's age. The risk in a 22-year-old mother is one in 1,600, the risk in a 28-year-old is one in 1,000. In a 35-year-old mother, the risk is one in 250 if the father is also 35, but one in 170 if the father is 40.

Do doctors discriminate?

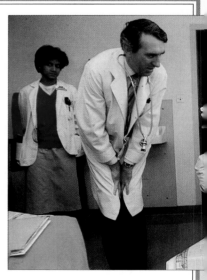

■ When men and women visit their doctor, they may find that the doctor's attitude to them differs. In particular, when men and women go to their doctor with similar vague complaints, women are more likely than men to be sent away with a prescription for tranquilizers.

There is an assumption among doctors (who are mainly male) that a woman's complaints may be neurotic and so she is treated accordingly. Moreover, some conditions found in women have been less thoroughly investigated than some found in men.

For many years women who suffered from painful periods were thought to be rejecting their female role or to have personality problems. Only with the discovery of the chemical causes of menstrual pain were such theories to some extent set aside. Similar attitudes persist with other disorders affecting women.

Attempts by some to show that women are less able to tolerate pain or that women complain more than men have been inconclusive. Others have argued that because women experience pain throughout their reproductive lives in terms of menstrual cramps and, for the majority, childbirth, they are to some extent toughened and more able to tolerate pain than men, although there is no actual evidence to support this.

depression. Although depression may have a biological basis, caused by changes in the body chemistry, social circumstances may determine its occurrence. Studies of women have shown a series of social factors which, when present in combination, are likely to lead to depression. For example, it has been found that the combination of being female, at home with small children and having sparse financial resources, is a high risk factor for depression. Women in this situation may experience social isolation and lack of control over their own lives, feeling cut off from the rest of the world. This makes depression more likely. Women who are in employment as well as being home-makers may fare better because their work offers a source of recognition, self-esteem and control, despite the burden of trying to fulfill two roles successfully.

Social pressures may also take their toll on men. For example, the feeling of being unable to fulfill his family's or society's expectations by providing material or emotional support may have a depressive effect on a man who is in employment, let alone one who is out of work or made redundant. Many men suffer feelings of depression and uselessness when they retire because they have devoted all their energies to their work for so many years. Even men able to provide adequately for their families and involved in satisfying work may succumb to mental or physical exhaustion from working too hard, commuting long distances each day, or having to work away from home for long periods.

What can you do for yourself?

The likelihood of developing a disease or illness changes with biological factors, exposure to a new environment and changes in lifestyle. Gender differences in response to those illnesses remain constant, influenced by sex hormones, which also influence our behavior and lifestyle. Women have benefited from advances in managing childbirth so that death at delivery is now rare. They have also been given more control over their lives by the widespread availability of reliable methods of contraception. The rise of feminism in the 20th century has given women more power in the community. Both men and women have benefited from safer and healthier working conditions and increased options for leisure.

In spite of gender differences, each of us can improve our mental and physical well-being through a healthy balanced diet, regular exercise and reducing stress. Stopping smoking, using alcohol in moderation and refraining from taking other drugs are also important. Other chapters in this volume contain suggestions how to do this. **AER**

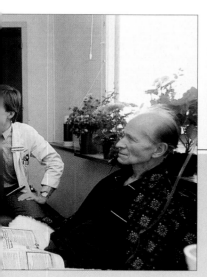

▲ **The doctor's bedside manner** *may vary according to the sex of his patient. This doctor's posture (standing) seems to indicate deference to his elderly patient. Many women, however, prefer to consult female doctors simply because they are more comfortable with them. Women doctors have also been shown in some studies to have a more sympathetic approach.*

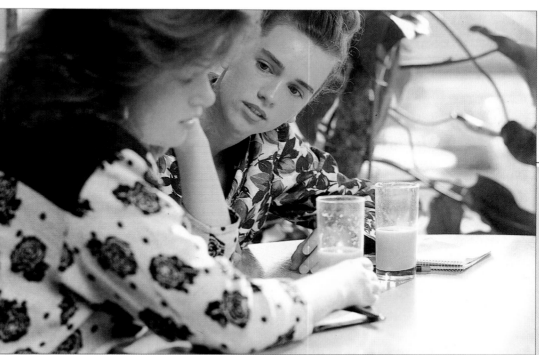

▲ **A friend of the same age and sex** *is often the best source of comfort. Having a network of emotional support is important to mental health and can help prevent depression, which is frequently influenced by feelings of isolation and loneliness.*

People who are in circumstances similar to yours can offer sympathy and sometimes practical help: a woman at home with small children may be freed to work part-time by a friendly neighbor who can babysit. Even if you do not want advice or assistance, it helps to talk things over with someone who will simply listen. Women ask for help more often from friends as well as professionals; men are more likely to act out their difficulties and to isolate themselves emotionally.

33

3

The Rhythms of Life

Staying alive from one moment to the next is a matter of heart and respiratory rhythm ● Our bodies also follow complex cycles day by day, month by month, and year by year ● Body-rhythms profoundly affect our psychology.

LIKE EVERY other living thing around us, human beings depend on and respond to fluctuations in natural rhythms. We have evolved so that our activities, moods and responses vary according to the changing amounts of light and heat around us. We now know that the human body is an extremely complex mechanism, and that our body-rhythms affect everything from the metabolism of the smallest of our cells to the way we sleep and how we perform difficult tasks. By understanding something about our bodyrhythms and the influence they have on our health and well-being, we can take steps to work with rather than against our natural rhythms, increasing our personal effectiveness and improving the way we do our jobs and make decisions in everyday life.

Your biological clock

Every one of us has a "biological clock" – a natural timekeeper regulating many of our physical and mental processes. In fact, it would be truer to say that we have a clock within a clock within a clock. The largest dial represents the life cycle itself – from birth, through adolescence and middle age to old age and death.

Elderly people may be most aware of the "life-span dial," but women can become particularly aware of the "ticking of the biological clock" when the question of whether and when to bear children arises in their lives.

The smaller dials are responsible for the rhythmic cycles of processes that involve much narrower measures of time. Most of the rhythms that rule our lives fall into one of two kinds. The first is known as the ultradian rhythm, which in adults has a cycle of 100 minutes. Research has shown that when we sleep (see *Ch 6*), we move from one stage of sleep to another about once every 100 minutes. There is an ultradian rhythm too in the way our attention span shifts from boredom to interest (in dull situations, we alternate between being more and less restless about every 100 minutes), in how often we nibble available food and in the way we fluctuate between alertness and drowsiness.

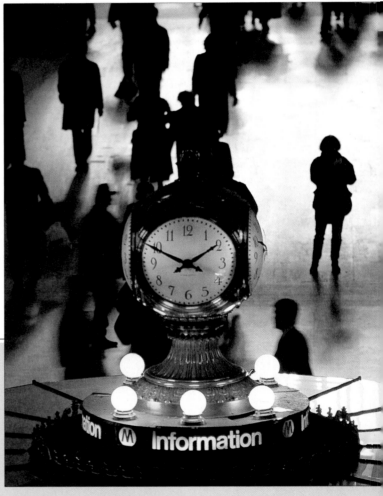

▲ **Time givers** *are an intricate part of our lives. We are aware of cycles in the world around us, such as the sunrise and sunset or the rotating hands of a clock. We are also aware of cycles in the way we feel: we notice hunger around noon, tiredness at the end of the day. The two ways of keeping time – by external and internal cues – are usually in harmony, but not always. Jet lag is a symptom of lost synchrony between our own internal rhythms and the external world. Chemical cycles in the jet-lagged body, responding to cues such as the changed cycle of light and dark, need to regain synchrony with the world.*

Rhythms of life minute by minute

■ At rest, the natural heartbeat for most people is between 50 and 100 beats per minute. If your heart beats 75 times per minute, for example, you must complete a full cycle every 0.8 seconds.

In one minute of rest, a complete blood supply of almost 5 liters (160fl oz) will circulate in an adult body. In that minute about 250cc (15 cubic inches) of oxygen are picked up from the lungs and transported through the tissues. This amount of oxygen can be increased four times for heavy exertion such as aerobic exercise.

A healthy adult can breathe in and out 30 times in a minute.

Normal breathing is at a rate of 18-20 exhalations per minute. The rhythms of breathing during heavy exercise are automatically regulated by the brain so trying to control it yourself will have no useful effect.

Nerve response cycles in the brain are among the fastest in our bodies. Cycles of 250 per second at rest occur in the cerebellum, which controls muscle contractions.

The timing, speed and direction of digestive contractions is controlled by nerve impulses directing esophageal, stomach and intestinal contractions with split-second precision.

Newborn babies, however, sleep and wake on a 50-minute ultradian rhythm. This means that they tend to rouse from sleep and cry for food every 50, 100, 150 or 200 minutes. It is only as they realize that they will have more attention from their parents during the day than at night that they tend to settle down into the other basic rhythm, the 24-hour cycle known as the circadian rhythm.

Understanding your body rhythms

Imagine one day as a 24-hour clockface. As you live through those 24 hours your body produces a regular pattern of quickening and slowing in your heartbeat, breathing, metabolism and temperature. On average your heart beats 70-80 times per minute and your lungs breathe in and out between 12 and 15 times per minute. However, your body functions do not maintain an average pace around the clockface but tend to fluctuate according to the time of day.

■ **Key body rhythms** – eg heartrate, breathing, brainwave patterns – speed up in a crisis, while others – eg digestion – slow down. However, the underlying synchrony between these rhythms keeps us alive.

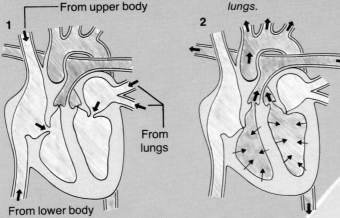

■ **The heart pumps** *blood to the lungs, where it picks up oxygen and transports it to the tissues, clearing them of carbon dioxide waste.*

1 *The walls relax and all four chambers fill with blood.*
2 *The heart contracts in order to pump oxygen-rich blood to the rest of the body, and to pump blood from the body into the lungs.*

From upper body

From lungs

From lower body

1

2

■ **Brain waves.** *The slightest activity, even opening your eyes, changes brain waves. Alpha waves (8-12 cycles per second) occur when you are awake but resting with eyes closed. Beta waves occurring at 18-25 cycles per second, accompany sensory and muscular activity. Delta waves, at less than 5 cycles per second, are found in deep sleep.*

Alpha

Beta

Delta

■ **The purpose of breathing** *is to prevent the buildup of carbon dioxide in the body. If there is too much, the nerves slow down; too little, and they become jumpy. To avoid these extremes, we rhythmically draw air into the alveoli (air spaces) in our lungs, where oxygen enters the blood. Carbon dioxide leaves the blood and is breathed out.*

Alveolar air space

Carbon dioxide

Capillary wall

Alveolar wall

Oxygen

Red blood cell

■ **Digestion** *rhythmically compresses food at the bottom of the stomach; it is then passed through the duodenum into the small intestine or, if too large, pushed back into the stomach for more grinding. Rhythmic contractions in the intestines help to mix in bile and pancreatic juices that break food down to make nutrients easy for the intestinal walls to absorb.*

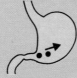

Many measurable body functions, such as metabolic rate and body temperature, have been found to reach a peak during the late afternoon or early evening. This is followed by a decline so that a minimum is reached in the early hours of the morning. Our pulse and breathing rate are both synchronized to our metabolic rate, temperature rhythm and sleep/wake cycle – and so they, too, slow down at night and speed up during the day.

It is likely that every body function has a rhythm of its own, with a peak and a dip at a time of day characteristic for that function. When the body is in equilibrium – each rhythm in time with the others – then we say that it is in a state of "internal synchronization."

The master clock

The body's pacemaker, or "master biological clock," is believed to be the hypothalamus, located at the center of the brain. It drives the rhythms of the heart, lungs and other organs, directly through the nervous system or indirectly through the release of hormones, and is responsible for activating the pituitary gland at the base of the brain. This, in turn, controls most of the hormones that affect other pacemakers in the body, such as those in the liver, in the sex organs and in the adrenal glands above each kidney.

The pineal gland, situated in the base of the brain, also exerts a major controlling influence over bodyrhythms. It has nerve links with the cells of the retina, the light-sensitive layer at the back of each eye, and with the hypothalamus. When the eyes register darkness, the pineal gland secretes the hormone melatonin. The production of melatonin usually reaches its peak about 2-3am. When the eye is exposed to high-intensity sunlight, production of melatonin slows or ceases altogether. At any one moment, the amount of this chemical messenger in the body allows each receptive cell to tell what time of day it is.

How we respond to time cues

Although we tend to be most aware of regulating our day according to clocks, watches, television and radio; it is the daily pattern of light and dark – day and night – that is the single most important external factor controlling our body-rhythms. All these external cues affecting our internal bodyclocks are known as zeitgebers ("time-givers").

Together they encourage us to sustain the normal 24-hour cycle, but without them that cycle begins to break down. In experiments where volunteers spent time isolated from the outside world in a bunker or cave without any time cues, most settled into a daily rhythm of between 25 and 27 hours, and a few even survived quite happily on 50-hour days.

In the absence of sunlight, the presence of other

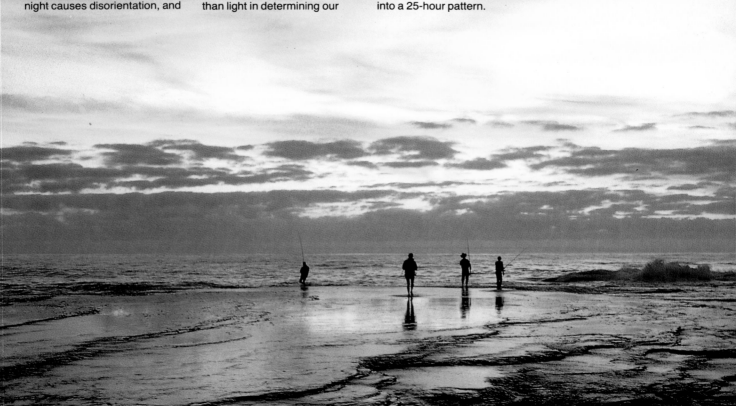

■ **Rhythms of life day by day.** Light is the most powerful external stimulus that affects our internal clock. A disruption of the normal pattern of day and night causes disorientation, and in some people the reduced amount of sunlight in winter will cause depression and lethargy. However, chemical patterns in our genes are more important than light in determining our sense of time. Experiments have shown that most people who are isolated from external cues such as light or dark, the arrival of the mail, etc, settle into a 25-hour pattern.

zeitgebers, social time cues, assume even more importance. This may explain why some people become confused as they reach old age. The development of cataracts may prevent sunlight from reaching the retinas, or the nerve pathways between the retinas and the pineal gland may deteriorate as may the effectiveness of the pineal gland itself. All this may disturb the secretion of melatonin, so that the body is not "told" what time of day it is. If this is combined with a rapid change in environment – admission to a hospital, for example – the new surroundings and routines can lead to a loss of familiar time cues and an increase in stress that, in turn, disturbs sleep and other normal bodyrhythms. The result is confusion and a lapsing from the state of "internal synchronization."

Are you a lark or an owl?

Our biological clocks not only affect the minute workings of our bodies, but also our effectiveness at different times of day. Most people classify themselves as either "larks" or "owls." Larks wake early, work well in the morning and need to go to bed early. Owls find it hard to face the day but, once they get going, can work efficiently into the night; they also tend to make the best shiftworkers (see *Ch 6*). Almost everyone, it seems, experiences a fall in performance and a subdued mood early in the afternoon, a "post-lunch dip"

that is evident whether or not you eat or drink at lunchtime.

Some psychologists claim that larks have quiet, introverted personalities, whereas owls are outgoing extroverts. There is no real evidence to support this, but there is, certainly, a close relationship between the rhythms of body temperature, sleep and mood. Generally, we are most anxious and depressed and slower mentally and physically in the early hours of the morning, when body temperature is at its lowest.

The phrase "the dead of night" has a macabre basis in truth. This is the time of deepest sleep when the body and brain are at their lowest ebb. Of all the points on the 24-hour cycle, death is most likely to occur at 4am when a person is asleep. However, staying awake and trying to work through this low point can also be hazardous: many of the worst industrial accidents have occurred after midnight, with human error playing a major role. For example, at 4am on 28 March 1979, one of the nuclear reactors at Three Mile Island in Pennsylvania developed a mechanical fault that shiftworkers failed to spot for some time. When they realized the danger, they made poor decisions and a disaster of world importance was only narrowly averted.

The effects of jet lag

When the internal synchronization of bodyrhythms breaks down, for any reason, it usually leads to sleep disturbance and confusion (see *Ch 6*). A rapid change in the body's external cues is the most likely cause leading to a

Bodyrhythms at the frontiers of medicine

■ As experts begin to learn more about the rhythmic nature of human life, their findings are beginning to have important implications in the diagnosis and treatment of physical illness. During every 24-hour period, the body's internal chemistry changes, making the symptoms of some illnesses show up more clearly at certain times of the day and, at the same time, altering the way the body will respond to drug treatment. For instance, research into leukemia has shown that at 6pm cancer cells are more susceptible to drugs, while normal cells are less prone to being poisoned by the same drugs. Another study has revealed that transplanted kidneys survive much longer if operations are performed at around 8pm – at this time of day the rhythm of the immune response is at its minimum.

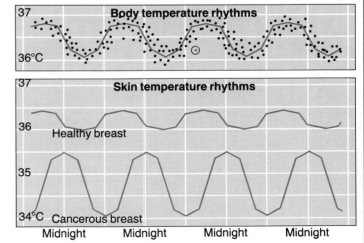

▲ **Understanding temperature rhythms aids diagnosis**. When time is taken into consideration TOP, it is clear that a normal temperature has a regular pattern of variation over 24 hours. A temperature that is normal at 3am would be abnormal at 3pm.

Experimental methods for early detection of breast cancer ABOVE *record daily, monthly and seasonal changes. Skin temperature is lower over healthy tissue and temperature changes are greater than over cancerous tissue.*

disruption in melatonin production triggered by the normal pattern of day and night. This occurs most dramatically when you fly over five or more time zones, in some cases arriving (by the clock) virtually at the same time you took off hours before (flying west on Concorde, you arrive before you take off). On landing, you find that you wake too early, begin to fall asleep at socially inappropriate times and suffer a general lack of energy and a loss of physical and mental performance. This will continue for a few days until your biological clock has had time to reset itself.

While this phenomenon – commonly known as "jet lag" – is experienced by all who fly, obviously people who travel regularly as a part of their job find it most difficult to cope with: an important meeting can begin to disintegrate simply because the biological clocks of those attending are telling them that it is long past their bedtimes. One way of trying to combat it is to schedule important meetings for when you would normally be awake at home. However, scientists may have come up with a better solution. In a recent study, experienced travelers who flew from New Zealand to Britain were given melatonin at 10am for three days before departure and at 10pm local time in Britain for three days after their arrival. They found that the symptoms of jet lag were substantially reduced, that they adjusted more quickly to the new time zone and reached normal energy levels faster than on previous trips.

The rhythms of illness

Short-term problems like jet lag are not the only outcome of disturbed circadian rhythms. The symptoms of certain types of mental and physical illness can be profoundly affected by the rhythms of the body, and a disruption of these may even, in some cases, be the cause of the problem in the first place.

Attempts are now being made to find a relationship between some forms of mental illness or other psychological disorders and disturbed daily rhythms. Abnormal hormone cycles, showing very little variation over 24 hours, have been found in anorexics (see *Ch10*) and abnormal temperature rhythms have been discovered in those with severe recurrent anxiety. It is well known that depressed

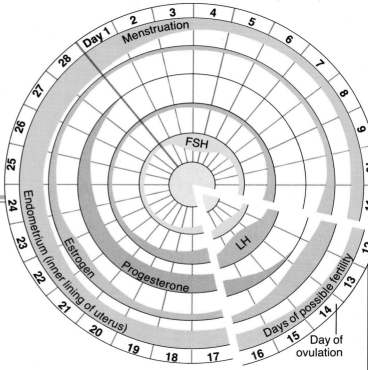

▲ **During the follicular phase,** *the ovary produces increasing amounts of estrogen (which causes the blood-rich lining of the uterus to grow in preparation to receive the fertilized egg), and the follicle-stimulating hormone (FSH) produced by the pituitary gland. When the secretion of estrogen peaks, the pituitary gland will release less FSH and start releasing the luteinizing hormone (LH). Midway through the cycle the sudden surge of LH causes ovulation.*

Rhythms of life month by month

■ A woman's menstrual cycle is one of the most familiar of human rhythms, a regular chain of biological changes happening across the span of a lunar month (approximately every 28 days) unless interrupted by pregnancy.

Menstruation (a woman's monthly bleeding or period) occurs on the first few days of this cycle and ovulation (the monthly release of the egg) occurs approximately half way through. The two-week build up to ovulation is called the "follicular phase," named after the follicle, the little sac of fluid in the ovary that grows to almost an inch (about 2cm) in diameter and bursts at ovulation, releasing the egg. During the following two weeks, called the "luteal phase," the burst sac is called the corpus luteum. It continues to have a central role – producing progesterone, the hormone that prepares a woman for the pregnancy she will have if the egg is fertilized.

Throughout the cycle the ovary produces hormones – natural chemical substances that act as messengers when released into the bloodstream by body organs (see diagram ABOVE RIGHT).

At ovulation the mature egg bursts from its follicle and passes into one of the fallopian tubes where it may or may not be fertilized. If the egg is not fertilized, the corpus luteum shrinks away, progesterone production ceases and the estrogen level drops. The uterus lining, no longer needed, starts to be shed, menstruation occurs and the cycle begins again.

While all this is going on, other cycles are occurring within a woman's body. Just before ovulation, her body temperature may drop slightly, and after ovulation it may rise a little above normal – a sign of the action of progesterone on the temperature-regulating center in the brain.

In addition, the mucus that is produced by the cervix (the neck of the womb) varies in consistency and quantity under the influence of estrogen, while the presence of progesterone is responsible for fluid retention, leading to weight gain and breast tenderness.

The emotions do not remain unaffected. Many women experience the symptoms of "premenstrual syndrome" (PMS), the lives of one in four being severely disrupted by them. These symptoms, occurring in the week or so leading up to menstruation, range from irritability, depression, tension and anxiety to restlessness and tiredness.

people tend to be inactive throughout the day and want to sleep a great deal, whereas manic-depressives become very active and require little sleep. One of the most common symptoms of depression is for sufferers to wake, depressed, early in the morning. Those suffering from neuroses, however, tend to be at their worst in the evening. Researchers have suggested that depression involves a shift of the circadian rhythms controlling the sleep/wake cycle, body temperature and hormone secretion, which is out of line with normal day/night variations. **KB**

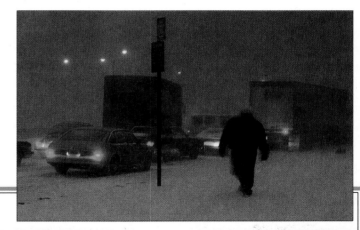

Rhythms of life year by year

■ The coming and going of the seasons may account for changes in mood. In general, people are more active and have a greater zest for life in the summer than in the winter. This may be because variations in the amount of sunlight can influence the emotions by indirectly regulating the amount of calcium available for nerve activity.

Some people suffer more acutely than others from the effects of this fluctuation in the amount of sunlight. They become tired and depressed during the winter, oversleeping, moving sluggishly and overeating. In spring, their spirits lift; and their sense of well-being soars during the sunny summer months. This condition is known as SAD – seasonal affective disorder. It seems to be due to an abnormality in the amount of melatonin secreted by the pineal gland. The amount of sunlight available during the winter is not enough for people affected by SAD to stop the production of melatonin during the day, so that it is secreted all round the clock instead of just at night.

SAD can be treated by extending the hours of daylight artificially: the person sits in front of a very bright (2,500 lux) full-spectrum fluorescent light for several hours during the morning before daybreak in the winter months. This is not as easy as it sounds. For the process to work, the person must look into this light, which imitates natural daylight, so that its rays enter the eyes and hit the

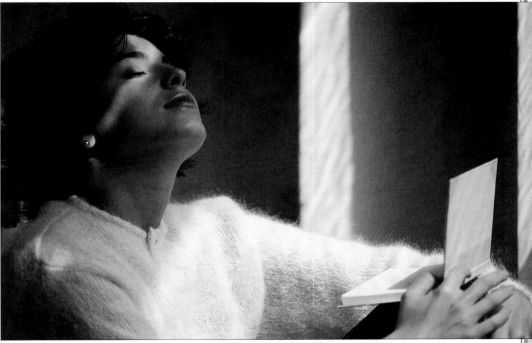

retina, sending signals to the pineal gland. Usually expert help is required to overcome this disorder. Working under bright lights at home or in the office will make little difference – as far as the pineal gland is concerned, the white light they emit is indistinguishable from darkness. Without doubt, in the future we will see the use of drugs and bright light therapy to allow us to reset our biological clocks. However, the importance of bodyrhythms remaining stable from day to day cannot be underestimated. For total body care, you must establish daily routines to help your body-rhythms cope with stress and anxiety and promote your health and well-being.

▲ **The dark of a winter storm** *TOP RIGHT may bring depression. Some people, mostly women, complain that during the winter months they feel tired, depressed and sluggish. This seasonal affective disorder (SAD) will begin to lift in the* spring, *but people who are affected only function normally in the long bright sunlight of summer. Direct natural sunlight ABOVE or very bright artificial light (10 100-watt bulbs) will improve SAD; ordinary lights turned on at night will not.*

▶ **Prolactin rhythms and breast cancer.** *Women in Kyushu, Japan, have less breast cancer than women in Minnesota. Their daily and seasonal production of prolactin, the hormone that stimulates milk production, is very different. Researchers are investigating the use of prolactin rhythms as diagnostic tools in assessing breast-cancer risk.*

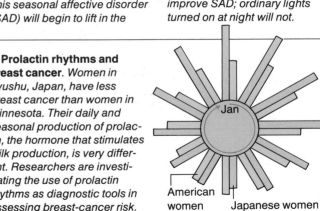

American women   Japanese women

39

4

Stress

Stress is a physical and emotional response to a challenge ● Are some people more prone to stress than others? ● Even positive events can be stressful ● How can we cope with stress so that our health is not affected?

TOO MUCH stress can contribute to a range of health problems, from poor performance at work to depression and serious physical illness. If stress is getting on top of you, coping with it better should be made a priority.

Does that mean managing things better "out there" – finding solutions to the pressures, annoyances and situations that are stressing you? This can well be part of the answer, but you should never overlook the fact that stress actually occurs *within*: it is the physiological and psychological arousal you feel when you react to a problem or some other stimulus. Too much stress can mean not only that your situation is burdensome, but that you are approaching it with beliefs and habits of mind that increase tension. Self-management skills can help you to feel less strain.

Demands, perceptions, responses

External events are certainly an important part of what causes stress, but the internal perceptions and responses of the person involved are just as important. An event causing one person extreme anxiety will not necessarily cause the same level of distress in another. What actually causes an excess of stress is not simply what happens, but the way a person handles it.

The demands made on your mental and physical resources – technically known as *stressors* – may involve major changes in your life. Losing a job, moving, divorce, the birth of a child or the death of a parent are recognized as highly stressful life events. More frequent stressors are day-to-day problems such as pressure at work, an unhappy

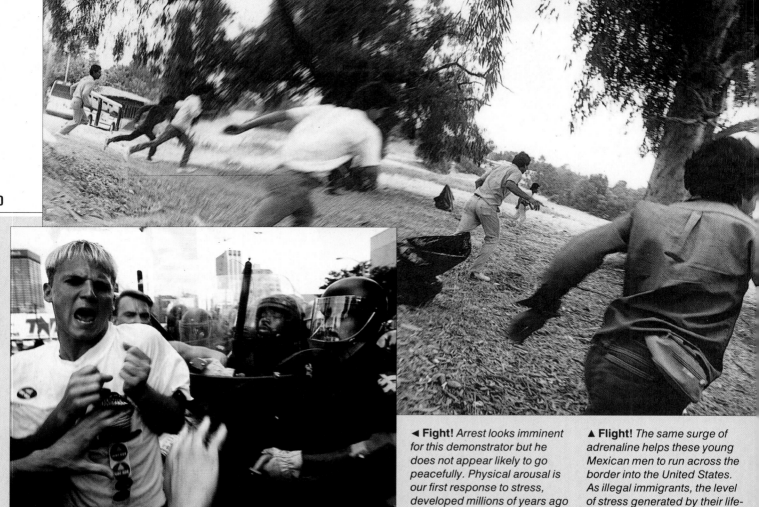

◀ **Fight!** *Arrest looks imminent for this demonstrator but he does not appear likely to go peacefully. Physical arousal is our first response to stress, developed millions of years ago as a survival mechanism.*

▲ **Flight!** *The same surge of adrenaline helps these young Mexican men to run across the border into the United States. As illegal immigrants, the level of stress generated by their lifestyle will be very high.*

relationship at home or financial difficulties. Our perceptions are the way we interpret these demands in terms of our assessment of what they mean to us and how well we will be able to cope. Finally, our responses are how we react, physically and mentally, to these perceived demands. An excessively stressed response is the result of an imbalance between how we perceive the demands and how we perceive our abilities to cope with them.

Why do some cope better than others?

We all know people who appear to sail unconcerned through situations which we feel sure would have turned us into nervous wrecks. Some people do not seem to be bothered by stressful events and may even appear to thrive on them. Others may be unworried by quite serious events such as a pile of unpaid bills, yet subject to fits of rage over traffic jams or other apparently trivial irritations. The element of perception makes an enormous difference to whether or not we are overstressed. An event is stressful according to whether or not we see it as threatening – whether we think it makes demands beyond our abilities to deal with them.

In one study, three groups of students were shown an exceedingly gory film, set in an industrial workshop. One group was told that the film was entirely fictional. Another group was told that the accidental amputations shown in the film were real, but that the film had been put together for safety purposes, as an educational guide. The final group was shown the film without any explanation.

While they watched, the viewers' physiological stress responses (such as heart rate and sweating) were recorded. Those in the first two groups were much less affected by the film than those who had not been given an explanation. They had been given a coping strategy to deal with the horrors of the film, either by denial – "This is not really happening" – or by intellectualization – "We are meant to learn from these mistakes." The third group had no such preparation to deal with the demands of the film.

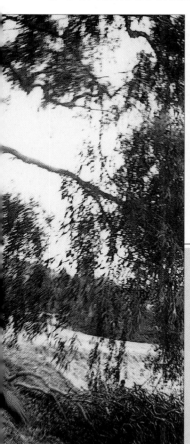

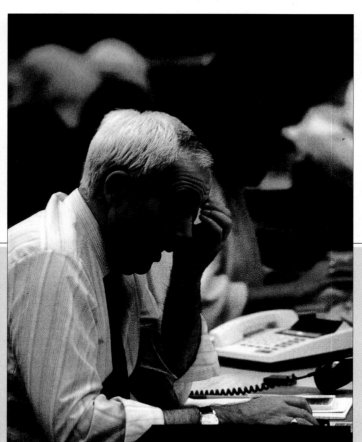

▲ **Trapped!** *The pressure of a demanding job may create a highly aroused state, but there is nowhere to run, although meetings may provide an occasional element of "fight." When there is no relief from pressure, the strain of long-term arousal appears. Headaches, exhaustion and hypertension may plague workers long after they finally leave their desks. Burnout may occur.*

Stress – a response of mind and body

■ Our earliest ancestors probably developed a physical stress response as a result of danger to life and limb. It is sometimes called the "fight or flight" state, when our bodies direct all our energies toward survival either by physical battle or by running away.

Today the cerebral cortex – the thinking and perceiving part of the brain – still sends stress signals to the hypothalamus, part of the lower brain, to prepare the body to fight or run, even though a physical response is not always necessary or even possible. The hypothalamus controls the body systems, particularly the systems not under our conscious control, like digestion or body temperature. If it receives stress signals from the cortex, it interprets these as signs of potential physical danger and prepares the body for "fight or flight." It does this even when there is no action that we can possibly take – for example, when you are faced with an awkward superior or traffic congestion. Your heart thuds, your blood races and your muscles involuntarily tense. You are feeling stressed. **PH**

41

Factors in stress management

Most people guard themselves against stressful events in similar ways, though their preparation may be less clear-cut than in the case of the students. Our natural defenses against stress seem to operate on three levels – physiological, psychological and social.

Basic physical health seems to be an essential buffer against stress. In addition, people who are regarded as psychologically hardy, who tend to assume control over situations, to show commitment to work, family and life goals, and to view negative events as a challenge, often cope very well with stressful experiences. They usually think about and prepare themselves for stressful life events, and their self-confidence and sense of control means that they generally have a high opinion of their own abilities to meet quite heavy demands. Others seem unable to develop adequate coping strategies because of their inability to perceive talent and potential in themselves. Finally, people with high levels of social support are less badly affected than those who have fewer friends and relatives to offer them help and reassurance.

Most people have developed coping mechanisms to deal more or less successfully with stress, sometimes even using it as a positive force for personal development. Stressful events happen to everyone, but we can choose to make them work for us rather than against us. **SW**

Do you get hostile?

Hostile and aggressive behavior is one means of defending ourselves in stressful situations. It is one facet of the "fight or flight" response our bodies adopt when we face a difficult situation, and it can be a useful, even necessary, response in some situations. However, hostility is often a coping strategy that backfires. If aggression is our only way of dealing with stress, it can lead to antisocial and even physically dangerous behavior.

Research has confirmed the role of anger and hostility in health and illness. Much of this evidence comes from recent developments in the study of what has become known as Type A behavior – an intense hard-driving competitiveness and a persistent sense of time urgency. When individual Type A characteristics are measured in terms of their effects on health, hostility emerges as clearly the most dangerous feature. Anger levels can be used to predict the development of heart disease and of early death from it.

Reducing hostile feelings

Can we reduce the chances of serious illness simply by avoiding aggression? For many people such avoidance means holding anger in and ignoring it, refusing to discuss or deal with their negative feelings. This is a poor solution to the potential problems posed by anger, because we need to reduce our feelings of hostility, not store them up.

42

▲ **Hostility is unhealthy.** *Screaming abuse is all in a day's work for this corrections officer, but if he cannot leave his work behind him at the end of the day, he may have a health problem. People who are chronically angry run a higher risk of heart attacks and strokes. Unexpressed anger can be even more damaging to your health and to your relations with the people around you, who may still sense it.*

How hassled are you?

■ Hassles are minor irritations that can build up into major stress factors, especially when the main ongoing pressures and crises in your life have used up your tolerance. Gauge how stressed you are on a scale of 1 to 3 for each problem according to how severe it has been for you during the past month (1 is minor; 2 is moderate; 3 is major).

- Trouble with neighbors
- Financial worries
- Disagreements at home
- Distractions from work
- Problems with colleagues at work
- Traffic jams
- Ill health in the family
- Transport
- Bad weather
- People breaking appointments with you

A score of 10 or more may indicate an excessive susceptibility to frustration and irritation. This may be a personality problem or it may reflect a particularly difficult set of circumstances – or both. Whatever your personal circumstances are, you should attempt to identify the main stressors in your life and develop new responses to them.

Other signs of too much stress are worth taking note of. Are you sleeping badly, smoking more or drinking endless cups of coffee? Do you feel lonely, inadequate or withdrawn, make silly mistakes or find it hard to make decisions? These are all common reactions to stress, and show that you need to develop new coping strategies.

Episodes of anger typically involve an unpleasant emotion, ranging in severity from mild irritation to rage. Accompanying this is the physical stress pattern, in chronically angry people usually geared to the "fight" response rather than "flight." Some useful treatments for anger focus on the process of physiological arousal. Relaxation techniques (see Ch 5) have been found to be effective in calming the anger response through controlling the body's physiological responses.

Other ways of reducing anger focus on the hostile thoughts themselves. Certain types of therapy assume that unrealistic interpretations of situations lead to inappropriate emotions. Anger is a typical response when you think that you have been mistreated or wronged, and chronically angry people have a general belief that they are treated unfairly. Therapy techniques can help these people identify the beliefs and attitudes that lead to hostility. Often personally insecure, hostile people defend their low self-esteem by blaming others. Improving their personal image and viewing others in a more positive, less defensive light can reduce their anger.

Another approach to reducing anger focuses on its function in interpersonal relationships. Anger is not just an emotional response to frustration or provocation. It is often a social communication – "Do not try to bully me." "Your behavior is unacceptable!" If people can be more articulate in their relationships, they may have less need to be angry. Social skills and assertiveness training have been found to reduce anger and hostility significantly.

Recognizing anger in yourself

Whether the chronically angry person uses self-help or seeks professional treatment, the first step is the most difficult. Hostile people often do not see themselves as having a problem. From their point of view, the problem lies in the fools, rascals and simpletons who cause so much irritation. Recognizing anger as a potential threat to health and accepting responsibility for reducing it is difficult, but essential.

Few people enjoy being angry. Changing a lifelong emotional habit can be hard, but the prospects of improved social relationships, reduced health risks and a more pleasant life altogether are strong incentives. **TWS**

How does anger lead to illness?

■ Chronic hostility leads in several ways to illness. Compared to more even-tempered people, angry and hostile personalities show larger increases in blood pressure when other people frustrate their wishes. Hostile people also seem to secrete a higher level of stress-related hormones during the course of a day than do positively assertive types. Particularly during the morning and early afternoon, hostile people demonstrate high levels of cortisol, a hormone released from the adrenal gland. Hostile people have also been found to have high levels of cholesterol in their blood. Hypertension (high blood pressure), excessive stress-hormone levels and high cholesterol can contribute to the narrowing of arteries, leading to strokes and heart attacks.

People who have narrowed coronary arteries (the arteries feeding the heart muscle its own supply of oxygen-rich blood) are especially vulnerable to heart attacks when under stress, either from strong emotions or physical exertion. A heart attack occurs when part of the heart muscle dies from oxygen starvation. This can happen when the heart is pumping hard to meet the whole body's increased oxygen demands during a stressful situation – at such times the heart needs much more oxygen itself than the narrowed coronary arteries can deliver. An angina attack is a less serious outcome of stress – enough oxygen is carried through the narrowed arteries to prevent any part of the heart from dying – but the shortage nevertheless causes heart-muscle oxygen shortages, felt as chest pains.

In addition to the medical dangers of hostile behavior, people who display anger openly to friends and colleagues often alienate them, and find themselves isolated in a crisis. During times of stress they may lack the helpful and caring contact with others that more friendly and assertive people enjoy. Hostile people also experience more frequent and severe conflicts with their families and coworkers. Chronic social strain and lack of support may increase the likelihood of illness.

"My life is at the mercy of any rascal who chooses to put me in a passion," reflected Dr John Hunter, an 18th-century pioneer in surgery and pathology. He suffered from chest pain due to heart disease, made worse by a ferocious temper. His words were sadly prophetic, as he died suddenly after a heated argument.

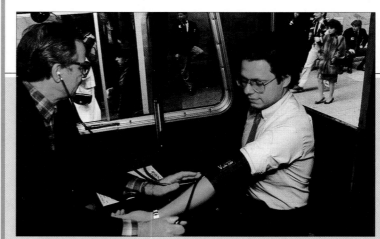

▲ **Time out for a blood pressure check**. *Then this stockbroker will return to the floor to resume his duties until the closing bell. Hypertension (high blood pressure) has been particularly identified with "Type A" personalities. They are more likely to suffer heart attacks and strokes because they will not or cannot slow down. If you frequently bring work home with you, lose your temper without much provocation and cannot bear to take a vacation, you should learn to relax – or find another job. A high-stress position is a threat to well-being when there is no relief through relaxation.*

When stress becomes depression

Each of us gets depressed from time to time – life seems to lose its luster, friends seem a little more distant, we are tired and listless and it takes more energy to do even simple tasks. Fortunately, the depression is usually mild and lasts only a few days. But one in four of us, at some time in our lives, will suffer a depression which will take us by surprise because of its severity or how long it lasts. Two situations in particular commonly cause depression.

The first is living under prolonged stress. Sometimes the demands of living exceed our capacity to cope. When this happens we can either pull the bedclothes over our head and hope the stress goes away, or we can try to find some extra energy from somewhere – we try harder, stay at work later. But if these attempts to cope fail, we are at risk of becoming helpless, of believing nothing we could ever do will help to solve our problems. The result is a draining of energy that in turn affects other aspects of our life that previously we were coping with quite well.

A second cause of depression is personal loss. It is not just the obvious losses, death or separation or loss of a job, that are important. When we move, change jobs or leave home, there are often changes in our roles and responsibilities. We are forced to let go something of ourselves. Psychologists have called this "role transition." Our role at work or in the family may be affected not only by what we do but also by other members of the family or other colleagues. When others take on new responsibilities or are ill or retire, it affects our roles too. Four aspects in particular need special attention: dealing with the loss of familiar social supports; dealing with the inevitable emotional disturbances (anger, resentment, fear) which accompany any change; dealing with the new job situation, the new baby, the new partner, etc; and dealing with the reduced self-esteem and increased self-doubt which may come from grieving for the lost role.

Stress feeds back

■ All of the physical processes involved in stress are connected by "feedback loops." The release of the stress hormone adrenaline into the bloodstream, for instance, encourages the nervous system to keep the body's automatic systems on alert. This in turn confirms the stressful situation to the brain, causing it to maintain stress signals to the body, including to the hormone releasing systems. A total body state like stress maintains itself in this way so that we can continue functioning appropriately until the perceived danger is past; but, especially when we feel helpless to cope with a situation, our perception of the stress the body is under-going may cause panic or depression. This in turn sends more stress signals to the body, creating a spiraling intensity of stress. **PH**

"If I feel like this, things must be bad." The physical symptoms of stress are themselves stress-ful. Feedback loops between the autonomic nervous system and the brain means that we perceive our own stress response as a reason to send out further stress signals. If we feel unable or unprepared to cope, depression sets in.

3 Stress centers in brain become further excited by messages from body

1 Stress signals from the brain tell hormone systems to speed body up

2 Signals from the body (eg fast-beating heart) tell brain that the body is facing a crisis

Fast-beating heart

Adrenal glands

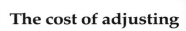

▲ **The happiest day of her life**
LEFT – and probably one of the most stressful. A major change in your life involves stress, even if the event itself is something you look forward to. On one scale of such changes, marriage is rated seventh out of 27 for its impact in creating stress. RIGHT Remembering someone you love is one way to adjust to bereavement. People who can cope well with a normal amount of stress are usually better equipped to handle extreme stress.

The cost of adjusting

■ The Social Readjustment Rating Scale was developed by Dr Thomas Holmes and Dr Richard Rahe, at the University of Washington School of Medicine. They gathered a list of stressful life events commonly preceding major illnesses from 5,000 case histories. Surprisingly, even wished-for events like promotion, marriage or having a baby could be major stressors. Marriage was assumed as a standard measure of major stresses, rated 50

Many symptoms of depression occur following loss of a loved one. This is perfectly normal. They will be at their most intense for the two to four months following the loss. Although the sadness and sense of loss will last much longer, there will be some return to a more normal lifestyle after this time. However, grief follows many patterns and it takes different lengths of time for different people to come to terms with the loss. If the grief still seems as intense, and the depression as severe, 12 to 18 months after the loss, then it might be worth seeking specialist help.

Catching it early

People have different "first signs" of depression. It may be a downward swing in mood, an increase in irritability, a physical pain such as a headache or heaviness in the stomach, a general feeling of slowness or a loss of energy. Or you may find that the first warning sign is when you start overreacting to small stressors. Try to identify what the first signs are for you.

At the very first sign that you recognize, before the depression becomes more severe, start taking preventive measures. While you still have some objectivity, try to make a list of things that you would like to do. The sort of things you may have on the list are phoning a friend to arrange to meet; deciding to do some small jobs that you have been putting off (for example paying a bill, writing a letter or hanging a picture). Appoint a definite time to do it within the next few days. Until the appointed time comes there is no need to think about it at all.

If the depression sets in, you may feel alone and that nobody wants to see you. Most likely, this is the depression talking. Answer it back. When you catch yourself thinking "I am alone: nobody could feel as badly as I feel," then try to answer back in your own way. Different people will find different answers but many people find it useful to tell themselves things such as: "A lot of people have similar problems and may be sympathetic. Just because everybody else seems to be getting on fine it doesn't mean they wouldn't understand. After all, I put on a brave face in public, yet inside I feel bad. Is there anyone who might need *my* company?"

If you feel "Nobody would want to spend time with me," then answer yourself with statements like: "Perhaps I've hidden myself away a bit recently. Perhaps that's why I haven't seen people around as much as I used to. Perhaps people think I have been busy and haven't wanted to bother me. Perhaps everyone has been a bit too busy to chat. Let me think of a specific person I could invite." **JMGW**

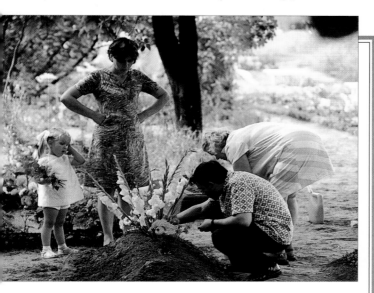

Event	Stress value
Death of partner	100
Divorce	73
Separation	65
Imprisonment	63
Marriage	50
Loss of job	47
Marital reconciliation	45
Retirement	45
Pregnancy	40
Sexual problems	39
Changing jobs	36
Taking on a large mortgage	31
Moving	23

on a scale up to 100, and other events were rated in relation to it. The list LEFT is a selection from 43 rated life events.

People with a high score (over 300 using the full list) reckoned over the course of a year seem to be more susceptible to illness and accidents. Those with healthy coping strategies, however, often withstand traumatic changes well. Life changes perceived as pleasurable are usually adjusted to with greater ease.

What is depression?

■ When we suffer severe depression certain changes take place in our bodies, in our behavior and in how we think about things. Recognizing that these changes are a normal part of depression can be a first step to recovery. Here are some of the most common changes:

- Depressed mood: feeling down, hopeless, crying, or wanting to cry but not being able to.
- Losing interest: getting little pleasure out of activities or relationships that used to please you.
- Changes in sleep pattern: either not being able to sleep enough or sleeping too much.
- Changes in eating pattern: either not feeling hungry or eating too much.
- Feeling guilty: blaming yourself for things you have done, thinking to yourself that you are a bad person.
- Thoughts of death or suicide: feeling that life is not worth living.
- Fatigue and loss of energy: you may tire easily, it is an effort to do anything.
- Reduced ability to think, concentrate or make decisions. You feel your memory is worse than it used to be.
- Agitation or slowing: you may be unable to sit still or you may feel as if you are living in slow motion.

These are the core symptoms of depression. Most of us experience each of these from time to time but we would not be considered "clinically depressed" unless we have four or five occurring at the same time and lasting weeks rather than days.

45

Learning to cope with stress

■ All of us have to deal with stressful situations from time to time; it is the way we manage them that determines whether or not we become victims of stress. Different personality types handle problems with varying degrees of success, so we will all find different situations stressful. Certain responses, such as depression and hostility, are common but essentially unsuccessful reactions to stress themselves – they create pressure, making people unhappy and antisocial.

Fortunately, there are many other possible ways of dealing with stress. Some of these methods are everyday coping mechanisms that many people use without even thinking about it. Others are strategies devised by psychologists specializing in stress reduction.

Of course, not every method will apply to every person or to every stressful situation, but by developing and using a number of coping patterns you can manage the pressured situations in your life more effectively and at less cost to your personal peace of mind.

Stress avoidance

Repression or avoidance is one way of coping with stress: usually the person refuses to face up to or acknowledge a problem, or goes to some lengths to avoid meeting it. Extreme repression and avoidance can be very damaging when the stressor is not something that will go away, but that can only be resolved through active problem-solving. Trying to ignore a painful or difficult task – giving up smoking, for instance – is a poor strategy for avoiding stress if the problem can be helped and is growing worse all the time.

Sometimes, however, repression or avoidance are perfectly reasonable coping activities, as when they are actually used to reduce stress. When there is nothing you can do to alter the situation, it is pointless to keep turning it over in your mind. Worrying about tomorrow's visit to the dentist, for example, is a fruitless exercise that may only make the actual visit more stressful. It is sensible in this sort of situation to try to forget about the appointment, by going out for the evening or finding a way to occupy yourself at home.

Certain stressors are best dealt with by avoidance rather than management if possible. Are you working too many hours in the week? Does a weekly lunch with an old friend always upset you? Decide firmly not to take work home at weekends, or look for a less stressful job. Stop your regular meetings with the person who upsets you. You do not have to be Superman – or Superwoman. Decisions like these can be positive steps to improving the quality of your life.

Sensitization is the flip side of repression. The stressor is not ignored or reduced, but carefully considered from all angles. Extreme sensitization can be damaging if it results in a feeling of being overwhelmed and unable to cope. Managed properly, sensitization can lead to careful consideration of a stressor, preparation in advance for dealing with it, and a lessening of its emotional impact as a result.

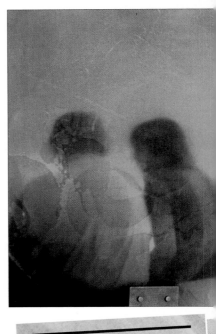

Some stressors appear overwhelming because so many issues are involved. It is useful to analyze the demands made upon you in order to break your response down into manageable steps. You can then rank each of these in order of priority and set about tackling them one at a time.

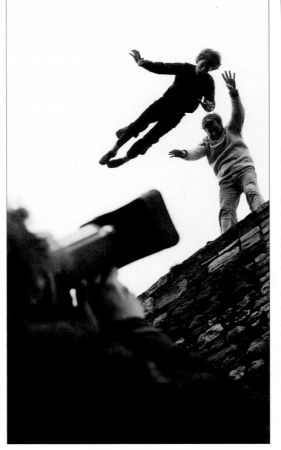

◄ **Stress inoculation** makes a person "immune" to a source of stress by gradual direct exposure to it. You may not need to learn how to cope with being flung from rooftops like this stunt boy. but whatever the stress you need to get used to, you will need to use the same principle of learning that he does: begin with small doses (this boy began by being thrown from a wall that was only a few feet high), and work up. If you are afraid of dogs, then approaching small, friendly dogs will help you to mobilize and practice coping responses that will then help to approach slightly larger dogs, and so on.

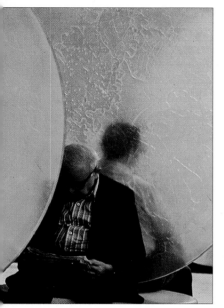

▲ **Avoid stress**. *Crowded settings promote stress, but one architect has decided to tackle this aspect of modern urban life by creating physical barriers in a waiting room. Reading is another method many people use to escape from stress in their immediate surroundings.*

Direct and indirect coping

Dealing with stress is usually either problem-focused or emotion-focused. Direct or problem-focused coping involves trying to change the situation itself – by avoidance, for example. Alternatively, the impact of a stressor may be minimized by prior preparation through increasing skills or knowledge, or by planning a response carefully. Emotion-focused coping strategies are concerned with softening the impact of a stressor once it has occurred.

Repression or denial – refusing to acknowledge the threat of a situation – is one form of emotion-focused coping. Intellectualization – trying to achieve emotional detachment – is another and more successful emotion-focused mechanism. It works best in arguments and disputes with others. Other emotion-focused strategies work on the way you act rather than on the way you think, trying to eliminate stress through its physical symptoms rather than through perceptions. Behavioral methods include relaxation techniques, while chemical methods include the use of alcohol and tranquilizers.

Preparing for stress

We are all asked to adapt continually to change. The people who tend to handle this best are those who can see such stress as a challenge, because they usually have support systems in place to deal with it when it happens. You can boost your emotional hardiness by taking regular exercise, eating a balanced diet, ensuring that you balance your work with the pursuit of active leisure interests, and taking steps to gain more control over your life. Although type A personalities may crave a high-pressure lifestyle, if they establish a pattern of work and play that reduces the number of opportunities for hostility and impatience it will in fact be easier to maintain over a long period.

Establishing good social contacts is also important. Talking about problems you are facing, "getting it off your chest," can be a very effective way of reducing tension, and you can also learn much from talking over other people's problems with them. Improving your general lifestyle in these ways will make individual stresses easier to deal with. **SW**

Passive, aggressive or assertive?

■ Which of the statements below best describes your behavior in stressful situations when dealing with others?

Passive people bottle up their feelings and adapt their behavior to others' demands. They may be very likable, but eventually they will be seen by others – and themselves – as inconsequential.

Aggressive people do not cope well with stress and they feel the need to control other people. Their behavior is likely to be hostile; they often explode.

Assertive people express their feelings without trampling on the needs and emotions of others. In a stressful situation, assertive behavior is more productive and less personally demanding.

Passive
- You avoid saying what you want, think or feel.
- You excuse your remarks with apologies and qualifications ("I'm sorry, but"..."I expect you think this is silly, but...").
- You are so busy listening for criticism you often fail to take in what others say.
- Your voice is weak, soft and hesitant, eyes downcast.
- You never know what to do with your hands.
- You appear uncomfortable, tense and inhibited.
- You want to be liked, and to please.
- You seldom get what you want, and repress your feelings to avoid expressing your anger.

Aggressive
- You say what you please at the expense of others.
- You use "you" statements that label or blame ("you're keeping information from me," "you're deliberately insulting me").
- You ignore, misinterpret or interrupt others.
- Your voice is tense, loud and demanding; you stare at others, or stand threateningly close to them.
- Your hands are in fists; you point with your fingers.
- You appear tense and angry.
- You want to dominate and humiliate.
- You usually get what you want, but by alienating others and stressing yourself.

Assertive
- You say what you think directly and positively.
- You use "I" statements to communicate points you feel strongly about ("I feel hurt by that comment" "I need to know more about...").
- You listen carefully to what others have to say.
- Your voice is firm and expressive; you look directly at others but do not stare.
- Your hands are relaxed.
- You appear relaxed and confident.
- You wish to communicate and to be respected.
- You often achieve your goals, are fair to others, and you feel good about your behavior.

5

Learn to Relax

People try to relax in all sorts of ways ● At worst they resort to alcohol, cigarettes or tranquilizers ● The safest and healthiest way of dealing with tension is to learn to let the body unwind itself mentally and physically.

A CAR WORKS best when it is humming along at a moderate pace, not stopping and starting in a traffic jam; or, at the opposite extreme, tearing around a race circuit at a phenomenal speed. In the same way, you are designed to perform at your best when all your body systems – the heart and blood circulation, muscles, nerves, state of mind and so on – operate more or less at the mid-point between too little and too much stress. Through relaxation, it is possible consciously to control your body's reactions to the stresses and strains of everyday life, to ensure that you remain on an even – and healthy – keel.

When tension becomes the norm

When you are confronted with something that is challenging or stressful, your body will suddenly become alert and your unconscious mind will ask, "Is it new?", "Is it dangerous?" or "Do I know how to cope with this?" If it is something you have experienced before and have learned to deal with, your body will return to its normal level of attention and you will simply cope with whatever it is. Otherwise, your defenses will remain on alert (see *Ch 4*).

In some circumstances, this stress response can be beneficial. Feeling under pressure can be extremely useful when you have to meet a deadline, take an exam or want to be assertive and put your point of view across at a meeting. In extraordinary cases, it can save lives – say, if you are being attacked or you have to react instantly to pull a child out of harm's way. However, if you are feeling stressed over long periods without adequate rest spells, the physical effects can take their toll in tension headaches, low-back pain, insomnia and tiredness. Stress has also been linked with more serious problems such as stomach ulcers, hyper-

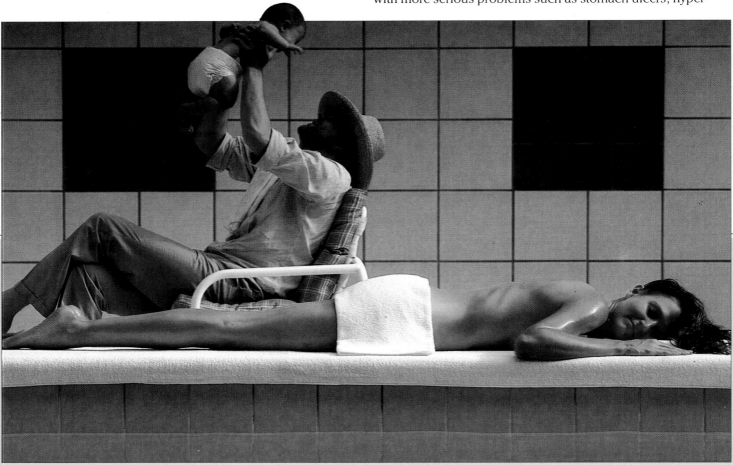

▲ **A little relaxation is easy** ... when you do not even have to think about it. If you feel confident and competent about playing with the baby, it will probably be a relaxing thing to do. It helps too to have a mind that is free of worries. On holiday, or in any situation where you are totally removed from the stresses of everyday life, most people find it easy to unwind mentally and physically. Holiday resorts, sports centers and health clubs are typical artificial environments where business or domestic worries can be excluded from your life for a while.

tension, heart disease and the worsening of asthma.

Over time, we teach our bodies how to react to stress by developing habits, both bad and good. Habits are usually linked to a trigger in the environment. For example, you may have unconsciously decided that driving is stressful, because you do not do it very often, because you have had a bad experience in your driving career, or because "everybody knows that it is." Consequently, each time you get behind the wheel (the environmental "trigger"), you may, without realizing it, hunch your shoulders, hold your arms rigid, sit forward in the seat and grip the wheel tightly. A few miles down the road and you are already tired and on edge. The whole experience is unpleasant (reinforcing your feeling that driving is stressful), and in this state, you are far more likely to have an accident – which would make the situation even worse for the future.

However, if you were to make a conscious attempt to break your bad habits and develop good ones – in this case, by changing your mind about driving and taking steps to alter your physical responses when you are behind the wheel – you can reduce dramatically or even eliminate unnecessary stress...and you might even come to enjoy driving.

How to control your autonomic responses

Almost everyone knows someone who never seems anxious. However, for the vast majority of us, being relaxed does not come naturally. It is a skill that has to be learned. One way is to develop your powers of suggestion and use them to influence your nervous system.

Experts often think of the nervous system as two separate parts: the part over which we have conscious control – the nerves that we can "instruct" to move the muscles of, say, our fingers – and the part that operates independently of our thoughts. This second part – called the autonomic (literally "a law unto itself") nervous system – includes the nerves that regulate the heartbeat, cause blood vessels to expand and contract, regulate digestion and are responsible for thousands of other body processes.

It was once thought that we could never have control of any part of the autonomic nervous system, despite stories of Indian yogis who seemed capable of dramatically slowing their heartbeats and performing other remarkable feats. However, in the 1960s, the American psychologist Neal Miller showed that, when rewarded by electrical stimulation of the pleasure center in their brains, rats could learn to control their blood pressure, gastric secretions, heart rate

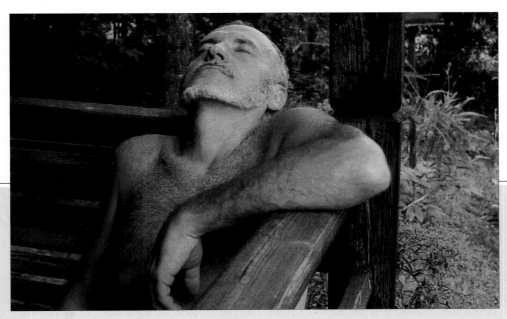

Devise a phrase that you feel comfortable with – for example "I am calm and relaxed" or "I am in control and feel confident." Say this phrase to yourself at different times of the day. With time and practice, just saying these few words will act as a trigger to relax your body.

49

◄ **Sometimes you have to make more of an effort** *to relax, but you can learn to control your level of tension by changing the way you behave and controlling the thoughts that run through your mind.*

Talking yourself into tranquility

■ "Autogenic" (self-generated) relaxation is the art of influencing your nervous system through what you think and say to yourself in order to produce soothing effects in the body.

Begin by making yourself comfortable. Take one or two deep breaths and focus your mind.

Now say the following phrases three times each, pausing after each repetition. Take your time, keeping your breathing slow and regular.
● I am at peace with myself.
● My right arm is heavy.
● My left arm is heavy.
● My neck and shoulders are heavy.

Now take another deep breath, and say to yourself:
● My right arm is warm.
● My left arm is warm.
● My right leg is warm.
● My left leg is warm.
● My neck and shoulders are warm.
● My heart beat is slow and regular.

● My stomach is warm and calm.
● My forehead is cool and calm.
Now take some time to enjoy the feeling of relaxation before saying to yourself:
● I feel refreshed and completely awake.

and other autonomic functions. If rats could do that, researchers asked, why not humans?

With the development of biofeedback machines which can detect minute changes in the electrical activity of skin and muscles, it was found that humans could, indeed, control body functions that had previously been thought uncontrollable. Researchers took these findings another step forward when they married this development with the system of mental exercises introduced by the German psychiatrist and neurologist Johannes Schultz in the 1930s, to arrive at "autogenic" (self-generated) relaxation.

Tapes and cassettes designed to help you relax usually work on the autogenic principle. Many of them focus on helping you to imagine feelings of warmth and heaviness. This is quite a clever prompt to your whole system. When the body's stress response is activated, one of the effects is to direct blood flow toward the major muscles and away from the hands and feet, which feel colder as a result. By focusing on making these parts become warmer, the blood flow returns to them and the autonomic system is cued to relax. And when muscles relax, they feel heavier.

Unwinding tensed-up muscles

A more direct method of relaxation is consciously to relax the muscles that tighten when you are tense. Before you can relax your muscles, you have to learn the difference

The simple stages of muscle relaxation

■ Set aside at least 20 minutes every day to relax. Take the telephone off the hook and let everyone know that you will not be available for a while. Make yourself as comfortable as possible in a supportive high-backed chair, or lying down either on a firm bed or on the floor. Many people like to lie with their head higher than their feet – 12 inches higher is ideal. To gain maximum benefit you should use a board for this, propped at an angle so that the body lies in a smooth backward slope. In this position the spine straightens out, and muscles that are normally tensed while you are standing have a chance to relax.

Tense and relax each of the following muscle groups, BELOW, each time holding the tension

- **Forehead**: raise your eyebrows as if very surprised.

- **Eyelids and eyebrows**: shut your eyes tightly.

- **Tongue and throat**: push your tongue hard against the roof of your mouth.

- **Neck**: press your head against a headrest or pillow, and then relax. Slowly bend your neck forward and back.

- **Shoulders**: lift them as if trying to make them touch your ears.

- **Triceps** (back of upper arms): straighten your arms as hard as you can.

- **Chest**: take a big, deep breath and hold it.

- **Hands and forearms**: make a tight fist.

- **Abdomen**: tense your stomach muscles as if someone were about to punch you there.

- **Biceps** (front of upper arms): bend your arms at the elbows and touch your shoulders with your wrists.

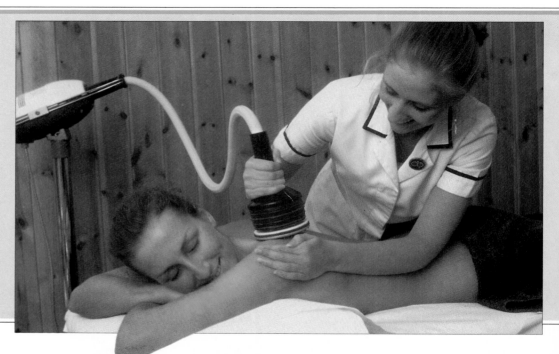

► **Body massage** is a deeply relaxing and soothing experience. Depending on the context and the techniques used, its effects range from the sensual to the therapeutic, and many practitioners of alternative medicine use massage techniques as part of holistic healing as well as to release tension. Professional masseurs use a range of equipment like the rotating disc shown above, but massaging by hand is equally effective using very basic stroking techniques.

between the sensations of tension and relaxation. This may seem quite self-apparent, but many people have been stressed for so long that they have forgotten what being relaxed feels like. To find out, concentrate on one muscle group – for instance, those in the shoulders – and simply tighten them as much as you can, in this case, by pulling your shoulders as close to your ears as possible. Hold this position for a few seconds and then relax: there really is a great difference. Continue by tightening and relaxing the rest of your muscle groups.

By being aware of which muscles are becoming tense and when, you can consciously relax them and so remove this part of your stress response. As a result, you can prevent

your body becoming more and more stressed as the day wears on. For example, you may spend a great part of the day either writing or typing at a desk.

If you write for long periods, you may well slouch and hunch your shoulders, and if your task is a particularly tedious or unpleasant one, you may tense other muscles as well – for example you may frown, grit your teeth or twist your legs around each other.

If you are typing, your shoulders and back muscles may be continually tensed over long periods. And if the phone should ring, this can trigger even more overall tension so that you grip the telephone and hunch your shoulders even more.

The result is a great deal of stress and physical discomfort, leading to even more stress. If, however, you occasionally stop working, relax your shoulders and adjust your posture throughout the day, you are unlikely to suffer the same consequences. You will be more able to do this if you are aware of your body state.

Take a deep breath

To achieve total muscular relaxation, it is important to pay attention to one particular muscle: the diaphragm. This muscular sheet lies between the lungs and the stomach and plays an important role in proper breathing. Rapid, shallow breathing causes an imbalance in the oxygen and waste gases in the bloodstream, making you feel dizzy and unwell. Shallow breathing is in itself a sign of stress; it can make you feel stressed even if you are not already. Normally, your breathing should be slow, calm, regular and not too deep, but in order to relax fully, try taking a few deep, "diaphragmatic" breaths – when you push the diaphragm

for about 3 seconds before letting go.

You may find that it helps to move the body part in order to release the tension – for example, wiggling your fingers after

tensing hands and forearms. If you have completed this exercise and any muscles still feel stiff and uncomfortable, simply tense and relax them again.

● **Hips and lower back**: arch your back and clench the muscles in your buttocks.

● **Feet and legs**: straighten out your legs and point your feet away from you.

The calming effect of deep breathing

■ A tranquil mind is often the product of a relaxed body. To achieve this, the diaphragm is the most important part of the body to learn to relax. This is the muscle beneath the lungs that controls breathing. To make sure that you are breathing properly using your diaphragm, practice this exercise:

● Lightly rest your hands just below your rib cage.
● Breathing gently through your nose, slowly fill your lungs. At the same time, push out your diaphragm and draw your shoulders up and back slightly. Your rib

cage should expand and you should see your hands rise.
● When your lungs are full, hold your breath for a count of three.
● Slowly breathe out – your rib cage and hands should fall. At the same time, relax the muscles in your chest and shoulders.
● Repeat these steps two or three times for effective relaxation.

A few deep breaths from time to time throughout the day can be an effective way of stopping tension from building up.

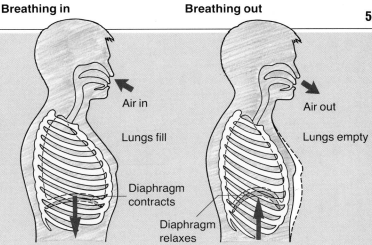

Breathing in   **Breathing out**

Air in   Air out

Lungs fill   Lungs empty

Diaphragm contracts

Diaphragm relaxes

▲ **Breathing is regulated** by the diaphragm, the sheet of muscle dividing the chest from the abdomen. When we breathe in, it contracts and flattens moving the ribs upwards and outwards. This increases volume in the chest and air rushes in to maintain the same pressure as before. When the diaphragm relaxes, air is expelled again.

51

down as far as possible and expand your lungs into all the extra space. This is also a very quick and easy way to relax in moments of stress – while sitting in a traffic jam, before an interview or sitting in the dentist's waiting room.

Thinking yourself relaxed

A third relaxation technique is simply to think relaxing thoughts. There is no point in trying to practice muscle relaxation or autogenic relaxation if your mind is churning with all your problems and fears. In relaxation, as with most things in life, your body and your mind must work together. To practice any form of relaxation you need to be able to

banish fears and problems. You may find that you can do this simply by listening to soothing music or by counting backward from 300. However, relaxation can be even more effective if your thoughts are not only free from invasion by day-to-day problems but also focused directly on relaxing images.

You may have come across a technique called "visualization." Sufferers from various diseases use it to turn their thoughts inward and "see" (visualize) the processes causing their illness. Then they imagine a means of stopping or destroying those processes. During relaxation, thoughts are also turned inward, but instead of destroying

Make yourself feel competent

■ It is relaxing to create scenes in your imagination that involve positive feelings of competency, control and achievement. Imagine that you are confident, comfortable and totally involved in what you are doing – for instance, you might imagine yourself doing an absorbing hobby.

You could also see yourself in a situation that you know you can deal with competently. Perhaps there is something you do at work that you enjoy because you feel confident in your ability to perform that particular task well.

Whichever imaginary scene you generate in your mind, enjoy the feelings it produces, taking as much time as you can. When you want to finish the session, it may increase your sense of control – and the relaxing effect that has – to count slowly backward from 5 to 1, gradually bringing yourself back to reality.

52

Identify the situations that cause you stress and use them instead as cues for relaxation. Some people stick colored dots in obvious places to remind themselves to unwind. A chiming clock or church bells are good prompts too.

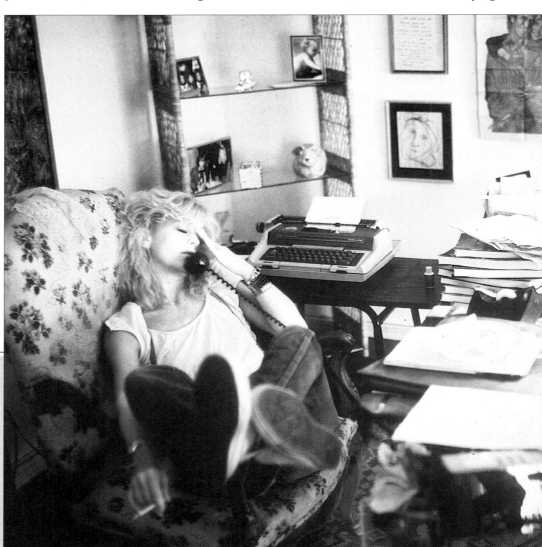

▲ **Mentally escape from a stressful situation** by picturing a beautiful and tranquil scene in your imagination. Many people find a green landscape with the sound of running water particularly peaceful, others prefer an image of themselves lying on a beach with the sun warming their body and the distant sound of waves.

Make the scene as comfortable and real as possible. Try to hear distant noises of birds or the wind blowing. Involve all your senses – imagine what the ground would feel like beneath you, the smell of the grass or the salt spray, or the feel of the breeze on your face.

You may like to picture the

the causes of stress, you simply ignore them, seeing your-self in an imaginary place similar to one where you have been relaxed before or in a situation that resembles one where you usually feel competent and sure of yourself. With practice, you will find that you can transfer the feelings of well-being experienced in these imaginary places and situations into the here and now.

Turning your enemies into your friends

Another useful mental trick is to transform stress triggers into relaxation triggers. Instead of regarding the ringing of a telephone, for example, as a cue for stress, the telephone

ring could be perceived as a trigger for relaxation, remind-ing you to shift position and relax any tense muscles. Stuck in a traffic jam? Instead of gritting your teeth and revving your engine, use the time to take a good look around you and enjoy the opportunity to be alone with your own thoughts, away from other people's problems...and from the ringing of the telephone.

Like most skills, the relaxation techniques outlined above will become more effective the more you practice them. Do not expect immediate results. However, once you have gained a measure of control and are able to relax more quickly and easily, you can begin to apply the skills you have learned to everyday situations, so that you can reduce your stress response and save it up for when you really need it. **PH**

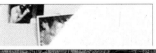

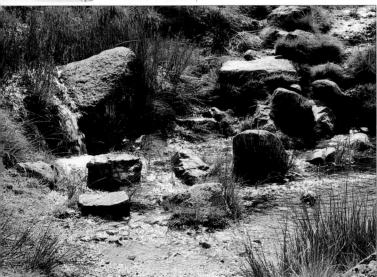

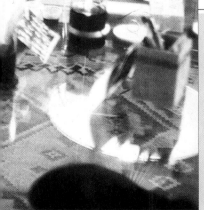

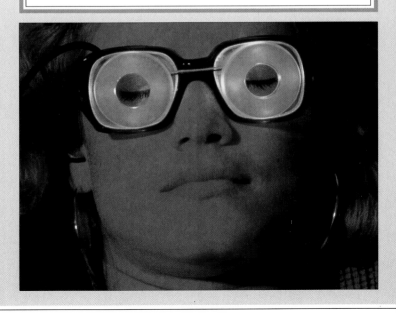

▶ **A gymnasium for the brain** *is the latest Hollywood trend in mental relaxation. These glasses are, in fact, a Whole Brain Synchro Energizer (also known as the Relaxman). They flash, at changing speeds and alternate rhythms, white lights through the wearer's eyes creating a 40-minute psyche-delic effect. The intended result is to leave the right (creative) and left (analytical) side of the brain in "sync" with each other. Experts recommend that after the "brain gym" clients should give themselves some time to re-orient before enduring the shock of entering the real world again.*

scene with friends who make you feel at ease. Stretch your imagination gently to build up a scene with all the elements that make you feel most content.

Massage for eyestrain

■ Stress and overwork can cause eyestrain, which in turn can result in a tension head-ache. Here is an easy and effective treatment.

● Place one thumb on the inner side of each eyesocket, on either side of the bridge of the nose, with the fingers resting on top of the head. Massage both eyesockets eight times, using small circular motions.
● Holding the bridge of the nose between the thumb and index finger of one hand, press up and then down eight times.
● Resting one thumb of each hand on either side of the lower

jaw, place the tips of the index and middle fingers of both hands on either side of the nose. Remove the middle fin-gers and massage under the cheekbones with the index fingers. Again, use circular motions eight times.
● Place your thumbs on either side of your forehead, curling your other fingers into loose fists. Gently rub these fists around each eye socket: start from the inner eyebrow out to the temple, then back under-neath the eye at the nose and out again to the temple. Do this eight times.

53

6

The Healing Power of Sleep

Did you have a good night's sleep? ● *Do you usually sleep well?* ● *How well and how long you sleep makes an important difference to your health and mental agility* ● *Sleep is probably much more complex than you think.*

GETTING enough sleep is fundamental to mental and physical health. It rests and revives the body, restores the mind and relieves tension. All too often, however, we underestimate its importance. In the midst of work, family responsibilities and leisure activities there is little time left to sleep and we try to get by with less than we need. Although a good night's rest promotes alertness and improves the quality of our waking lives, sleep is often the first casualty in a crisis or during periods of ill health. Why does the body need regular sleep? What can you do to ensure that you get enough? And what goes on during that third of our lives that we spend unconscious?

After you turn out the light and let your thoughts drift away, your mind and body continue to work. The eyelids close, the pupils shrink, breathing becomes slower and deeper, heart rate and temperature drop and the flow of digestive juices and saliva decreases. You lose consciousness for a time, but a noise, a sudden movement or a light can bring you back to consciousness immediately. The brain still registers sound and touch.

Researchers have identified two main kinds of sleep: rapid eye movement (REM) sleep; and nonREM sleep which is more tranquil. NonREM sleep may be anything from dozing to a deep slumber, so experts often divide it into four stages, each deeper than the one before. As you begin to doze you enter stage 1 sleep: your thoughts wander and you may drift in and out of sleep, experiencing a sensation like dreaming. Eye movements become slow and rolling, and breathing becomes more even.

No matter what age you are, about half of each night is spent in stage 2 sleep (light sleep). Stage 3 is a period of deep and restful sleep; muscles relax and blood pressure drops. Stage 4 sleep is the deepest of all, and on some nights sleepers may not achieve it. Most stage 3 and 4 sleep occurs during the early part of the night.

Sleep cycles during the night

During a typical night's sleep we change from one stage to another, often in cycles moving from light to a deeper sleep (stages 1-4 of nonREM sleep) followed by several minutes of vivid dreaming (REM sleep). The first period of REM sleep usually happens between 70 and 90 minutes after falling asleep, and on average we complete five cycles every night. REM sleep occurs in four or five episodes of increasing length. The first period may last 15-20 minutes, and the final one 30-60 minutes in the early morning.

The stages of sleep

■ A good night's sleep, typical, as seen here, for a young adult. Four or five distinct cycles of sleep occur in a single night. The sleeper usually falls first into a light and then a deeper sleep before ending with several minutes of dreaming.

A postural shift often occurs after stage 4, but not during dreaming – our muscles seem to be paralyzed to prevent us from acting out our dreams.

Deep sleep phases are much longer in the first half of the night than in the second. We often wake briefly but in the morning we seldom remember having done so.

The brain wave patterns drawn along the bottom of this chart are not to scale. They indicate typical changes in depth and frequency of waves.

Major change in body position

Muscles "paralyzed"

△ Vivid dreams likely

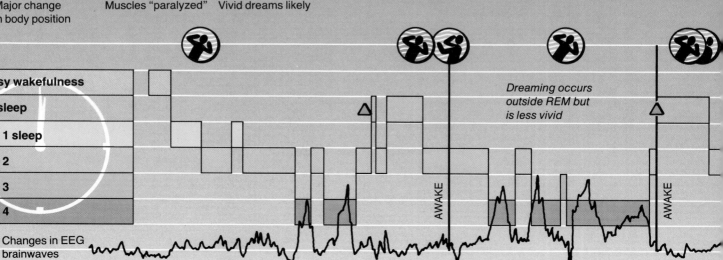

Drowsy wakefulness

REM sleep

Stage 1 sleep

Stage 2

Stage 3

Stage 4

Changes in EEG brainwaves

Dreaming occurs outside REM but is less vivid

AWAKE

AWAKE

The last third of the night is dominated by REM sleep, while most of the deep sleep of stages 3 and 4 takes place early in the night. We change posture between stages and may wake up several times without remembering later. NonREM sleep is often described as "an idling brain in a movable body." By contrast, REM sleep is a period of considerable mental activity but the body is effectively paralyzed, which stops us trying to act out our dreams. Accompanying the rapid eye movements that give this phase its name, the heart rate increases and becomes more variable, blood pressure fluctuates, and both oxygen consumption and blood flow to the brain are higher than when we are awake. Everybody dreams during REM sleep, though dreams are not always remembered. REM imagery is very vivid and sometimes bizarre, often incorporating colors and sounds. Men experience penile erections during this phase, and women engorgement of the clitoris.

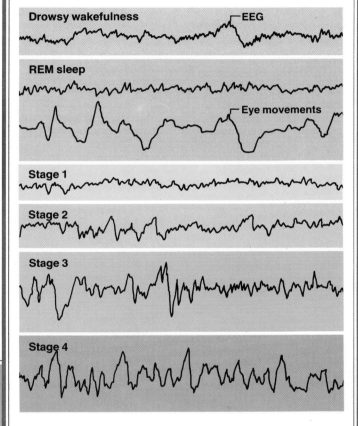

Brain waves and sleep

■ Brain waves, eye movements and muscle activity can tell researchers how we proportion our sleep. When we are drowsy, the electroencephalograph (EEG) shows alpha brain waves. In rapid eye movement (REM) sleep, when we dream, brain waves are faster and deeper and, except for muscle twitches, the body is paralyzed with loss of muscle tone. During stage 1 sleep (dozing), the eyes are still. In stage 2 brain waves speed up. Stages 3 and 4 (slow-wave sleep) show deep and slow brain waves. There is a higher proportion of slow, deep delta waves in stage 4.

Drowsy wakefulness — EEG

REM sleep — Eye movements

Stage 1

Stage 2

Stage 3

Stage 4

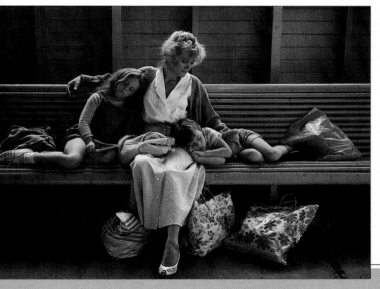

▲ **How much sleep do they need?** *Newborns are highly variable, but they typically sleep 16-17 hours per day, one-year-olds 13-14 hours. Between 5 and 15, children sleep between 9 and 10 hours per day.*

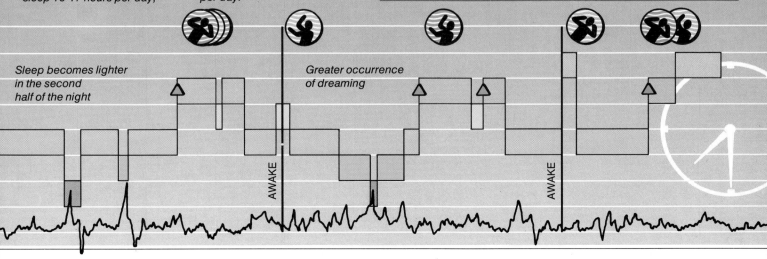

Sleep becomes lighter in the second half of the night

Greater occurrence of dreaming

AWAKE

AWAKE

Why do we need sleep?

Sleep is a form of active regeneration of the mind and body. NonREM sleep seems to play a greater part in restoring physical energy while REM sleep seems to have more effect on the functions of the mind. When people are deprived of deep sleep (stages 3 and 4) they complain of aches and muscle stiffness in the morning. Interference with REM sleep affects the memory of recent events, suggesting that REM sleep plays a role in helping us to retain material newly learned during the day. It seems that we need a certain amount of each kind of sleep: if we get less deep sleep or REM sleep on any night, we automatically make up the deficit on following nights.

Many clues about why we need sleep emerge when we experience the effects of sleep loss. The occasional few hours makes very little difference. It may lower our motivation to do things the next day, or make us irritable. Prolonged loss of sleep, however, affects alertness, performance and mood. People deprived of sleep have difficulty concentrating and are poor at tasks needing sustained attention. They are irritable and depressed, their powers of perception may be affected, and in extreme cases they may hallucinate. Surprisingly, depriving people of sleep has been used as a treatment for depression. This treatment works in the short term, but for obvious reasons it cannot be sustained.

How much sleep is enough?

Not everybody needs eight hours of sleep each night. The most important thing is to sleep for as long as you need in order to feel refreshed in the morning and alert throughout the day. There is, however, some surprising evidence about the link between how much sleep a person needs and both their life expectancy and psychological well-being.

A survey of the health and lifestyle of over one million Americans showed that the average length of time they slept was a reliable predictor of their longevity. Between 7 and 7.9 hours of sleep per night was associated with the longest life-

Snoring can be a medical problem

■ Is snoring just an annoying noise? While most people realize that having a partner who snores can put a tremendous strain on a relationship, fewer are aware that it is, potentially, a serious medical problem. According to surveys over 19 percent of the population snores habitually, often driving their bedfellows into separate bedrooms.

Men tend to snore more than women, and the likelihood is increased by obesity, age, alcohol and sedatives. It is more frequent during nonREM sleep, and is made worse when the person lies on their back.

The noise that we hear is caused by a vibration of the soft tissue in the back of the throat. It is often linked with hypertension

(high blood pressure) and can be a sign of a more serious disorder known as apnea.

Typical symptoms of apnea include intermittent snoring with quiet pauses followed by a loud snort, or periodic pauses in breathing accompanied by very loud snoring.

What is actually happening is that the sleeper stops breathing up to two or three hundred times during the night, but without being aware of it. This leads to a fragmented night's sleep and to extreme difficulty in staying awake during the day.

The sleeper's partner may also suffer a severely disrupted night's rest. Often the solutions are weight loss, breathing devices and surgery.

Coping with shiftwork

■ About one worker in five spends some hours on evening or night shifts – it is standard requirement for nurses, police officers, doctors, pilots, truck drivers and many others. Often they work in rotating shifts, on duty during the day for a set period of time, then working an evening shift for a similar period, followed by a night shift. A schedule like this requires constant resetting of the biological clock, and has inevitable effects on the health and well-being of the person concerned.

Shiftworkers suffer more complaints affecting their sleeping patterns than people following a normal daytime working schedule. On average, night-workers sleep 5-7 hours per week less than dayworkers and they often have difficulty falling asleep during the day and staying awake at night. As a response to this they consume more sleeping aids and more stimulants. Although most attempt to catch up on sleep

during their days off, night-workers, particularly, function in a constant state of sleep deprivation which can alter mood and impair performance.

One of the greatest problems is the strain on marital and social relations, and on the worker's role as a parent. Our society is organized to suit the conventional working day, and it may become impossible for a shiftworker to see friends locked into a different timetable, or to take part in community activities.

Social isolation is a real problem, so is childcare. In addition, the sleeping time of a shift-worker is not as protected as that of other workers – telephones, doorbells, electrical appliances, noises from the street and hundreds of other disturbances go on constantly during the daytime and die down at night. Shiftworkers need to expend considerable extra effort to minimize disruption.

How age affects sleep

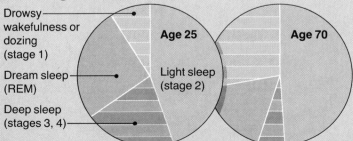

Drowsy wakefulness or dozing (stage 1)

Dream sleep (REM)

Deep sleep (stages 3, 4)

Age 25

Age 70

Light sleep (stage 2)

▲ Compared with a 25-year-old, a 70-year-old spends only one-quarter as much time in stages 3 and 4 of sleep, but almost four times as much time awake in bed or in stage 1 (dozing). Dream sleep remains the same from young adulthood to old age.

expectancy. People who slept for a significantly shorter time (4 hours) or a longer time (10 hours) had a higher incidence of heart disease and strokes. This does not necessarily mean that sleeping for a short time causes disease, many have led long and productive lives on 3-4 hours of sleep per night. In fact, psychological research has shown that people whose natural tendency is to need little sleep are more energetic and active, and better adjusted socially.

Age is a significant factor in how much sleep we need. Newborn babies sleep on average 16-18 hours per day, but as the child grows older this figure diminishes rapidly. Elderly people sleep an average of only 6.5 hours per night. Sleep needs vary substantially among adults, from as little as 4-6 hours per night to 9-10 hours, but two-thirds of adults sleep between 7-8 hours per night. **CM**

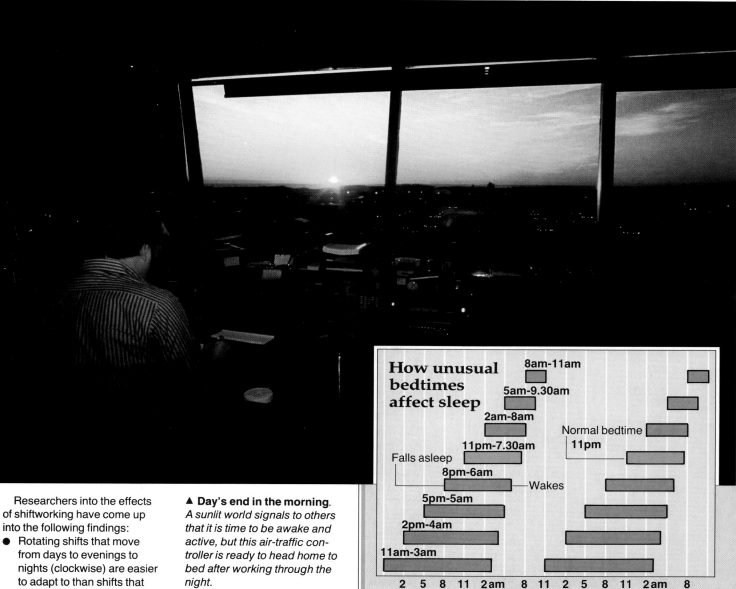

How unusual bedtimes affect sleep

Normal bedtime 11pm

Falls asleep — Wakes

| | 2 | 5 | 8 | 11 | 2am | 8 | 11 | 2 | 5 | 8 | 11 | 2am | 8 |

8am-11am
5am-9.30am
2am-8am
11pm-7.30am
8pm-6am
5pm-5am
2pm-4am
11am-3am

Researchers into the effects of shiftworking have come up into the following findings:
- Rotating shifts that move from days to evenings to nights (clockwise) are easier to adapt to than shifts that rotate in an anticlockwise direction.
- To help your biological clock adjust, shifts should rotate every two or three days, or else remain the same for a period of three weeks.
- It is easier to establish a regular sleeping pattern if

▲ **Day's end in the morning.** *A sunlit world signals to others that it is time to be awake and active, but this air-traffic controller is ready to head home to bed after working through the night.*

you maintain the same schedule on days on and off work.
- People who tend to be more awake at night are better suited to shiftwork than people who are at their best in the morning.

▲ *How long you sleep does not just depend on how tired you are. Sleep is also controlled by the body's natural rhythms. If you go to sleep earlier than usual you will probably take longer to fall asleep and wake earlier, but sleep longer. If you go to bed late you will fall asleep quickly and wake late but get less sleep in total. Occasionally, when you stay up very late you may run into a period of your body's natural cycle that lets you sleep for as many as 16 hours.*

Troubled sleep

■ After the common cold, difficulty in sleeping is the most frequent health problem in our society. About one-third of the population of the United States complains of lack of sleep, and sleep clinics have been set up to examine the problem.

Over 50 percent of those who decide to visit a sleep clinic struggle constantly to stay awake during the day. They have found themselves falling asleep at the wheel of their car, at work, in meetings and in a variety of dangerous or embarrassing situations. Often these sleep-deprived people talk about sleep the way starving people talk about food, but they still feel unable to get enough of it.

Most are carrying a large sleep debt through not being able, or not allowing themselves, to sleep at night. Typically they work long hours during the day and try to sleep for short periods at night. Often the weekends are used for catching up on sleep, but the debt mounts again by mid-week. Most often they say they suffer from insomnia. In some cases the problem is sleep apnea, a breathing difficulty during sleep. More rarely, people who suffer from sleep disorders are getting a normal amount of sleep at night but still feel drowsy during the day. They may suffer from a condition called narcolepsy, characterized by sudden and irresistible sleep attacks; but

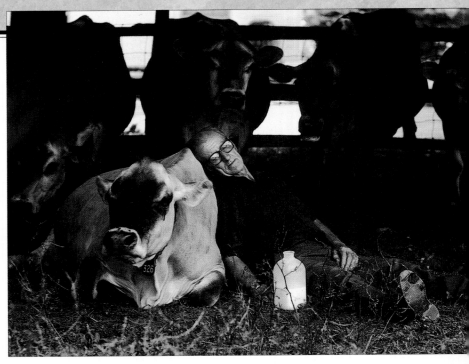

alcohol, prescribed drugs or over-the-counter medicines can also cause excessive daytime sleepiness.

What is insomnia?

Strictly speaking, insomnia is the total inability to fall asleep, but it is often used as a general term for difficulty in falling asleep, waking during the night or waking too early in the morning. Persistent lack of sleep undermines your physical and mental health, leaving you tense, drained and exhausted.

▲ **Does daytime napping rob you of nighttime sleep?** *If you find that it leaves you restless and unhappy at night then try to break the napping habit – but a midday nap can for some be part of a healthy lifestyle. Milking cows involves intense work early in the morning and late in the afternoon, with a quiet period between. In hot countries, a siesta at midday allows activity in the coolest parts of the day.*

58

The hazards of sleeping pills

■ Sleeping pills are prescribed to 4.3 percent of the American population every year, and an even greater number use over-the-counter aids. Bensodiazepines, one of the most popular kinds, induce sleep quickly, cause fewer awakenings, and prolong sleep, but these benefits are short-lived, wearing off after a few weeks of constant use. There is always a price to pay for taking sleep-inducing drugs. They alter the normal sleep cycle so that, although the total number of hours slept is increased, there is less deep sleep and less REM sleep. They have side-effects including day-

time clumsiness and confusion, and some impairment of the mental facilities on the day after use. Elderly people taking long-acting medication for insomnia have a higher incidence of falls and hip-fractures. Those on short-acting drugs seem to have greater difficulty remembering what happened after taking the medication.

The most dangerous situation is when a person takes a sleeping pill at bedtime, wakes up in the night not remembering the first pill, and takes another. If this happens too often, the risk of becoming dependent is high. The body develops tolerance to

the first (prescribed) dose and a larger dose is needed to have the same effect. Many of those who use sleeping pills for the first time find that they are unable to sleep without them when the bottle is empty, and they continue to take them for months or even years. Drug-dependent insomniacs are convinced that they cannot sleep without medication, yet research has shown that their sleeping patterns are no different from those not taking drugs – in effect their dependence is psychological, not physical. Dependence is most frequent in people who have a tendency to

abuse other substances too, including alcohol.

Coming off sleeping pills can be a painful process. Often it leads to rebound insomnia – a temporary worsening of the situation, or to excessive REM sleep, possibly causing nightmares. Placebo pills (having no active medical ingredients) can often be a solution, since they provide psychological reassurance without having any other effects. In practical terms the over-the-counter aids have little more than a placebo effect. They may produce drowsiness, but rarely sleepiness.

Most of us suffer from loss of sleep at some time, often triggered by stress, anxiety, pain, noise or jet lag. A family death, divorce, pressure at work or impending surgery are common causes. "Sunday night insomnia" is also frequent after sleeping late over the weekend. Most people can establish their normal sleeping pattern again after adjusting to these changes, but for 15-20 percent of the population insomnia becomes a constant or recurring problem.

A host of different factors can lead to insomnia – medical, psychological, environmental, or directly linked to lifestyle. It is more common in women than in men, and it becomes more likely in both men and women as they get older. Understanding what is at the root of the problem is the first step toward relieving it. People prone to insomnia tend to focus on sleep loss rather than on the fundamental cause. After several nights of poor sleep they may associate going to bed with fear and worry about being unable to fall asleep.

Often people who have reached this state sleep better away from home where the surroundings do not remind them of recurring difficulties. Similarly, they may find it easier to sleep at home when they are not trying to sleep – while reading or watching television, for example. Often they may become very sleepy in the living room, but become wide awake and anxious as soon as they go to bed.

The psychological causes

The things we do, think and feel during the day influence how we sleep at night. Poor sleepers tend to be more sedentary, spend more time alone and worry more about their problems than good sleepers. On the whole, people who suffer from anxiety are more likely to report difficulty in falling asleep, while people who tend to be depressed report more difficulty in maintaining sleep. The results of research, however, have called these judgments into question. Experiments using electroencephalographic recordings which monitor brain wave patterns show that many people's perception of how badly they sleep is not at all accurate. Often they overestimate the time it takes them to fall asleep and underestimate the total number of hours spent sleeping. Some patients who had slept 6-7 hours in a sleep laboratory, for example, felt certain that they had only been asleep for 2-3 hours.

The physical causes

Apart from the obvious factors like excessive noise or bright lights, pain is the most common reason for lying awake at night. Breathing difficulties (sleep apnea) and leg twitches (nocturnal myoclonus) frequently disrupt sleep, although the sleeper may not actually wake. The sleeper's partner is often the only one consciously aware of the disturbance. Alcohol consumption is likely to disrupt sleep; so is caffeine (too much coffee, tea or cola) or nicotine which acts as a stimulant. Several prescribed drugs, especially those intended for the treatment of asthma or hypertension, have side effects which may keep you awake. In addition, you may be kept awake by unfamiliar surroundings, an uncomfortable mattress, or by being too cold or too hot. Older people may find that they are much more sensitive to these factors than when they were younger. Sleep difficulties or disruptive nighttime behavior are two common reasons for putting elderly relatives into care.

What are the effects on health?

Insomnia is not a trivial complaint; prolonged lack of sleep can diminish the quality of life, causing considerable distress to the person concerned and to the whole family. It impairs judgment, increases reaction time and decreases alertness. At the very least it leads to poor performance and low motivation. Many insomniacs become concerned about their sleeping patterns to the extent that sleep becomes their central concern. Sleeping pills are often more dangerous than lack of sleep itself. Apnea (a breathing disorder during sleep) can reduce oxygen levels to the brain, lowering alertness and affecting the memory. If untreated, the long-term consequences include irritability, depression, sexual problems, hypertension, and, in the most serious cases, damage to the heart or lungs. Excessive daytime sleepiness can cause fatal accidents on the road and serious human error in situations where lives or environmental safety are at risk.

Help yourself to a better night's sleep

■ There is more to getting to sleep than counting sheep. See what combination of the following strategies works for you.

● Allow yourself one hour before bedtime to unwind.

● Use the time to follow a bedtime ritual, perhaps have a bath and read.

● Do not rehash the events of the day or plan tomorrow.

● Only prepare to go to sleep when you are drowsy; going to bed when you are not sleepy only gives you time to worry about sleep.

● If you do not fall asleep quickly, get up again and do something else. Do not go back to bed until you feel ready to sleep. Following this routine will help you associate your bedroom with falling asleep quickly.

● Maintain a regular rising time, set your alarm clock and get out of bed at the same time every morning (weekdays and weekends) regardless of how much sleep you have had the night before. This helps regulate your biological clock.

● Use the bedroom for sleep only, do not work, worry, eat, or watch television there during the day or evening.

● Do not spend too much time in bed when not sleeping.

● Ideally you should avoid daytime napping – at very least try not to nap after midafternoon – to ensure sleep at night.

● Avoid caffeine, nicotine and alcohol before bedtime.

● Eating a heavy meal usually hinders sleep, though a high-carbohydrate snack or milk may help.

● Exercise during the afternoon usually aids sleep, though vigorous exercise before bedtime may stimulate you too much.

7

Sexuality

A healthy sex life requires mental and physical health ● *Good sex is in turn beneficial to our well-being* ● *Discovering our sexuality means dispelling false beliefs* ● *Understanding your partner's needs is crucial to a relationship.*

EVERYONE is interested in and curious about sex. It is a compelling drive and a major source of pleasure and gratification, but it is fuelled by psychological as well as physical needs and feelings. Having a good sex life requires a healthy body, an ability to relate to others and a sense of self-esteem.

Human beings think about sex a good deal – for most people, several times a day. Whatever our individual circumstances, sexual drive and interest permeates and colors our attitudes, thoughts and actions. Advertising companies know this only too well – the promise of sexual attraction attached to a product frequently acts as a ploy to increase sales. Such advertising techniques work because much of our thinking about sex involves worries about our desirability and performance.

Understanding your sexuality

Leading a healthy sex life needs more than an understanding of the basic mechanics of sex. Our attitudes to other people, the relationships we develop and our feelings about ourselves are just as important. In addition, stress and anxiety in other areas of our lives can make us feel vulnerable and nervous about sex.

Physical and mental well-being enhance a good sex life; but our overall health is also improved by satisfying sexual experience. Sex can make us feel loved, loving and lovable, and if we find understanding and sensitive partners it will improve our self-confidence and self-image too. Because there are so many factors involved, good sex is not dependent upon specific physical attributes, and it can be learned and improved upon, whatever your age or condition.

The physical response

The sexual response in men and women is remarkably similar despite anatomical differences. Sexual stimulation causes an increase in blood flow to the penis or the blood vessels surrounding the vagina. This causes erection in a man, and swelling and lubrication of the vagina and clitoris in a woman. Arousal is not under our conscious control. The chain of reactions is regulated by the parasympathetic nervous system, the system that controls our involuntary body functions such as heartbeat and breathing, so it can

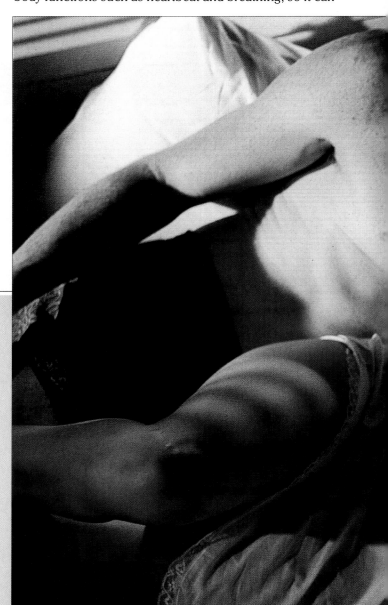

Thought, feeling, fantasy

■ Uninhibited sexual pleasure depends on both partners feeling free from anxiety and trusting each other. Fantasy may also contribute to the enjoyment of sex, with the nature of the fantasy differing between men and women. Males tend to imagine themselves as dominant and are very responsive to the visual stimuli of pornography. Women tend to fantasize quite complicated narratives in which touch rather than images are paramount, and may invoke scenarios involving submission. This does not mean that women enjoy or secretly want this in reality. A sharp distinction needs to be drawn between sexual fantasy and preferred sexual practices.

Perfection can be daunting – handsome men and extremely beautiful women can invoke sexual fear. If you are an ordinary-looking person, you will engender less anxiety in potential partners. Friendly and easygoing people are just as sexually desirable as the stunningly attractive.

occur when it is unwanted and is difficult to produce intentionally.

Once arousal has reached a sufficient peak, orgasm may occur, with or without sexual intercourse. Orgasm is a series of rhythmic contractions of the muscles at the base of the penis or surrounding the vagina. These muscles can be controlled by the voluntary nervous system, so that it is possible to delay an orgasm. In a man orgasm is signaled by ejaculation, followed by a period of rest before another climax is possible. Called the refractory phase, this resting time lengthens over the lifespan. Studies have shown men to be most responsive at around 18, with the refractory phase extending progressively over the years.

The female orgasm has been the subject of considerable debate in influential studies such as those by Masters and Johnson and Shere Hite. Is vaginal or clitoral "best"? In fact scientists now feel that there is only one sort of female orgasm, caused by stimulation of the head of the clitoris, but this may be experienced in the muscles of the vagina. The female orgasm can be caused by direct stimulation or by the thrusting of intercourse. However, women may fully enjoy sex without an orgasm.

Why are we so anxious?

If sex were as simple as its basic functioning, we would not spend as much time as we do worrying about it. Satisfactory sexual arousal and response is associated with an upsurge of well-being and a discharge of tension. It can make you feel better. Yet physical or mental stress, either associated with sex or in quite another area of our lives, seems to inhibit our responsiveness and can lead to even more stressful feelings of anxiety and rejection.

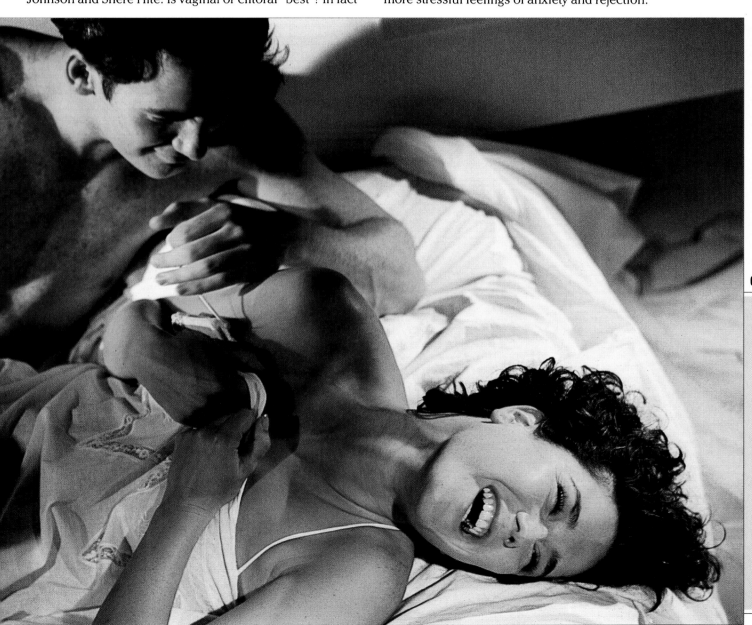

Perhaps because we are so physically and emotionally vulnerable during sex, we seem to need to feel at our most secure before we can enjoy its benefits. Understanding the relationship between sexuality, physical health and mental stability is one step towards a good sex life.

A troubled body, a troubled mind

Sexual drive is sensitive to many factors and is easily reduced by ill health. It usually returns when health recovers, though some conditions, and certain medications, can result in a chronic state of low or inhibited sexual desire. Sex can be improved by basic good health and by exercise, to a limited extent. Exercise can improve cardiovascular conditioning, which may increase your breathing and cardiac capacity during love-making, giving you greater energy and stamina. Women may benefit from exercising the muscles surrounding the vagina. These can be toned by repeated tensing, and may increase the ease with which a woman achieves orgasm. These muscles also apply pressure to the penis, and if they are strong a man may receive enhanced pleasure from intercourse.

Stress-reduction and relaxation techniques, however, remain the most useful physical preparation for sex, as they make you feel less distracted and less self-involved, able to immerse yourself in a sexual experience and to respond emotionally to your partner. Too much emphasis on the physical technique of sex can make it cold and mechanical.

Sometimes the inability to have intercourse is due to physical causes. Sex requires adequate hormones, intact nerve endings and a working vascular system, and problems can arise with any of these. Testosterone, the male hormone, appears to be responsible for sexual appetite in both women and men (with estrogen contributing to a woman's sexual response), and hormone treatment can be given if this proves to be the problem. A man's difficulty in achieving erection may be due to the veins in his penis being unable to dilate properly; implants and injections can treat this.

Breaking the anxiety cycle

Problems with sexual response are much more likely to be psychological than physical. Anxiety inhibits both desire and the capacity to respond. Men may be fearful about achieving an erection -- and their very fears may be self-fulfilling. Women who are apprehensive about intercourse, whether due to fears of pain or inadequacy, may experience vaginismus, a painful contraction of the vaginal muscles that can make intercourse uncomfortable or even impossible.

Women take longer to become aroused and may have problems achieving orgasm because of inadequate stimulation or foreplay. Men should be sensitive to this and women can make sure that their partner is aware of their need for more time. Often men rush intercourse because of a fear of premature ejaculation; once again, stress and anxiety usually make the problem worse, so relaxation is vital to good sex.

Sometimes it is intellectual defenses or barriers that prevent arousal. Sex requires immersion in the experience. A tendency to observe what is happening, rather than simply to enjoy it, can have unwanted inhibiting effects. Self-consciousness and embarrassment, as well as over-concern with the mechanics of sex, can contribute to this "outside-looking-in" syndrome.

The ordinary stresses and strains of life also can spill over into your sexuality. Anger, tension and unhappiness inhibit the sense of freedom and security necessary for good sex. People suffering from depression, alcoholism or drug

Common sense or fallacy?

■ Our society places great pressure on us to sustain a good sex life, but it has also produced a number of false ideas that get in the way of a healthy sexuality. Most of these ignore the complexity of our sexual feelings and concentrate on a mechanical view of sex. Psychologist Bernie Zilbergeld in his book *Male Sexuality*, lists a number of common sexual

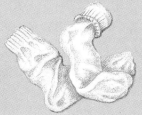

myths. Do any of them sound familiar?

● "Men should not have or express certain feelings." Our society does not encourage men to relate sexual release to emotional expression, but arousal is closely tied to our emotional needs.

● "Performance is what counts." A lover who is busy counting a partner's orgasms or demanding assurances about his technique does not encourage the security required for good sex.

● "A man is always ready and wants to have sex." Since

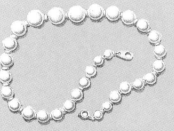

sexual arousal is involuntary, this is simply not true and can lead to feelings of inadequacy in men and of rejection in women.

● "All physical contact has to culminate in sex." This belief discourages us from physical intimacy for fear of arousing expectations. We need to learn ways of communicating what we

want while being mutually open and supportive.

● "Sex equals intercourse." Good sex can take many forms. Kissing, cuddling and mutual stimulation are all part of the enjoyment of sex. Absence of an erection only prevents penetration by the penis. Everything else is still possible.

● "Sex ends with an orgasm." Usually for men this will be the case, but women frequently enjoy sex without an orgasm and men can too. The closeness after intercourse is just as much a part of sex as the arousal beforehand.

addiction rarely have satisfactory sex lives. Everyone finds that tension can lead to an unhappy sexual experience occasionally, and this in turn can trigger further anxiety about performance, leading to more difficulties. Relaxing usually leads to a better sexual experience and sexual confidence because it relieves the symptoms of stress and encourages a calm and positive outlook. Sex itself is accompanied by the release of tension and a feeling of happiness, and may even actively improve health by relieving excess strain in the cardiovascular system and enhancing the body's immune system. If stress or anxiety is affecting your sexuality, learning some relaxation techniques (see *Ch 5*) may be of benefit to your sex life and subsequently to your total health.

Securing a warm relationship

Sexual harmony and happiness is most often reported from within the context of a satisfying relationship. Despite a moral climate that allows for divorce and for a degree of sexual experimentation with a number of partners, most people actively search for steady relationships, even if these do not last for life.

Long-term relationships improve your sex life in a number of ways. Couples who are faithful to each other avoid some of the dangers of disease transmission through sex, while maintaining an active sex life. Knowledge and experience with your partner's body, emotional and physical needs and desires can be built up in the context of a relationship – it is easier to please and be pleased by someone you know rather than a stranger. Most important of

all, lack of self-consciousness, relief from tension and a sense of security come more readily when we are with those we like and respect.

Sex counseling

A poor relationship can be worse than no relationship at all. Unhappy couples do not have good sex; their problems follow them into bed. Problems with sex usually lead to the deterioration of a couple's relationship outside the bedroom. Sometimes the only solution is to part. Very often, however, if the problem is rooted in the sexual aspect of the relationship, seeking a new sexual partner is not an answer – the same problems may be repeated.

Sex counselors are often called in as objective outsiders to help troubled couples. Some of their techniques can be used by couples before trouble starts:

Be open to variety and new ideas. The familiar old routine can become dull and weary for the most ardent lover. With the same stimulus, arousal may diminish, even though appetite is unchanged.

Talk about sex. Express your desires and disappointments openly, without becoming critical of your partner. Just knowing what your partner has always wanted or what they find worrying can improve your sex life and make you both more confident of pleasing and being pleased.

Give up sexual intercourse for a while. Couples can become obsessed with sexual performance and fears of inadequacy. Forbidding intercourse in favor of cuddles and caresses can encourage two people to relax again in each other's company.

Be prepared to adapt. No one remains sexually the same throughout life. Our natural bodily changes influence sexual appetite and level of arousal. It appears to be easier to cope with these changes in the context of a good relationship.

63

Sexuality and self-esteem

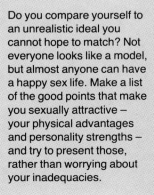

■ Sexual appetite is influenced by your sense of yourself. A good sexual relationship requires an absence of guilt and anxiety and a sense of comfort about your body. If you are self-conscious about your appearance, you will be tense and anxious and you will not project yourself as a lovable person. Luckily there are a number of things you can do to improve your self-image.

● Look after yourself. Are you embarrassed about your weight? Do you think your body is not attractive enough for sex? You can lose weight and improve your figure by a sensible diet and exercise.

Regular exercise in particular will tone your muscles and will help your overall health, which in turn will make you feel more confident about your body. Changing the way you dress or other aspects of your appearance can also make you feel and look better.

● Concentrate on your good points. Try to be less self-critical and more accepting.

Do you compare yourself to an unrealistic ideal you cannot hope to match? Not everyone looks like a model, but almost anyone can have a happy sex life. Make a list of the good points that make you sexually attractive – your physical advantages and personality strengths – and try to present those, rather than worrying about your inadequacies.

Find time to enjoy your relationship

■ When so much of the rest of our lives is planned and organized, sex may be also, and it should be none the worse for that. A deliberately seductive dinner is, after all, a common sexual fantasy. The notion that sexuality will look after itself can result in frustration and disillusionment.

Patterns of sexual desire

In women, sex hormones fluctuate over the menstrual cycle. Studies have shown no conclusive relationship between cycles of hormone levels in women and sexual desire, perhaps because sexual interest is complicated by so many social factors for women, such as fear of unwanted pregnancy or gaining an "easy" reputation.

After childbirth a woman's sexual interest may be low. Following delivery there is a rapid fall in the female hormones, and if a woman breast-feeds her baby, the milk stimulant prolactin will continue to lower estrogen levels.

Sex during menstruation can be messy, and some men and women find it uncomfortable or embarrassing. It is certainly perfectly safe, and some women find it relieves menstrual cramp. Menstrual blood itself is not "dirty" or "impure", but if either partner has a sexual disease it *may* be more easily communicated during menstruation – research is still going on concerning this. Sex during pregnancy is usually safe, though partners may have to work out more comfortable positions as the pregnancy advances. Couples are usually advised to refrain from sex for the first three months if the woman has a history of miscarriage, and for the last month before the baby is due.

Sexuality across the lifespan

Following menopause, a woman's estrogen levels show a further decline, and women subject to mood swings at this time may reject sex; others find their desire increases. Most commonly women find vaginal dryness a problem, making the use of lubricants necessary during sex. Women in a

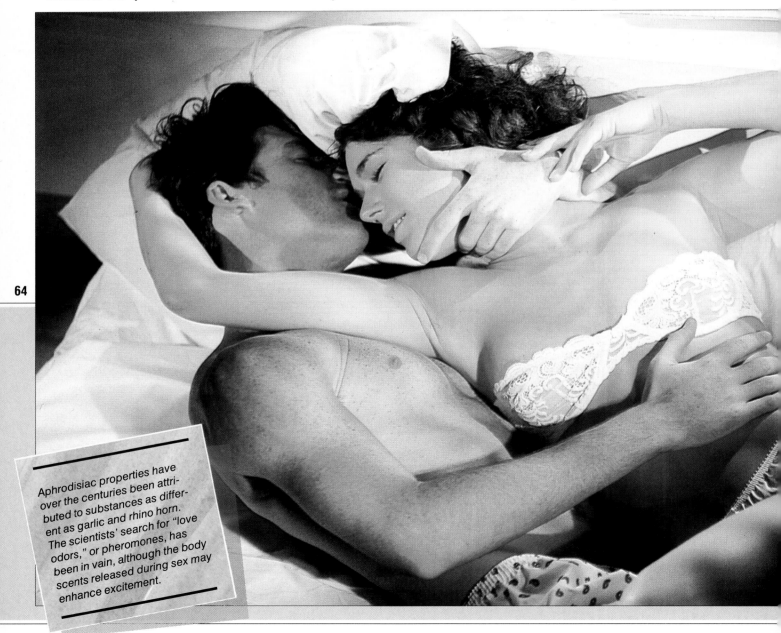

Aphrodisiac properties have over the centuries been attributed to substances as different as garlic and rhino horn. The scientists' search for "love odors," or pheromones, has been in vain, although the body scents released during sex may enhance excitement.

64

Contraception

■ For many couples the birth-control pill is ideal because it is easy to use and 98 percent reliable. However, some women find it can cause headaches and weight gain, and some research suggests that long-term use of certain types may increase the risk of breast cancer. A woman who has completed her child bearing may prefer the IUD (intrauterine device), a coil inserted in the uterus which prevents implantation of the ovum, but this can increase the risk of pelvic inflammatory disease and increase menstrual pain and bleeding. Condoms limit the risk of sexually transmitted disease, but along with other barrier methods like the cap, diaphragm or vaginal sponge, they are often felt to impair sexual enjoyment. Make your choice of contraception on the basis of medical advice.

regular sexual relationship appear to maintain higher levels of estrogen and show less atrophy of the vaginal lining. Regular sexual activity may influence hormone levels, thereby forestalling menopause and retarding the physical changes associated with aging.

Men are also affected by aging. The refractory phase, the length of time between male orgasms, increases steadily from about 18, as does the force of the ejaculation. Older men may take longer to become aroused and may require more stimulation to achieve and maintain an erection.

20th century thinking on sex and health has been dominated by Freudian theory. This assumes that health and happiness require a satisfying sex life. However, our definitions of what constitutes good sex need to be continually re-evaluated. The key is to establish a satisfactory sexual relationship where stress and tension are released and where you and your partner feel free to be open and secure. This may require emotional effort, even risk, but the results will be worth it. **AER**

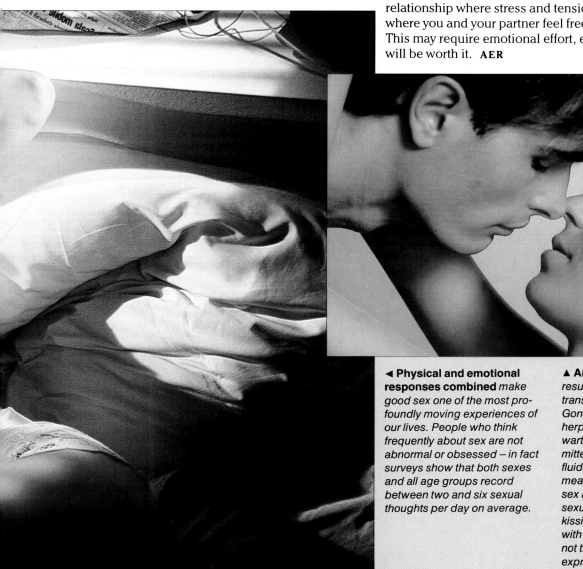

65

◄ **Physical and emotional responses combined** *make good sex one of the most profoundly moving experiences of our lives. People who think frequently about sex are not abnormal or obsessed – in fact surveys show that both sexes and all age groups record between two and six sexual thoughts per day on average.*

▲ **Anxiety about sex** *may result from the fear of sexually transmitted diseases. Gonorrhea, syphilis, genital herpes, chlamydia, genital warts and AIDS are all transmitted by exchange of bodily fluids. Disease avoidance means refraining from casual sex and engaging in safe sexual practices such as dry kissing and genital stimulation with the hands. Penetration is not the only form of sexual expression. If penetrative sex is preferred, it should never be practiced casually without a condom.*

8

Good Nutrition

Our established eating habits are seldom the healthiest ● By keeping a check on what we eat we can improve our nutrition and still enjoy our food ● Healthy eating means paying attention to our bodies' needs for a balanced diet.

HEALTHY eating is a subject of considerable concern, but we are often puzzled by how to go about it. We are bombarded with information and suggestions from health experts, the press and television and the advice of friends – some of it contradictory – which we try to fit together with cultural, family and social eating patterns and with our personal food preferences. More and more people live in households where all the adults are working, making it increasingly difficult to take time over shopping and cooking. Additionally, our choice of foods varies with where we live, the time of year and how much money we are prepared to spend. Preparing healthy meals can be complicated and confusing, and in a busy world many people decide just to eat what they want and ignore all the mixed messages about what is good or bad for them.

Unfortunately, many convenience meals are made up of foods that are high in fat, calories, salt and sugar. These foods appeal strongly to human tastebuds, but do little for your health. An understanding of the basic principles of nutrition may help you and your family to eat both for good health and for pleasure.

What is good nutrition?

Until recently our primary concern about nutrition was simply the consumption of enough food to fill stomachs and sustain lives. In developing countries this is still the case.

Why do we need protein?

■ Protein is required by the body for growth, maintenance and repair of cells and tissues. Named after the Greek word meaning "first importance," most proteins are manufactured by the body. But of the 20 amino acids that make up protein, nine cannot be manufactured by the body and must be supplied by food. Foods that supply these nine essential amino acids in sufficient quantities to promote growth and repair are high-quality protein sources.

Foods of animal origin – meat, dairy products and eggs – are good sources of high-quality protein. Vegetables and grains contain some of the nine elements but must be eaten in combination with other foods, to provide all the essential amino acids.

Vegetarians, who abstain from eating meat, often combine milk or cheese with grains. Vegans, who consume no animal products, can receive sufficient high-quality protein – by combining grains with legumes or beans at a meal, for example. A diet high in meat-based proteins may also contain too much fat, so gaining some of your protein by food-combining is recommended, even for those who eat meat.

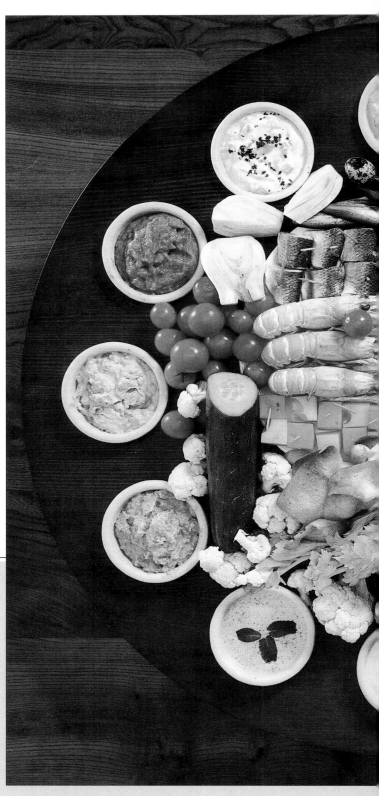

▲ **Variety is the key to healthy eating.** *The functioning of our bodies depends on the right combination of proteins, carbohydrates, fats, vitamins, minerals and fiber, and a varied diet is the best way of ensuring that all the elements are present. One of our worst habits is the consumption of too much*

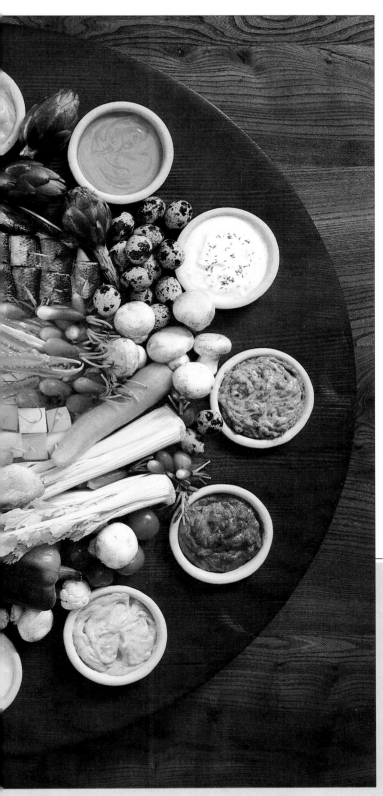

Western societies today have an abundance of food, and most of us are much more likely to suffer nutritional problems related to an excess or imbalance of food intake rather than too little. While serious malnutrition does not often occur in well-fed people, a diet poor in necessary vitamins and minerals is certainly possible in those who fail to eat a balanced range of foods, and vitamin deficiencies may contribute to a great deal of low-level ill health (such as a tendency to colds, flu and infections).

Excess calories, fat, salt, sugar and alcohol increase the risk of the primary killer diseases of our time: heart disease, hypertension, cancer, diabetes and liver disease (cirrhosis). Chronic, serious overweight (obesity) is also associated with a higher rate of some of these illnesses, especially diabetes and hypertension. As a result, health professionals and the public alike have developed an increased awareness of the relationship between our health and what we eat. Nutritionists concentrate on how the body utilizes the elements contained in our food. The major nutrients in food which are essential to life include protein, carbohydrate, fat, vitamins, minerals and water. Making nutrition work for us involves knowing how these food components function to give the body health, strength and energy.

The benefits of a good diet

Good nutrition requires a balance of major nutrients as well as the appropriate amount of calories. A well-nourished person is generally healthier and better-equipped to meet the physical and emotional challenges that life brings. Research suggests that the ill effects of unavoidable stresses and demands on your body may be offset somewhat by a consistent, well-balanced diet. A good diet prevents or reduces fatigue, increases our resistance to illness and enhances a general sense of well-being.

67

fat. The foods in this picture tend to be low in fat, with other necessities in plentiful supply. Raw vegetables are high in fiber and certain vitamins and minerals, while other essential vitamins and minerals are present in seafood.

Why do we need water?

■ Water is the most vital of all essential nutrients. It makes up about 60 percent of total body weight (though this varies with age and body composition) and is essential for vital functions – you can survive for up to a month without food, but seldom longer than three days without water. Most adults require at least two quarts of water or other fluid per day to maintain the body's water level and to replace daily fluid losses through urination and sweat.

We obtain the majority of our fluid requirements through beverages and some through solid foods. Depending upon its source, water can be a significant source of certain essential minerals. Spring waters are often sold on the strength of their mineral content, but even ordinary tap water may provide for some of our basic mineral needs. Unfortunately, water can also contain toxic elements from the environment. Constant monitoring of the water supply is necessary to safeguard public health.

Often the time, energy and inconvenience involved in changing their eating habits stops even the most well-intentioned people before they begin. To make a change in your diet, the first step is to recognize the benefits and reasons for the change you intend. The next step is to increase awareness of your current eating patterns. It may help to keep a food diary of what you eat, how much, why and at what times. Then you can analyze your food intake using the charts and tables provided in this chapter to determine where your diet needs improvement. You may consume a reasonable amount of calories, for instance, but find that the level of fat in your diet is unacceptably high. A registered dietitian or your doctor can give further advice.

Men, women, children, the elderly

The basic nutritional needs of all human beings are very similar. Children do not need quite as many calories as adults because they are smaller, but they are also growing and that requires energy. Balanced nutrition is especially important because of their developmental needs. If you want to change a child's diet radically you should always consult a doctor first.

The effect of aging upon nutritional requirements is currently an area of great interest in the scientific community. It is not entirely clear how or if our needs for vitamins and minerals change as we grow older. The elderly need fewer calories, but this is largely because of reduced activity, not the physical changes that accompany aging. Older people may not absorb nutrients as efficiently as when they were young, making a high-quality diet even more important. Nutritional supplements may also be beneficial.

Men generally need to eat more than women because they are bigger, weigh more and have a higher proportion of muscle; all three factors increase their need for calories. Women need more iron and calcium. Blood loss during menstruation can lead to iron deficiency (anemia), and after the menopause reduction in the blood levels of the hormone estrogen can lead to a loss of bone mass if calcium intake is low. Pregnant women also require a particularly good diet rich in vitamins and minerals. Taking these differences into account will allow you to "fine tune" your dietary plans to provide the healthiest eating for you and those you feed.

How to form good habits

Certain general guidelines are commonly agreed to lower the risk of disease and promote health, providing vigor and the ability to meet the demands of your life.

Improving children's eating habits

■ Parents' anxiety about their children's eating habits can turn the table into a battleground. Here are some ideas for encouraging healthy eating in children:

● Sit at the table with children – keep them company even if you are not eating at the same time.

● Do not bribe with desserts, etc – children will think that ice cream is delicious and broccoli is boring.

● Follow a schedule for meals and snacks. If a child leaves the table without eating and is hungry five minutes later, be firm about waiting until the next regular snack or meal. This is not punishment. It is reinforcement of good eating habits.

● Do not pressure children about eating – what they eat, how much, how little and whether their appetite changes from day to day. Let them choose from what is on the table (try for a varied menu, not just reliable favorites). Do not try to force them to try something new; they will experiment at their own pace.

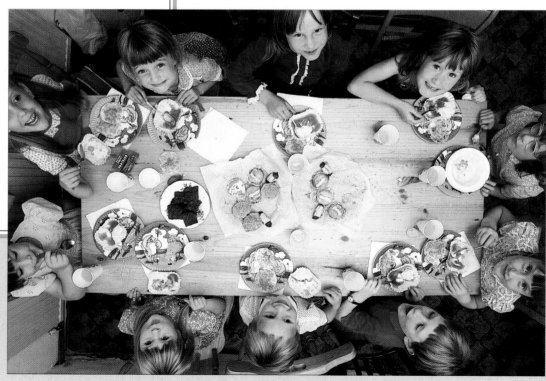

▶ **A treat for children** *often involves unhealthy sugary foods. Often children acquire from their parents the idea that unhealthy food is the most desirable food. Given more choice from early on, they could well establish healthy eating habits on their own.*

Why do we need fats?

■ Fats are the most concentrated source of energy or calories in our diet. They contain essential fatty acids and fat-soluble vitamins, so some fat is necessary in a healthy diet. However, the amount of fat most Westerners consume is typically two to three times the level recommended by health experts.

The kind of fat we consume has health implications as well. Fats made up of a majority of saturated fatty acids are known as saturated fats; fats made up of a majority of polyunsaturated fatty acids are polyunsaturated fats; and fats made up of a majority of monounsaturated fatty acids are known as monounsaturated fats.

A diet high in saturated fats like butter and most animal fats seems to increase the risk of cardiovascular diseases, while unsaturated fats, including vegetable oils and most margarines, may lessen the risk. Evidence suggests that some unsaturated fats in oily fish like mackerel and salmon may actually be beneficial. All fats are high in calories, however, and should be used in moderation.

■ **To help reduce your intake of fat**

Use...	Instead of...
skim or low-fat milk	whole milk or cream
plain low-fat yoghurt	sour cream or cream
sherbet or ice milk	ice cream
half the fat in a recipe	regular amount of fat
lean, trimmed meats	marbled cuts with untrimmed fat
poultry without skin	poultry with skin
fresh fish, broiled, baked, poached, or steamed	fried or frozen breaded fish
low-fat sauces and marinades	high-fat sauces and marinades
unbuttered popcorn, pretzels	chips, snack crackers, peanuts
bagels or toast with jelly	doughnuts, pastries
mustard, ketchup	mayonnaise, tartar sauce
fresh fruit.	high-fat cakes and desserts.

The first aim to keep in mind is to include a variety of foods in your daily diet. Consuming a variety of foods from all the major food groups should ensure that you get all the vitamins and minerals you need. It is also the best way of obtaining the proper mix of protein, carbohydrate and fat in your diet. Do not worry about vitamin supplements unless you are pregnant, breastfeeding or elderly – concentrate on eating a wide range of foods instead.

The next essential is to achieve and maintain a healthy body weight. In the industrialized world most people do not have to exert much physical effort to perform tasks that at one time required considerable time and labor. We generally sit for a living. Only 2 percent of modern occupations require enough energy use to keep our hearts healthy and our bodies trim, yet many of us still eat as if we were farm workers. Our diet is often high in fat and low in carbohydrates as well.

The key to managing weight is balancing food intake with the amount of energy we use. Regular exercise and a permanent reduction in fat consumption will burn more body energy and reduce calories, gradually decreasing body weight and increasing the ratio of muscle to fat in our bodies. Obesity provokes a number of minor and major health problems, so maintaining weight at a reasonable level is an important part of a healthy lifestyle.

Why you should eat less fat

If you were to make just one change in your diet, it should be to eat less fat. Reducing consumption of foods high in fat and preparing foods in a low-fat way (ie baking or broiling instead of frying) is the surest way of reducing the amount of cholesterol and saturated fat that you eat. High levels of these substances in the diet are strongly linked with an increased risk of heart disease. When you do use fat in

69

Why do we need vitamins?

■ The body needs vitamins to perform virtually all of its chemical processes and functions. Foodstuffs can supply all of our vitamin needs, as long as we eat a wide variety of food types in adequate amounts. Vitamins are classified either as fat- or water-soluble. Fat-soluble vitamins, including those known as A, D, E, and K, can be stored in our fat reserves; overconsumption can lead to toxic levels. Water-soluble vitamins include all the B vitamins and C; our bodies can store only a tiny reserve of these so we need a daily supply.

Vitamin	Sources	Benefits
Vitamin A	Liver, broccoli, carrots, pumpkin, apricots, butter.	Good for eyesight, healthy skin, bones, and teeth; fights infection.
Thiamine Vitamin B1	Pork, liver, lean meats, whole grains, pulses, nuts.	Helps the body obtain energy from food; good appetite and digestion.
Riboflavin Vitamin B2	Dairy products, liver, green leafy vegetables, grains.	Helps tissue repair; good for eyesight and healthy skin.
Niacin	Lean meats, poultry, fish, dark green vegetables, grains, peanuts.	Required for healthy nervous system and skin.
Folic Acid	Liver, pulses, green vegetables.	Helps use protein and form red blood cells.
Pyridoxine Vitamin B6	Lean meats, poultry, fish, green vegetables, grains, pulses.	Helps the body use protein and fats; essential for normal growth.
Vitamin B12	Lean meats, poultry, fish, dairy products.	Necessary for producing red blood cells and building new proteins.
Vitamin C	Citrus fruits, strawberries, cantaloupe, tomatoes, potatoes, peppers, green leafy vegetables.	Helps bond cells and tissues together; heal wounds and fight infection; good for healthy teeth, gums and blood vessels.
Vitamin D	Dairy products, egg yolk, fish oils – also direct sunlight.	Helps build strong bones and teeth.
Vitamin E	Vegetable oils, green leafy vegetables, pulses, nuts.	Thought to help form red blood cells and muscle tissue.
Vitamin K	Green leafy vegetables, cauliflower, egg yolk, liver.	Promotes normal clotting of blood.

cooking, it is healthier to use unsaturated vegetable oil.

At the same time as you reduce the levels of fat in your diet, increase your intake of foods high in complex carbohydrates and fiber. These foods are rich in vitamins and minerals and provide valuable energy without unnecessary calories. Fiber is an important aid to digestion and is associated with a lower risk of some cancers. A baked potato with low-fat cottage cheese, broccoli and fruit instead of a steak, french fries and chocolate mousse will provide you with sufficient energy, fiber and protein as well as all the vitamins and minerals you need, and will be far better for your health.

Beware of SACS

We should all try to limit our use of SACS – sugar, alcohol, caffeine and salt. Sugar contains few nutrients – ordinary cane sugar has none at all – and no fiber, and is relatively high in calories. Alcohol is a concentrated source of calories. It has no nutritional value and may actually interfere with the absorption and use of certain minerals by the body. Caffeine is a stimulant, although we do not fully understand exactly how it affects the body. Health experts recommend limiting your intake to the equivalent of two cups of coffee a day – remember that tea, cola and chocolate contain caffeine as well. Salt is an essential mineral, but

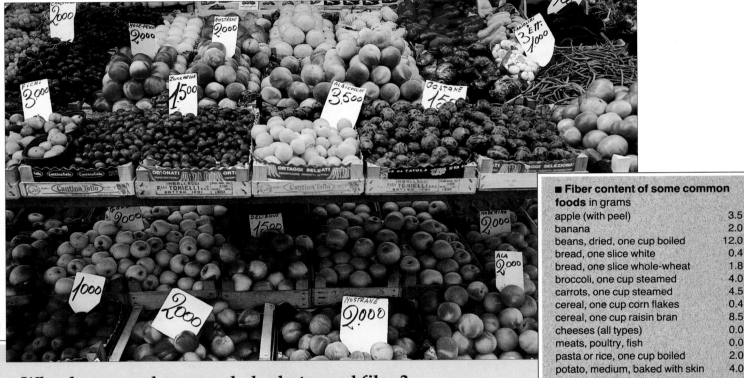

■ Fiber content of some common foods in grams	
apple (with peel)	3.5
banana	2.0
beans, dried, one cup boiled	12.0
bread, one slice white	0.4
bread, one slice whole-wheat	1.8
broccoli, one cup steamed	4.0
carrots, one cup steamed	4.5
cereal, one cup corn flakes	0.4
cereal, one cup raisin bran	8.5
cheeses (all types)	0.0
meats, poultry, fish	0.0
pasta or rice, one cup boiled	2.0
potato, medium, baked with skin	4.0

Why do we need more carbohydrates and fiber?

■ Carbohydrates include starches, sugars and fiber. Found in foods of plant origin, they are the major source of energy in the world's diet. Complex carbohydrates, generally thought of as starches, are found primarily in whole grains and vegetables. They are an important source of dietary fiber. Fiber, though it passes through the intestine undigested, is vital to a healthy diet. It reduces the risk of certain forms of cancer and may help prevent heart disease, diabetes and obesity.

Simple carbohydrates, including sugars, are often high in

calories but foods that contain them, for example, fruits and vegetables are rich in vitamins and minerals. The sugar that we use at the table, sucrose, is high in calories but has no other nutritional value, so it should be used in moderation.

▼ **More carbohydrates.** *Carbohydrates were once condemned as "fattening," but health experts now realize that a diet high in complex carbohydrates and low in fat would be a healthy improvement in the average diet.*

▲ **Eating more fruit** *is one way of improving our dietary fiber intake, which in most Westernized nations is well below levels recommended by nutritionists. Most people consume about 10-15 grams a day. Health experts suggest no less than 20 grams, preferably 30 grams or more. A switch to a low-fat diet that is high in complex carbohydrates, the main source of fiber, would result in an increased intake. Use the chart to determine how much fiber you usually consume in a day, and to plan for a higher-fiber diet.*

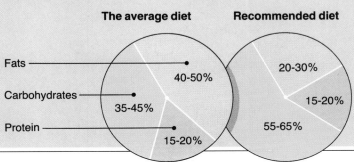

The average diet

Recommended diet

Fats — 40-50% / 20-30%

Carbohydrates — 35-45% / 55-65%

Protein — 15-20% / 15-20%

most of us consume at least ten times the recommended amount; and high-salt diets are associated with high blood-pressure and strokes, although the exact relationship is not precisely clear.

We can all see how much coffee we drink, and our intake of alcohol can be watched fairly simply (see *Ch15)*. We can cut down on the amount of salt and sugar we put in our food, but many processed foods contain large amounts of both – read the labels carefully.

Enjoy your food in good health

With all the recommendations, fads and food scares that bombard us, it is easy to become overconcerned about food. For many of us, our preferred eating patterns and social lives do not always make it easy to eat a diet that is low in fat, high in fiber and rich in nutrients. There are many positive changes we can make, but as we begin to become more selective about what we eat it is important to remember that there are no "good" or "bad" foods: all foods have something to offer. Chocolate cake is only bad when it

is eaten in excess as part of a diet already high in fat and calories. Consumed occasionally as part of a balanced diet, it is not harmful. Bran cereal is good as a source of dietary fiber, but if you ate nothing else you would become ill. No food on its own is perfect; it is the range and balance of foods eaten that make a diet a healthy one.

There is no need to be a puritan about food. If you want to eat a low-fat diet but your cupboards are stocked with high-fat foods, it may be a good idea to clear out some of the things that tempt you to eat poorly and to customize your kitchen to the type of diet you want to follow. But there is no need to cut out desserts, snacks and high-fat foods completely. An occasional treat is a reasonable part of a healthy diet and prevents the high-fat cravings that can sabotage your eating plans. If you are too rigid or strict with yourself, you will inevitably violate your own rules about food and end up feeling a failure. Food can become an obsession if you treat it as a panacea or cure-all; it is only one part of a healthy lifestyle. Food is health-giving and nutritious, but it is also meant for us to enjoy. **JP-C**

Why do we need minerals?

■ Certain minerals present in our food supply are essential for life, growth and reproduction. Minerals are present in higher concentrations in, and are more readily absorbed from, foods of animal origin. Even with our abundant food supplies, a deficiency of certain essential minerals (mainly iron and calcium) is quite common and remains a health problem. This may be because our diet often relies on processed foods, which have often lost their natural mineral content in the preserving process. Eating a wide variety of all types of foods, including as much fresh food as possible, should provide you with a full range of essential minerals.

Sodium is a constituent of common table salt. We need about 500 milligrams a day – less than one-fifth of a teaspoon of salt. Most of us consume far more than we need in processed foods even without adding salt at the table.

Calcium	Dairy products, green vegetables broccoli, tofu, figs.	Builds and maintains healthy bones and teeth; aids in blood clotting, important in wound healing and fighting infection.
Copper	Green vegetables, seafood, whole grains, dried fruits.	Needed for formation of blood.
Iodine	Iodized salt, salt-water fish and shellfish.	Needed for formation of hormones made by the thyroid gland.
Iron	Lean meats, liver, egg yolk, enriched whole grains, pulses, dried fruits, dark green vegetables.	Necessary for production of red blood cells and the transport of oxygen in the body.
Magnesium	Whole green cereals, soybeans, nuts.	A must for strong bones and teeth; helps with muscle contraction; necessary for transmitting nerve impulses.
Phosphorus	Dairy products, nuts, whole grains, pulses.	Works with calcium to keep bones and teeth healthy; involved with proper use of fat in the body; needed by the "energy" enzymes.
Potassium	Lean meats, dried apricots, avocados, bananas, pulses, potatoes, most fruits.	Keeps nerves and muscles healthy; helps to maintain fluid balance.
Sodium	Table salt, processed foods, luncheon meats, pickled foods, most cheeses.	Preserves water balance in the body.
Zinc	Green vegetables, shellfish, liver.	Used for building proteins in the body.

How safe is your food?

■ There are frequent scares about food contamination. How concerned should we be, and how does this affect what we should be eating?

It is impossible to make the food supply completely safe and even if it could be done, it might even be harmful: decreasing one risk may increase another.

It may be good to be exposed to some bacteria. This is the principle on which vaccination is based – it helps you to build immunity. Exposure is especially beneficial to women as preparation for pregnancy. Some infections, if a pregnant woman has not been exposed to them before, can kill an unborn child while causing the mother only minor illness. A pregnant woman who has eaten many different foods in her life is more likely to be immune to food-borne infections that could damage her child.

It is more important to pick fresh food for nutritional value than to worry about possible dangers. By eating a variety of foods you will maintain good nutrition and avoid a concentration of any substance found in one particular food.

71

9

The Diet Dilemma

Overweight is not the same as "fat," or vice-versa ● *What is the "right" weight, and how hard should we try to achieve it?* ● *Obesity is a health risk, but a lifestyle of crash diets will cause more problems than it solves.*

WE LIVE in a society that puts a high value on thinness in the midst of culinary plenty. This is something new: in older cultures and in those with a deficiency of food, good fortune is equated with being fat.

We have retained many features of that old equation. We encourage children to clean their plates and praise them for being "good eaters." Providing food is a sign of nurturing and eating it is a form of acceptance, comfort and reward for us. But we do not accept the results of consuming food.

Many affluent societies now favor an extremely slender bodyshape that contradicts the abundance and ready availability of food as well as the high fat and sugar content of modern foodstuffs. It is not surprising that many people, men as well as women, are thoroughly confused about food and often tend to alternate bouts of eating well with periods of dieting.

Everyone knows that it is "common sense" that people who are overweight should go on a diet, but sometimes "common sense" is not so sensible. The idea behind dieting is simple. If you eat fewer calories than your body burns up, you will lose weight. In actual practice, however, dieting is not as simple as it sounds, and many people find it difficult to establish whether their weight is too high, too low or just right. Losing weight healthily and successfully entails being aware of some basic facts and avoiding certain common pitfalls.

Is your eating out of control?

You may feel convinced that you need to change the way you eat. One of the most important considerations in evaluating your eating patterns is how much you care about health as opposed to appearance – how the body feels and functions, not just what it looks like. Before you even try to diet, you should assess what is really wrong with the way you eat now. Perhaps you could keep records of how much and what kind of food you eat over a "baseline" period, during which you make no changes in your daily routine. The purpose of this is to get a current and detailed picture of your normal diet including the circumstances and times of day when you usually eat. Is your normal diet random, unbalanced and high in junk food, or are you following a healthy regime which does not result in your being as thin as you would like?

Is it just your eating or weight that is a problem, or do other aspects of your life seem out of control as well? Eating often reflects emotional and stress-related problems. You may overeat when you feel tense and then be overrestrictive when less stressed. To change, you need to achieve a balance. Eat only at planned times. At first, eat as much as you want at these times. Control of amounts and types of food can be introduced later if your weight increases.

If it is just your eating that feels out of control, you may be seeking an unrealistic weight goal and find yourself swinging between periods of very high and very low caloric intake. If your overeating tends to occur at a specific time (at night or at the weekends), try to eat more at the times when you have been eating less (for example, at lunch or supper). This will help you stabilize your habits and your weight.

Keeping a food diary

■ To establish an informed picture of your eating habits, set yourself a "baseline" period – say two weeks – when you will keep a diary about them. Making no conscious changes in your eating, record the types and amounts of all food and drink that you consume. Record the time, place, moods and events associated with your eating.

It might be helpful to count your calories and daily fat intake and to record information such as the level of hunger, anxiety and guilt you feel before and after eating. Weigh yourself once a day at the same time and keep a record.

When the record is complete, ask yourself these questions:
● How do I feel about my weight?
● Can I eat this way for the rest of my life?
● What effect would it have on my weight and health?
● Do I use food to handle stress?

If you decide that changes are necessary, make a list of the specific ones you would like to make. Be positive – describe the new eating habits you want to acquire, not the ones you want to lose. Be sensible. Design a healthy diet that you can really live with.

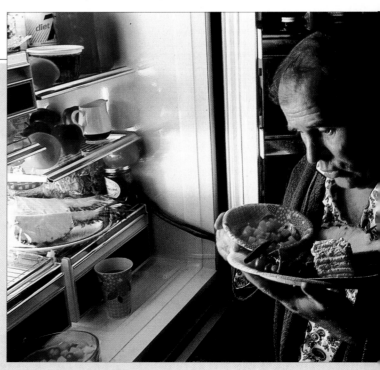

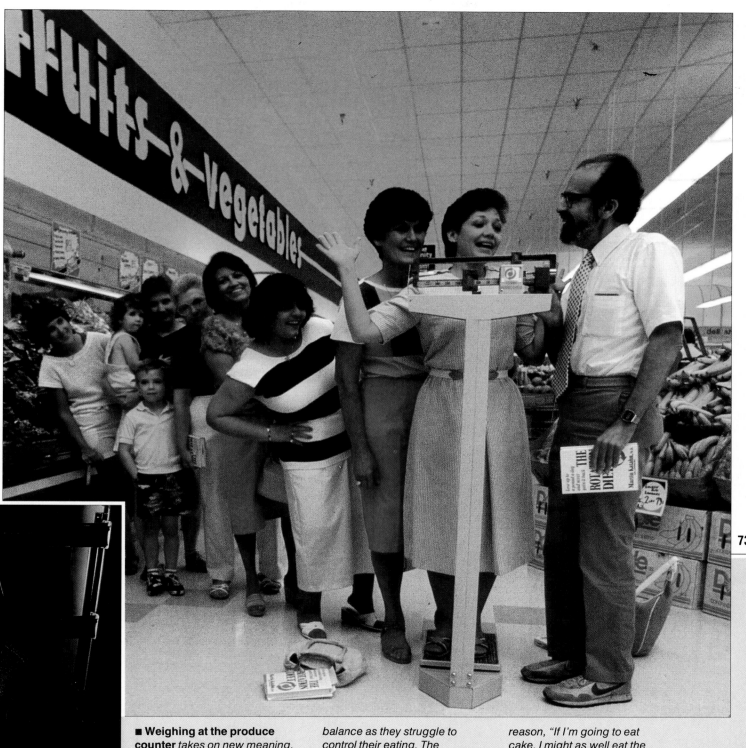

■ **Weighing at the produce counter** *takes on new meaning, further evidence of our cultural obsession with weight and food. The strict dieter is like an acrobat on a tightrope: strong emotions, special occasions and even the sight or smell of forbidden food can upset their* balance as they struggle to control their eating. The extreme self-denial involved in many diets can contribute to overeating and even binge eating as normal hunger and frustrated appetite inevitably assert themselves. When the diet is disrupted, the person may reason, "If I'm going to eat cake, I might as well eat the whole cake since tomorrow I will have to go back on my diet and I can never eat cake again."

Food obsession is a symptom of an unbalanced diet. Decide how much weight you could tolerate gaining in order to lose this feeling, and gradually increase your meals or snacks until you have reached it. If you still feel obsessed, or are unable to tolerate any weight gain, you may have a body-image problem or an eating disorder and you should seek professional advice. If you have a specific food craving, indulge it for a while as part of a planned meal or snack.

Many people who worry about their weight feel that external pressures are causing them to eat more than they should. These pressures are much less severe if you are at your natural weight. Research indicates that people who habitually restrain their eating tend to overeat from time to time and on these occasions they will eat with total dis-

regard to hunger or recent eating patterns – a condition known as disinhibited appetite. Try to be honest with yourself about these occasions. Do you look forward to them as a break from your customary eating pattern? Perhaps your ordinary food intake is too restricted. If you are going out to dinner and fear that it will be an occasion for disinhibited eating perhaps it would be better to eat before and have very little while you are out. The occasional party cannot hurt you very much, but if you have to eat out frequently remember that party foods are often very high in calories.

Satisfied with your eating, but gaining weight?

A yearly gain of only two or three pounds translates into 40-60 pounds over 20 years, so this situation should be taken seriously. Assuming that none of the symptoms of

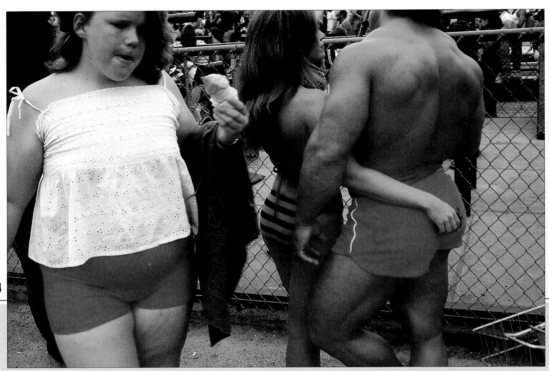

Some fat is good

■ Some body fat is necessary for survival. Ideally, men should have less than 25 percent body fat and women less than 30 percent to be considered healthy. Men who are very athletic, especially runners, can get down to 10-15 percent fat, while athletic women may drop to 13-18 percent. Such low levels may cause infertility: women often cease having periods and men may suffer a reduced sperm count. This is probably the body's reaction to what it perceives as starvation. When fat reserves are restored to normal, fertility is restored fairly quickly. **DGS**

Women are shaped like pears – they tend to have more fat on their hips; men are shaped like apples (broad around the middle). Research has shown that "apples" have lower levels of "good" cholesterol (HDL-2).

▲ **Fat takes up more space** *than muscle but weighs less. Women have a higher normal percentage of body fat than men (22.5 percent at age 22 compared to 16 percent in men), but more women than men are both overweight and too fat. However, a lifestyle of crash dieting promotes fat. Exercise is the best way to get rid of it. Many diets that promote rapid slimming through very low calorie intake do nothing to reduce actual fat, and weight is usually regained rapidly.*

▲ **Jane Fonda, actress**, *producer and author of several workout videos, took up exercise because she felt "too fat on screen" at 115lb. She is now 15 or 20lb heavier than she was when she took up exercising, but improved muscle tone means that she looks thinner, feels more firm and muscular – and no longer worries about her weight. Weight and fat are not always related; often it is better to judge by the eye than by the scale.*

starvation are present, you can easily rectify this. You could cut calories (a little, not a lot), increase exercise (gradually) or lower fat intake (without further lowering calorie intake). This should allow you to maintain your natural weight easily and will improve your health generally.

If your weight is stable and you do not feel hungry, you may already be at the best weight and reducing it may be harmful. If you do attempt to reduce, resign yourself to a slow rate of weight loss and expect to reach a plateau where your weight will not change. Slow weight loss is more beneficial in the long term and allows you to look for changes in eating patterns that bring about losses big enough to make the sacrifice worth it; what is more, they are generally patterns that you can live with comfortably for the rest of your life and maintain without great effort. **OWW**

What matters is body composition

Many of us have had the experience of going to the doctor, stepping on the scale and being told that we are above our "ideal weight." Alternatively, many of us have found out this disconcerting news for ourselves by consulting a chart of "ideal weights" in a book or magazine. These standards were set up by life-insurance companies based on the study of the age of death of hundreds of thousands of people. Ideal weight was defined as the weight for each height that was associated with the lowest rate of death; it has since been modified by the recognition of different ideal body weights for different body types.

These weights are considered ideal by insurance companies because people at or near their ideal weight appear to live longer, so delaying the payment of life-insurance

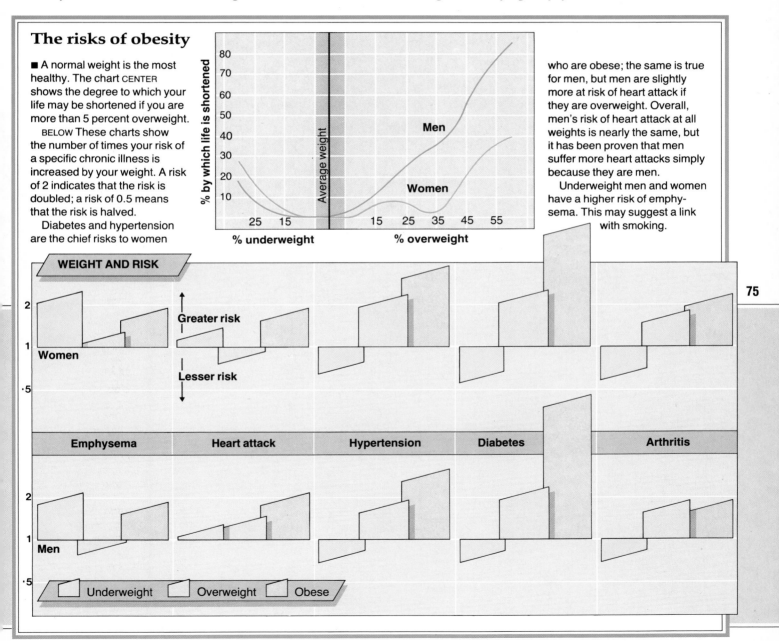

The risks of obesity

■ A normal weight is the most healthy. The chart CENTER shows the degree to which your life may be shortened if you are more than 5 percent overweight.

BELOW These charts show the number of times your risk of a specific chronic illness is increased by your weight. A risk of 2 indicates that the risk is doubled; a risk of 0.5 means that the risk is halved.

Diabetes and hypertension are the chief risks to women

who are obese; the same is true for men, but men are slightly more at risk of heart attack if they are overweight. Overall, men's risk of heart attack at all weights is nearly the same, but it has been proven that men suffer more heart attacks simply because they are men.

Underweight men and women have a higher risk of emphysema. This may suggest a link with smoking.

WEIGHT AND RISK

Greater risk

Lesser risk

Women

Men

Emphysema   Heart attack   Hypertension   Diabetes   Arthritis

Underweight   Overweight   Obese

75

benefits. The findings of other studies have shown that being either below or above ideal weight is associated with death at an earlier age. However, other factors are involved in the correlation between weight and life-expectancy, and they need to be considered in order to determine the "ideal weight" of any person.

Being overweight is not the same thing as being fat. People who are very muscular or who have a large frame (heavy bone structure) can be "overweight" without being too fat. It is also possible to be at your ideal weight yet carry too much fat. Your body is made up of many different kinds of fluids and tissues. In evaluating a person's health, the body is divided into two parts, fat and lean. Your health is evaluated by measuring the percentage of your body weight which is fat. Some body fat is necessary for survival. Women generally have higher body-fat percentages than men.

Body composition is measured in several ways. The best way is called underwater weighing. This method compares your weight in air to your weight underwater. Since fat floats, the difference between these two weights is used to estimate your body-fat percentage. Another method uses calipers to measure how thick the layer of fat under your skin is at different places on the body. This sort of measurement is much more accurate than ideal weights in determining a person's

health prospects and provides some interesting statistics. Twenty-three percent of men between 20 and 74 in the United States are at least 20 percent over their ideal weight, but only 55 percent of these men are too fat. Unlike men, 30 percent of women in the United States are 20 percent over their ideal weight, but 74 percent of these are also too fat. Of the men and women who are technically normal weight, 9 percent have too much body fat.

What creates a body's size and shape?

Children often look very much like their parents. This is true not only of facial features but also of body size and shape. It used to be thought that this was a result of learned eating patterns and how they affected weight. Certainly, we do pick up many of our parents' eating habits during childhood, but even if we change those habits in later life many elements of body size and shape are inherited. The length of the long bones, the proportion of muscle, the size of the rib cage and centers of fat storage (around the stomach or on the hips and thighs) are all controlled by the genes inherited from parents, and not much can be done to change this basic body shape. Fundamentally, your appearance and weight are determined by the combination of your genetic potential, your normal eating pattern and how much exercise

FINDING YOUR "IDEAL" WEIGHT

Underweight / Healthy/normal weight / Overweight

2.0m (6'7") 1.9m (6'3") 1.8m (5'11") 1.7m (5'7") 1.6m (5'3") 1.5m (4'11")

40kg (88lb) 50kg (110lb) 60kg (132lb) 70kg (154lb) 80kg (176lb) 90kg (198lb) 100kg (220lb) 110kg (242lb)

▲ **Healthy weight** *is determined by height and sex. This chart follows the "ideal weight" system developed by insurance companies.*

◄ **Pinch an inch.** *A simple way to determine whether body fat is excessive is to pinch the fold around your waist between thumb and finger. If you can pinch 25mm (an inch) or more, you probably need to lose some fat.*

Your ideal weight – does it exist?

■ The difficulty in deciding whether you are underweight or overweight is working out how much you should weigh in relation to your entire body composition. A large, heavy bone structure weighs more than a small one.
● For men: Allow 106lb for the first five feet of your height plus 6lb for every inch above that. For instance, if you are 5ft 8in, add 106 + 48, giving an ideal weight of 154lb.
● For women: Allow 100lb for the first five feet of your height plus 5lb for every inch above that. If you are 5ft 4in, add 100 + 20, giving an ideal weight of 120lb.

76

you take throughout your life. Your genes will set a definite limit on how diet and exercise will influence your weight and appearance. A short, stocky person will never be able to look like a fashion model; similarly, a thin, gangly person will never become either voluptuous or a professional weightlifter.

Adjusting your "natural weight"

If you weigh yourself every day, you will find that your weight fluctuates around an average. In fact, there is more variability in your food intake from day to day than there is in your weight. All people have a typical weight which the body returns to when they are not trying to diet. This is known as natural weight. Maintaining weight above or below this point requires a sustained and considerable change in food intake. Set-point theory accepts this basic fact and proposes ways of resetting the body's natural weight to reduce or increase weight.

Your set point can be changed in two ways. High-fat diets contribute to the development of a high set-point weight, while low-fat diets result in a lowering of the body's set point. This seems to work by raising or lowering the body's fat percentage, which appears to be directly linked to body metabolism and consequent "natural weight." This is not a matter of calories, but of the amount of fat in your food. Cutting your intake of fat down to 40-60 grams per day, about half of the standard amount of fat that is consumed in the United States, can reduce your body's set point by approximately 5-6 percent.

Exercise can also change your set point, both by reducing body-fat percentage and by increasing muscle mass. Sedentary people can usually reduce their set point by 5-6 percent by beginning an exercise program involving 45 minutes per day, four to five times a week. Fat reduction and exercise will not only help you lose weight and keep it off; it will make your body healthier.

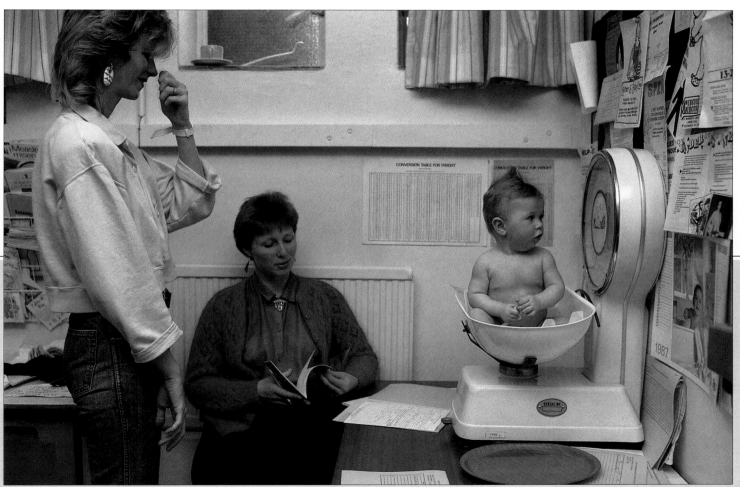

▲ **Blissfully unconscious of her weight** – *but not for long. Prejudice against obesity is learned at a very early age, and is especially feared in girls even* as young as 9 or 10, who may go on diets (sometimes prompted by their anxious parents) because they are "too heavy." Eating normally and not being obsessed with weight is very important for children because they require plenty of food in order to grow. Studies have shown that depriving children of food is more likely to cause obesity in young adulthood than allowing them to eat as their natural appetite demands.

What weight is best for you?

Assessing your own ideal weight involves three factors. You need to establish your correct height – many people were last measured at school and assume their height to be as much as several inches below what it actually is. Second, take a good look at your body in a full-length mirror. Are you muscular, stocky, small-boned, wide-hipped, long-bodied? Where does your body fat tend to settle? These are things you cannot change, and an ideal weight based on an unreasonable image of yourself will never be achieved. Finally, "pinch an inch" – how much of your body is composed of fat? If you are fairly lean you are probably the right weight, even if you do not fit the "ideal weight" charts. If your weight is "normal" but there is a great deal of fat on your body, you may in fact need to lose some weight, or exchange some of your fat for lean muscle through exercise. Actual weight is far less important than your muscle/fat ratio.

Yo-yo dieting

Dieting means adopting a set of rules that tell you what you can and cannot eat. Many of our favorite foods become "no-nos" when we are on a diet. In an effort to control our eating and lose weight quickly, we often grasp at bizarre diet fads which may restrict not only what but when, how often and in what combinations food can be consumed. Special diet foods are produced by manufacturers, some of them genuinely useful low-fat alternatives, which encourage us to make a distinction between "diet" food and "real" food. Distinctions like these also set up cravings and feelings of deprivation. Most of us learned as children that food is both a reward and a source of comfort. As adults, however, we developed a confused relationship with food as it remains both rewarding and comforting but has now become "bad" because it is fattening.

Am I a chronic dieter?

■ How many of the following statements are true of you? If the number is 5-10, you are probably a chronic dieter. If more than 10, you may be a "yo-yo" dieter.

- Before I eat a food, I think about the calories.
- I have tried many diets.
- Losing weight is easy for me; keeping it off is hard.
- I often overeat when I am upset or depressed.
- There are certain foods I love, but I consider them forbidden.
- I sometimes skip meals in order to lose weight.
- When I go off my diet, I tend to indulge myself.
- My life would be better if only I could lose my extra weight.
- When I am on a diet, I never seem to lose weight quickly.
- I know which foods are fattening and which are not.
- I tend to forget my diet when with others who are eating.

- I am afraid to have even a taste of some foods because I might lose control.
- I sometimes use food as a way to make me feel better.
- When I eat I feel guilty.
- If I ate whatever I wanted, I would get very fat.

An eating pattern that alternates between strictness and excess can damage your health. It may maintain or even reduce weight, but it encourages the rapid creation and storage of fat, called hyperlipogenesis. So you may not be overweight, but you may be too fat.

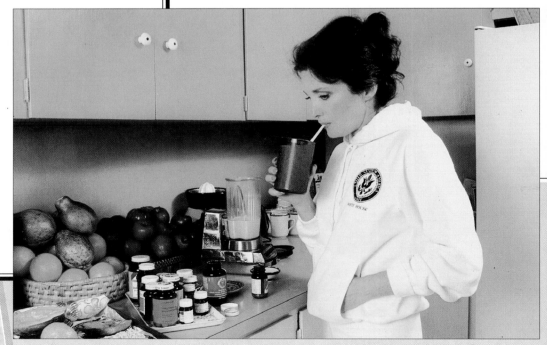

▲ **Breakfast and exercise** fit into the lifestyle of people who feel as good as they look. By contrast, the starvation approach to weight loss may mean that you lose little weight in spite of not eating since the body's reaction to an inadequate supply of food is to slow down its metabolism (the rate of burning calories). "Yo-yo" dieting – alternating strict dieting with overeating – actually contributes to the build up of fat, and a diet of less than 800 calories per day can cause the loss of lean muscle. A less severe regimen combined with exercise is most likely to produce the desired result.

78

Strict dieting is easily interrupted by the rewarding or comforting properties of food. "Blowing your diet" relieves the deprivations and provides temporary comfort, but at the same time leads to feelings of guilt or despair. We feel good about not eating and want to be rewarded, so we eat, then we feel bad, so we forbid ourselves to eat. Alternating periods of dieting and overeating, called yo-yo dieting, result in repeated cycles of weight loss and weight gain that can be difficult to break. This pattern is a vicious circle and it can damage health by leading to the development of a high body-fat percentage, even when the losses or gains are only moderate.

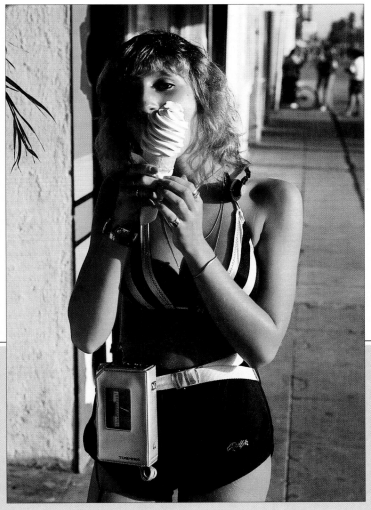

▲ **One treat will not ruin every-thing**, *especially for people who exercise. Compared to dieting, exercise does have some drawbacks. It will take time out of your day; weight loss will be slower; and it demands as much discipline as a diet (dropout rates from exercise are high). However, a long-term* *program of regular exercise is much more beneficial than chronic dieting. Your body will be firmer and trimmer even if you do not lose a spectacular amount of weight. Your health and general fitness will improve much more rapidly, and you will be able to eat normally without counting every calorie.*

Developing a more healthy eating plan

Dieting should mean a sensible change of lifestyle rather than denial, discipline and deprivation. The mistake most people make is to be impatient to lose weight. They cut back on food intake by establishing a set of rules that are too strict to be followed for any period of time, let alone for an entire lifetime. This quickly induces yo-yo dieting. Ideally, dieting involves restricting your calorie intake a little bit, so that you burn up 500-1,000 calories a day more than you take in, leading to a slow, steady weight loss of 1-2 pounds a week. Often simply reducing the level of fat in your diet to a healthy level will do this.

Do not cut out any food entirely – especially your favorite; eat less of it as part of your whole diet. Try to eat regular, planned meals. Overeating is often the result of "snacking," and if you eat well at meals you are less likely to be tempted with extras. Vary your diet as much as possible – this will ensure your diet is nutritionally sound and prevent bore-dom, another common cause of overeating. Develop a regular exercise program that you enjoy and can keep up. Finally, once your new, healthy lifestyle is a habit, *forget about dieting*. If you are living in a healthy way your weight should take care of itself. **DGS**

After dieting

■ People on extreme diets often experience alarming symptoms when they come off them – but do not use this as a reason for continuing with a severely restrictive diet. A rapid weight gain of 5-7 pounds is not unusual. Weight gained immedi-ately after a restrictive diet is usually water that your body has shed in reaction to its "starvation." Your weight should level off once your body becomes rehydrated, providing you are eating moderately.

Bloating and constipation sometimes result. Your diges-tive system has been under-worked and needs some time to return to its normal functioning. Your appetite may be alarmingly acute as well.

Foods that you ignored may have enormous appeal as you go back into a normal eating pattern. This soon subsides as long as you do not binge and then restrict your food. Eat what you want at planned meals and your digestive system and body state will soon return to normal. **OWW**

Slow weight loss allows your body image to keep pace with your body. Research indicates that people who lose weight quickly tend to feel just as fat afterwards as before. A gentler pace allows you to observe and enjoy the changes in your body as they happen, and removes the emphasis of the diet from food to feeling good.

■ **What is a calorie?** A calorie is a standard unit that measures the energy value of foods. Technically it is the amount of energy needed to raise the temperature of one gram of water by one degree Centigrade. Spelled with a capital C, a Calorie is 1,000 calories, or a kilocalorie (a Kcal). It is normally Calories, not calories, that dieters count, whether or not their charts insert the capital C.

10

Weight Control and Self-Image

Gaining or losing weight is central to most people's self-esteem ● Feeling comfortable about your body shows in the way you move and relate to others ● Unrealistic expectations can spoil your sense of self-worth.

IN 1984, *Glamor* magazine's body-image survey found some depressing statistics about the way American women regard their own bodies. 75 percent of women who responded to the survey felt "too fat," including 45 percent of those who were underweight by an objective standard. The dissatisfaction begins young. A study conducted in 1986 found that 50 percent of 9-year-old girls in San Francisco schools, and 80 percent of 10- and 11-year-old girls, had put themselves on diets because they felt "too fat." Insecurity drives women in

particular to seek out instant help. In 1986, for example, there were 313 diet books in print in the United States.

Nearly all women and many men want to be thinner. This is mostly because of concern over appearance, not health. In a society less obsessed by weight than our own, slimming down might be quite straightforward. After all, if your clothes no longer fit and you have recently acquired a "spare tire" around your waist, maybe it really is time for you to lose some weight. But is there really a roll of fat around your middle? Have your clothes really got tighter? Can you trust what you think you see in the mirror?

Many of us have friends who complain about the size of

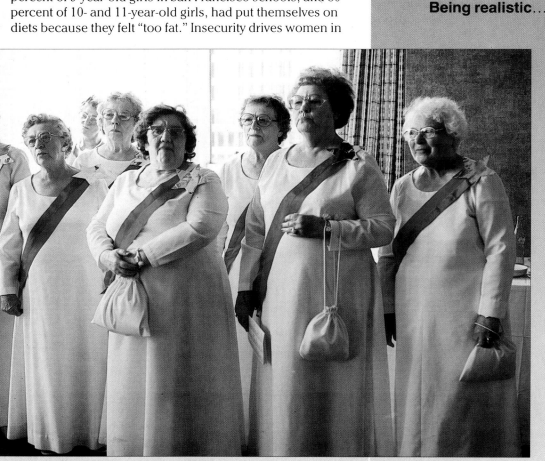

Being realistic...

▲ **Being "overweight"** *is a state of mind as well as a physical condition. Most of these ladies are above the weight given for their height on typical ideal weight charts. However, when they are socializing together they will not make each other feel unacceptably fat. Whether consciously or subconsciously, each of them* *can feel reassured that she is within the average range established by her peers. On the whole, people tend to take their cues from each other, and enjoying an active social life with friends who look similar goes a long way toward making us feel accepted and acceptable.*

▶ **The "ideal" figure** *is often dictated by fashion rather than good health. Today most men and women admire a body shape that is sleek, streamlined and only delicately curved – a far cry from the voluptuous ideal of other eras. In reality few are born with this shape or can ever achieve it.*

their legs or the thickness of their waists; yet to us they look perfectly normal, even slender. When they look in the mirror, they do not see a reflection of the person they are but of someone they do not want to be. That person's real problem may not be weight at all, but weight has become such an obsession in our society that other dissatisfactions are often focused through it.

What do you see in the mirror?

If you are not happy with your weight regardless of what you eat, or are only happy if you are losing weight regardless of what you weigh and of how you have to eat (or not eat) to make this happen, you have a body-image problem. Most people have trouble viewing their bodies objectively, but this problem exists in varying degrees of severity and changes according to feelings and situations. Some people feel mildly dissatisfied with their bodies or certain aspects of them, but on the whole they live happily, realizing that not everything can be changed. Other people are deeply unhappy with their physical selves and would (and sometimes do) try anything to change it. On the whole, people are more likely to be dissatisfied with their bodies when they are feeling bad about something else – often work or personal relationships.

If your body image is seriously distorted you may need professional help. But the first step you need to take, whether your body-image problem is serious or minor, is to recognize its existence, to acknowledge that you may not be seeing your body as it really is, and that you would not be happy with it whatever it was like. Distortions of body image are quite common, and there is often no relationship between a person's weight and the degree to which they are satisfied with their body. This means there are many heavier-than-average people who like their bodies, and,

...about how your body looks

◄ **A distorted body image** *is often the result of striving vainly to achieve the impossible. Unreal expectations can generate such anxiety that even when people have trimmed their figures to a personal best they fail to recognize any improvement, and continue to feel "fat" and dissatisfied.*

Do you have a body-image problem?

■ If you answer yes to more than seven of the following questions you have a poor body image. If you answer yes to all of them, you may have a serious body-image problem.

- Do you sometimes feel panicked about not losing weight?
- Does the idea of people seeing your body naked or in a bathing suit make you feel nervous or upset?
- Do you hate the way your body is shaped?
- Do you check yourself in the mirror to make sure you are not getting fatter?
- Do you insist on having sex with the lights off?

- When you walk into a room, do you automatically compare your weight to the other people in the room?
- After you have eaten a big meal, do you find yourself worrying about gaining weight because of it?
- Do you often find yourself envying other people and wishing your body looked like theirs?
- Are you sometimes convinced your scales are mistaken?
- Do you sometimes weigh yourself more than once a day?
- Do you wear loose-fitting clothes to hide the parts of your body that you think are too fat?

A recent study of schoolgirls in selected areas of the United States found that 60 percent of average-weight girls were trying to lose weight as well as 18 percent of girls who were already underweight. Some of them, as young as nine years old, were on severe and potentially dangerous regimes.

81

sadly, many more who dislike their bodies even though they are ideal even by current standards of slenderness. It is disconcerting to realize that you cannot trust the evidence of your own eyes. What can you trust then? Fortunately there are objective questions you can ask yourself to determine whether you have a distorted body image, and some simple exercises that can help you come to terms with your body and your expectations of it. **oww**

Anorexia nervosa

The world of the chronic dieter becomes one of extreme contrasts. Dieting is good, eating is bad. Lettuce is good, bread is bad. Losing weight is great, gaining weight is horrible. Dieting is deprivation, eating is pleasure. Most of all, dieters come to believe that their own goodness or badness comes to depend upon eating or not eating.

"Yo-yo dieting" – a pattern of strict dieting followed by chronic lapses, followed by more strict dieting – is a common pattern contributing to lifelong weight problems and the medical, social and psychological consequences associated with being overweight. The same kind of thinking that causes yo-yo dieting can get out of control and lead to the development of an eating disorder.

There are two major kinds of eating disorder: anorexia nervosa and bulimia nervosa. Anorexia occurs when a person is too successful at dieting and reduces down to less than 85 percent of their ideal body weight. Even though the anorexic is very thin, body-image problems create the feeling of being "too fat." Anorexia occurs mainly in adolescent girls and young women and is fatal in about 10 percent of cases. Anorexics may not menstruate, and often suffer from insomnia, constipation, extreme sensitivity to heat and cold, and excess hair loss due to hormonal disruption. Heartbeat, circulation, blood pressure and perspiration may become sluggish. Some anorexics diet until they literally starve to death.

Many ideas have been put forward to explain why anorexia occurs and why it is mostly found in women. The advertising and fashion industries are often blamed for promoting a prepubescent body standard for women which leads to unrealistic expectations about womanliness. Conversely, anorexia is also thought to be a pulling-back from the responsibilities and difficulties of womanhood by retaining a childlike body. Anorexics generally express self-hatred and a sense of rejection, feelings that may lead to their attempts literally to disappear. Susie Orbach, in her study *Fat is a Feminist Issue*, relates all these explanations to the search for control. By refusing food, an anorexic establishes one area of life that is not confusing or threatening, and also apparently reconciles the tension between accepting and rejecting current models of femininity.

Bulimia nervosa

Bulimia is more common than anorexia, and also occurs mostly in young women although men are also prone to this "secret" problem. It is often known as binge/purge disorder, which describes the symptoms very well. Bulimia is closely related to the eating patterns of the yo-yo dieter and distin-

How do you feel about your body?

■ People who dislike their bodies tend to have poor self-esteem, suffer from depression and are more prone to becoming chronic dieters, anorexic or bulimic. Developing a body-image problem in the first place, however, is usually caused by having unrealistic expectations. To form a realistic view of how well your body meets your ideal, try the following exercise. First, establish what your ideal is. Go through some magazines and cut out pictures that represent how you think your body should look at its best. Using the pictures as a guide, sketch the outline of your ideal body on a plain piece of paper. Make some photocopies of this sketch so that you can draw and mark on it without destroying the original.

■ Using the sketch of your ideal body size while standing in front of a mirror, rate each of these parts of your body on a four-point scale:
Face
Shoulders and neck
Arms, especially upper arms
Chest (includes the breasts, for women)
Stomach
Hips
Thighs
1 I am extremely happy with this part of my body
2 I am satisfied with this part of my body
3 I dislike this part of my body
4 I hate this part of my body
   If you add up the ratings, this score will reflect your overall level of satisfaction or dissatisfaction with your body. Scores above 20 indicate that you are unhappy with your body while scores above 25 indicate a severe problem with body satisfaction.

■ Now find some photographs of yourself from different periods of your life. Look in particular for ones that reveal your body shape and size. Pick out three: one that shows you at your highest weight, another at your lowest weight and finally one that is most recent and reflects your current weight.
   Using the photograph as a guide, sketch your current body shape on top of a photocopy of your sketch of your ideal body shape. Be careful to make the relative proportioning of the body parts match the photo-graph – if your legs are shorte than the legs on the ideal ima make sure that the legs on the sketch of your actual body siz look like the photograph. Usin a different color each time, sketch the outline of your larg and smallest body sizes.

■ How much difference is the between your smallest body . size and your ideal? What pa of your body are shaped very differently from your ideal dra ing? Is there a relationship between the differences in yo actual and ideal sizes and yo satisfaction ratings? Are thes differences due to fat – or the shape and size of your bones and muscles? Comparing you current body size to your larg and smallest sketches, what

guishing between the two is a matter of degree. Bulimia is the result of a severe body-image problem when the person is extremely afraid of gaining weight and is very anxious to lose weight. Unlike anorexics, bulimics are not very successful at dieting and will frequently go on eating binges. These binges leave the bulimic feeling guilty and afraid of getting fat. Bulimics differ from chronic dieters in that they will regularly "purge" after an eating binge in order to avoid becoming heavier.

Purging may take the form of inducing vomiting, taking an overdose of laxatives, going on an extended fast, or exercising excessively and to the point of exhaustion and injury. Once bulimics begin to use purging as an antidote to binging, they often completely lose control over their eating behavior. The typical person with bulimia nervosa binges and purges two to three times a day. Vomiting and laxative abuse cause many medical complications, from tooth decay due to the corrosive effect of stomach acid in the mouth after vomiting, to gastric ulcers and ruptures, to heart attacks brought on by the loss of potassium caused by purge methods. Complete loss of control over food intake can lead to severe depression or suicide.

Unlike anorexics, bulimics are usually at or only slightly above normal body weight (though they usually see themselves as repulsively fat). Many of their preoccupations with food are shared by people with much milder eating problems, and bulimics often follow their cycle of binge and purge for years without anyone suspecting that there is a serious problem. Like anorexics, bulimics seem to suffer extreme confusion and frustration about their sexuality and use food in an attempt to gain control over their lives. They often dislike themselves and still suffer from unresolved childhood traumas and rejections.

Treating eating disorders

Ten years ago anorexia and bulimia were seldom recognized as serious problems even in their most acute and obvious forms. Today such problems are swiftly diagnosed. Treatment includes drugs, psychoanalysis, behavioral therapy and group discussion, but the chances of successful treatment are low unless the person with the eating disorder recognizes the problem and wants to solve it. It may take years for a person with a severe eating disorder to break the cycle of self-loathing and body torment.

Awareness of the dangers and possible causes of eating disorders is one way of preventing them occurring at all. If you fit the pattern of a chronic dieter you should begin to work on your body image and eating patterns now. Eating disorders are the bottom of a spiral of unrealistic ideals, distorted body image, self-disgust and poor eating habits. While most people do not have the underlying mental problems that result in full-blown eating disorders, even minor problems with food can cause a great deal of personal unhappiness. Learning to like yourself and your body is much healthier and happier than dieting. **DGS**

changes can you realistically expect to make by diet and exercise? Are there parts of your body that probably cannot be changed by diet and exercise? Do you need to change your expectations of what your body should look like for any of the body parts?

■ Think hard about these questions and try to answer them honestly. Try the exercise at different times – when you are feeling depressed, and when you are feeling good about yourself – and see if and how much the answers differ. Keep track of the situations where you feel bad about your body. This will alert you to a distorted body image, and give you help to correct it. **DGS**

▶ **Danger signs**. *Teenage girls, in particular, are highly susceptible to anxiety about what they eat and about being "too fat." Signs of a severe eating disorder include refusing to eat in public, secret eating, sudden weight gain or loss, expressions of distaste toward others who are "fat" (particularly if they are not really) and either constant discussion about food or a refusal to mention it at all. If you think that someone close to you has an eating disorder the best thing you can do is to encourage them to recognize that they have a problem and to seek professional help.*

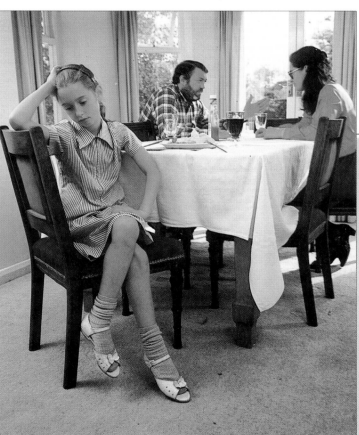

11

Exercise and Physical Fitness

*Suppleness, strength and stamina are the rewards
of spending time on your physical fitness
● Exercise tones the body, sharpens the mind
and contributes to overall confidence and
self-awareness ● It makes you feel better too.*

THE INDISPUTABLE connection between health and exercise means that, for all of us, choosing and developing a regular fitness program that we can follow for the rest of our lives is of major importance. Whether your specific motivation is a trimmer figure, weight loss, fear of heart disease or relaxation, you should make exercise a habit. Few of us get enough exercise, or the right kind, in the course of our work, so we have to make a conscious effort to achieve optimum fitness.

Understanding what exercise is and how it works is the first step toward exercising your way to better health. The general term is used to describe various forms of physical activity that are undertaken to improve or maintain physical fitness. Different kinds of exercise are defined by the type of physical activity and the primary energy system used for it. There are two major groups, aerobic and anaerobic. These terms are used frequently in exercise classes manuals and videos and the difference between them needs to be clearly understood as they affect us physically in separate ways.

Anaerobic exercise

Some exercise puts a great strain on our muscles but not on our lungs and heart. This is called anaerobic exercise and common examples include sprinting and weight-lifting. It is usually performed at a high intensity level in which the oxygen demands of our muscles are greater than the body's ability to deliver oxygen to them. Anaerobic exercise relies on immediate and short-term access to energy stores that produce energy rapidly, fueled by the compounds adenosine triphosphate (ATP) and cretin phosphate (CP). These compounds are stored within the muscles.

During intense activity, the stores of ATP and CP are depleted quite rapidly (in as little as 10-20 seconds). Enzymes in the muscles can break down some of the sugars present to produce further ATP (a process called anaerobic glycolysis), but this produces a waste product called lactic

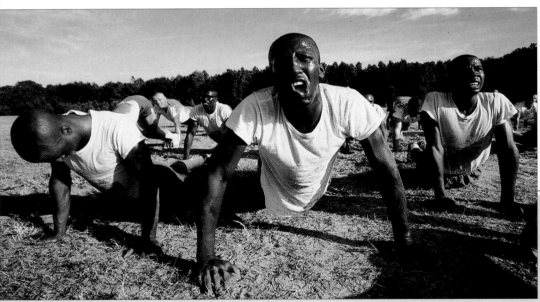

■ **Total fitness** *is a healthy balance of strength, flexibility, speed and endurance. The potential benefits of anaerobic exercise ABOVE and aerobic exercise RIGHT complement each other, and combining the two has much to offer in terms of health and physical performance. The first offers increased strength, the other greater stamina. These Marines training on Parris Island are doing pushups to increase* *strength in their upper bodies; the joggers are building endurance through toning their cardiovascular systems (increasing the efficiency of the heart and lungs). Whether you are training for a particular sport, or just keeping fit, you will benefit from both types of exercise. Weightlifting, for instance, is an anaerobic activity, but a healthy heart and lungs developed through aerobic exercise can give the weightlifter an extra* *edge by improving endurance. Cycling is primarily an aerobic sport, but it needs strong muscles which can be built up more readily in an anaerobic exercise such as sprinting.*

acid that limits the ability of the muscles to sustain high-intensity activity for longer than 1-2 minutes. This explains why anaerobic exercise can only be performed for very short periods before excessive muscle fatigue sets in.

As well as sprinting and weight-lifting, anaerobic activities include the movements performed on most fitness machines, many calisthenics, and the rapid bursts of exercise required by very energetic sports like squash and fencing. Exercise of this sort can help to improve muscular strength, endurance, agility, power and speed, all qualities important to overall fitness. Anaerobic activities will have some effect upon your heart rate and breathing, but to really improve your cardiovascular system you will need to undertake some aerobic exercise.

Aerobic exercise

Aerobic exercise uses large muscle groups, is repetitive, rhythmical, and can be sustained for a long period of time. It is performed at a low enough intensity to allow the body to provide a sufficient supply of oxygen to the exercising muscle – sufficient ATP is produced without the production of excessive lactic acid. Because aerobic exercise can be maintained for a long period, it exercises the lungs and heart by raising the amount of oxygen required, forcing the lungs to take in and process more air, and the heart to circulate the blood faster.

For an activity to qualify as aerobic it has to be continuously sustained for at least 15 minutes, with a substantial increase in heart rate (at least 75 percent of the maximum recommended heart rate). Popular forms of aerobic activity include walking, jogging, swimming, bicycling and aerobic dancing. Aerobic exercise burns calories at a significant rate and improves coordination, flexibility, endurance and muscle tone (though not necessarily muscle strength). Most importantly, aerobic activity produces significant improvement in the efficiency and capacity of the cardiovascular system which, in turn, greatly improves overall health.

Physical activity and regular exercise have numerous health benefits, but perhaps the greatest and most far-reaching is the improvement to cardiovascular health.

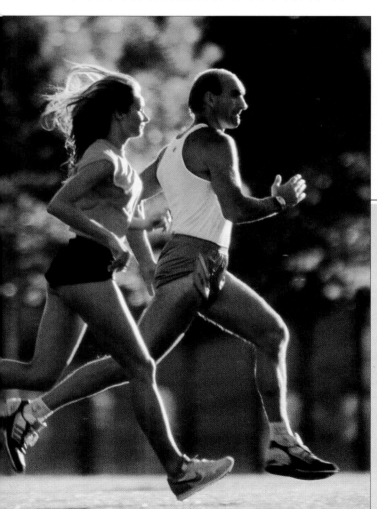

Which exercise is right for me?

■ Now that more and more people work out in the gym, experts are turning their attention to developing the perfect exercise machine. Training with free weights and barbells will certainly produce results, but only after dedicated hard work over a period of time. So much of the benefit depends, too, on how carefully the exercise is done – poor technique can sometimes do more harm than good. The ideal machine works the muscles you want to exercise evenly and at their maximum capacity. With free weights, however, the effort you can put in is limited by the weakest part of the movement.

● If you are trying to lose weight you should take part in lower-intensity, high-frequency and long-duration activities to use up the most calories.
● If you do not have much time to spend exercising, a program of high intensity and short duration done three times a week is enough to produce health benefits.

Exercise	Type	Benefits
cycling	aerobic	heart, lungs and thigh muscles
swimming	aerobic	heart, lungs and all muscles
weight lifting	anaerobic	strengthens all muscle groups
jogging	aerobic	heart, lungs and leg muscles
rowing	aerobic	heart, lungs and leg and arm muscles
sprinting	anaerobic	leg muscles
aerobic dancing	aerobic	heart, lungs and general muscle tone
situps	anaerobic	abdomen and lower back muscles
pushups	anaerobic	chest and arm muscles

Everyone can benefit from a program of sustained aerobic exercise. There is an inverse relationship between exercise and the incidence of fatal and nonfatal heart disease – regular exercisers are less likely to develop heart disease and are more likely to survive it if they do.

Working against heart disease

One of the earliest studies examining the link between people's occupations and the average rate of death from heart disease examined the work habits and health of 3,686 longshoremen over a 22-year period, in the days before mechanization and containerized cargo shipping.

Those whose work involved the greatest expenditure of energy (8,500 calories or more per week) had significantly less heart disease at any age than those men whose energy output was less than this. In addition, the association between hard physical labor and a low risk of heart disease occurred independently of other risk factors such as a family history of heart disease, smoking or high blood pressure.

A study of 16,936 male Harvard alumni between the ages of 35 and 74 showed that the most sedentary alumni were 25 percent more likely to have a heart attack than the next most active group. Among very active participants, those who regularly played a vigorous sport were 38 percent less likely to have heart disease than those who rated themselves as very active but did not play any vigorous games. Men who expended less than 2,000 calories per week in exercise were at a 64 percent greater risk of heart attack than those who exercised more. In fact, heart disease among the alumni would have been reduced by 23 percent if all had exercised away more than 2,000 calories per week.

Heart attacks were rarer among active alumni regardless of their exercise habits as students. Former athletes who discontinued their physical activity were at a substantially higher risk for heart disease than inactive students who had developed active lifestyles later in life. Exercise has to be maintained in order to provide any advantage to health.

Improving your cardiovascular health

The greatest physiological changes improving health and decreasing the risk of heart disease are the result of a lifetime of participation in regular exercise. However, cardiovascular health can improve quite rapidly after you begin a regular program. Research demonstrates that improvements in general heart and lung functioning and a reduction in the factors that cause heart disease can occur after six to eight weeks of beginning a new routine.

Regular aerobic exercise works by improving the cardiovascular system's ability to transport and use oxygen. This

High-impact or low-impact

■ Aerobic dance, commonly known simply as aerobics, is excellent cardiovascular exercise and very enjoyable, but it can cause stress injuries to the joints, back and feet. In many dance studios, "high-impact" aerobics with a great deal of jumping and high kicking has been supplemented by "low-impact" movements, in which one foot is always touching the ground. This usually lessens the risk of injury. However, low-impact aerobics may not always allow people who are very fit to reach their desired heart rate. "Middle-impact" aerobics attempts to combine the benefits of low and high impact by keeping one foot in contact with the floor but increasing the amount of arm and upper body movement. Most gyms and fitness clubs now hold classes in all three types of aerobics and will advise you on which type suits you best.

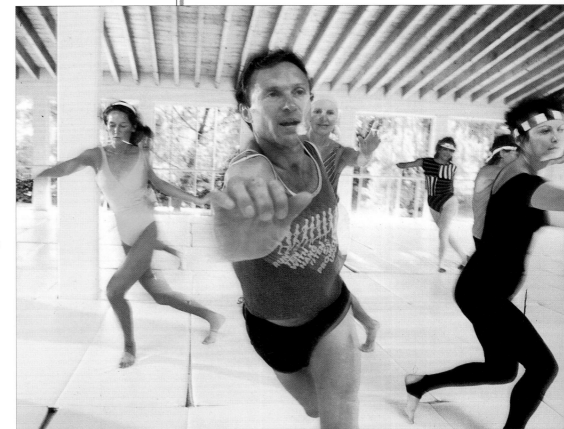

means that over time the body has to work less and less hard to maintain itself, either at rest or when active. This increase in cardiovascular endurance (also known as aerobic capacity) is often termed the "training effect." The body becomes more efficient and able to do more work, so the heart rate tends to slow down and consequently blood pressure is lower, both at rest and during exercise.

Lowering blood pressure and cholesterol

The connection between regular exercise and reduced blood pressure has been of particular interest to experts, because hypertension (high blood pressure) is known to be a significant risk factor in the incidence of heart disease. The causes and effects of high blood pressure are still not entirely understood, but it does appear that active people

How hard should I exercise?

■ Choose an activity that increases your heart rate, but not too much.

Your heart rate is a simple and effective measure of how intensely you are exercising. It is easy to monitor and beginners are well advised to check their progress in this way.

To determine your highest safe heart rate, subtract your age from 220. This will give you the maximum number of beats per minute that a person of your age should demand of their heart. Exceeding 85 percent of

this figure will quickly lead to fatigue, especially in people unused to exertion, and can be dangerous for those at risk from heart attack.

Your exercise program should be based on a fixed percentage of your maximum safe heart rate, called the "training range."

After warming up, you should try to maintain your heart rate within your training range throughout your exercise period.

To measure your heart rate,

take your pulse. Wrap the fingers of one hand around the back of the wrist of the other. Press your middle and index fingers (not your thumb) on your wrist until you can feel your pulse. Using a watch with a second hand, count the number of pulses during 15 seconds and multiply by four. This is your present heart rate.

Your heart rate decreases rapidly once you have stopped exercising, so take your pulse immediately after you stop, or even while you are exercising.

■ Rating your exertion.
The figures given below are known as a Rating of Perceived Exertion (RPE). An RPE of 13 is roughly the exertion that would make your heart beat at 70 percent of its maximum safe rate (ie, it is at the lower end of your ideal training range). Maintaining an RPE of between 10 and 12 is considered to be ideal for beginners, and may be increased to 13-15 over time. If you are suspicious of your subjective judgment, measure your heart rate.

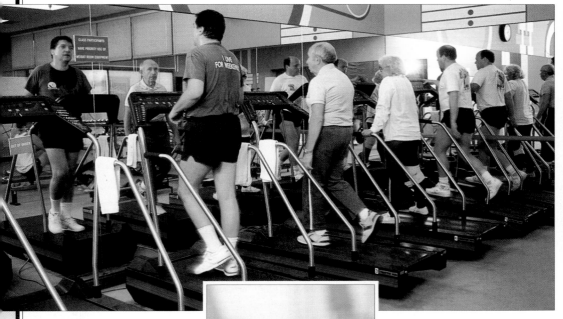

20	
19	exertion producing nearly your maximum safe heart rate
18	very, very hard
17	exertion
16	very hard exertion
15	
14	hard exertion
13	exertion producing
12	about 70 percent
11	of your maximum safe heart rate
10	fairly light exertion
9	
8	very light exertion
7	
6	very, very light exertion

▲ Joining a health club or fitness center can be very helpful in beginning and maintaining an exercise routine. Instructors will help you devise a safe and sensible program, and many people enjoy the camaraderie of exercising alongside others with similar problems, goals and motivations.

◄ Maintaining your ideal heart rate during aerobic exercise is much easier if your trainer or instructor links you to a heart monitor like this one. Most people are fascinated to see how dramatically their heart rate responds to jumping higher or bending lower as they work out.

Your training range is from 70-85 percent of your maximum heart rate. If you are 32 years old, your maximum is 188 beats per minute. Your training range is between 132 and 160 beats per minute.

87

display lower blood pressure, and that participation in a regular aerobic exercise program may lower blood pressure regardless of how much you weigh (another determining factor).

Some studies have shown that regular exercise lowers the levels of cholesterol and other fats (or lipids) in the blood. Only aerobic activity appears to have this effect.

Until recently, researchers have focused on the total level of cholesterol in the blood serum, but this emphasis is changing. We now know that there are different kinds of cholesterol, some of benefit to the cardiovascular system and others potentially dangerous. High-density lipoprotein (HDL) actually forestalls the dangerous buildup of fatty deposits in the arteries by carrying fats away to the liver to

be broken down. Low-density lipoproteins (LDL), however, carry cholesterol into the arteries. Aerobic exercise seems to increase the amount of HDL and to decrease the amount of LDL.

Toning the whole body

Regular exercise has many other health benefits besides cardiovascular improvement. Obesity as a result of over-eating and lack of physical activity is a serious health problem associated with diabetes, hypertension and heart disease. Exercise burns up calories that might normally be converted into fat, and it also alters your body composition, promoting the formation of muscle rather than fat. Regular exercisers exhibit a lower percentage of body fat and greater muscle mass than sedentary people regardless of their diet. Combined with a sensible eating plan, exercise can help you maintain a healthy weight and body composition. The aging process also contributes to increasing fatness and decreasing muscle mass; exercise can slow this process.

Aerobic exercise produces the greatest health benefits, but anaerobic activities such as strength training can also

Pumping iron

■ Exercising with weights is now popular as part of the regular fitness program of both men and women, but opinion is divided between the benefits of free weights or fixed weight machines.

Free weights (dumbbells) do not always allow you to get the most out of an exercise movement: at certain phases you may be using your muscles to the full, at others not at all. You can also injure yourself by using a weight that is too heavy or by

lifting it with poor posture.

Exercise machines ensure that you stand or sit in the correct position, and are designed to make all your movements work the muscle targeted by the machine. They are expensive, however, and to get a full workout you need to use a whole set of them. Most exercise programs now include both free and fixed weight activities. Whatever you use, the amount of effort you put in determines how good the results are.

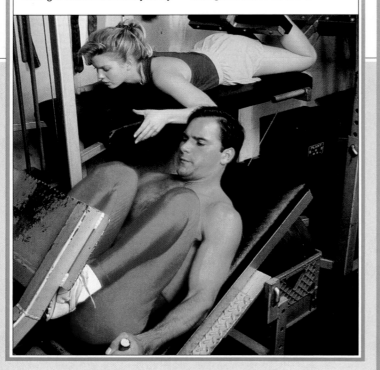

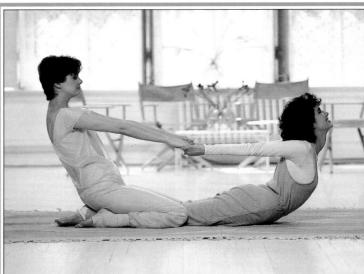

Stretch – and loosen up

■ In the simple tasks of everyday living, we often use our bodies in strained or awkward ways, creating stress and tension. A kind of muscular rigor mortis can set in, leading to reduced range of movement. If you are not used to exercising, you can start by taking 10 to 15 minutes every day to stretch and flex your body gently. This will offset tension and rigidity so you can use your body with greater ease. These stretches

are also a good way to start off your exercise program, to "warm up" your muscles before engaging them in strenuous activity, and to "cool down" your body gradually after a workout. Warm-ups and cool-downs are necessary additions to an exercise program because they prevent strains, cramps and more serious injuries that can occur if the body is not gently prepared and recovered from strenuous exercise.

significantly improve health and well-being. Both inactivity and aging can make the body lose muscle mass and flexibility in the joints. In addition, they contribute to a stiffening of the connective tissues (cartilage, ligaments and tendons). Loss of physical agility can result in pain, a reduced range of movement, and eventually chronic musculoskeletal problems such as low-back pain and permanently stiff joints. A nonaerobic strength and flexibility program can improve flexibility, range of motion, muscle mass and strength. These improvements can relieve musculoskeletal problems, contribute to overall fitness and make aerobic activity more pleasant and profitable.

Both aerobic and anaerobic exercise of any kind will improve your coordination, flexibility, balance and agility. Exercise makes you concentrate on your body and as you come to know it better you will recover some of the grace and confidence that children have naturally, but which adults lose all too soon. One of the earliest benefits regular exercisers report is this sense of confidence and assurance, and researchers have long been interested in the psychological effects that exercise seems to have.

Exercising the mind

Numerous studies have detected a range of mental benefits arising from regular exercise, especially of the aerobic kind. Research in this area has been plagued by difficulties due to the problem of evaluating what people say they feel

---

How long should I exercise?

■ No matter how hard you work, your system will not benefit much if you do not sustain the activity for at least 20 minutes — it takes at least that long for your body to respond by working more efficiently rather than just by depleting energy supplies. If you are very unfit you may only be able to sustain an exercise program for 15 minutes at first, but you may work up to as much as 60 minutes of strenuous exercise.

Duration is related to intensity. If you are happier doing a low-intensity exercise you will need to sustain it over a longer period than for a high intensity one to attain the same results. But improvements in aerobic capacity come more readily with longer duration programs whatever the intensity.

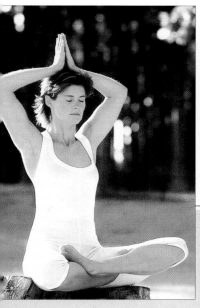

▲ **Yoga** is often practiced purely as a system of exercises to increase flexibility and improve body tone. Stretching into and holding a posture for several minutes will not necessarily improve your strength or contribute to your cardiovascular fitness. However, combined with other activities, yoga can make an enormous difference to your coordination, agility and posture. Most people also find that it induces feelings of relaxation and well-being.

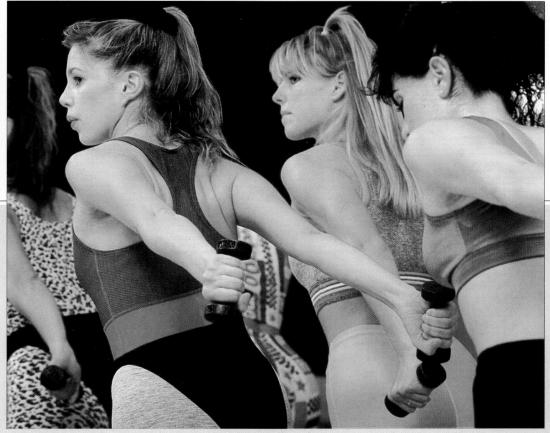

▲ **Working out with weights** is becoming increasingly popular with women. Exercises using low weights and high repetitions can shape and tone specific areas like flabby upper arms that can rarely be improved through dieting. Since women have around thirty percent less upper-body muscle than men, and rarely want to train with such heavy weights, this "tricep kick-back" exercise will never result in bulging shoulder muscles.

before and after exercise, which are very difficult to assess objectively. However, several studies do seem to show fairly conclusively that regular aerobic exercise has the effect of improving mood and diminishing feelings of anxiety and depression.

Duke University Medical Center in the United States recently ran a study of people undergoing a 10-week program of walking and jogging, balanced by a control group of people maintaining their usual sedentary habits. Both groups completed a range of psychological tests, which included the State-Trait Anxiety Inventory (STAI), so called because it is designed to measure both current mood states (how you feel now) and general traits of personality (how you feel most of the time). Test scores revealed that the group taking exercise improved significantly in both their general and specific moods and were less prone to be anxious and depressed. The scores for the comparison group not taking exercise remained the same and in some cases actually got worse.

Responding better to stress

Exercise also seems able to reduce any harmful physical responses to mental stress. A controlled study to test the effects of exercise on a group of people classified as "Type A" personalities (see *Ch 4*) was held at Duke University Medical Center. Type A people are hard-driving, competitive and aggressive. They are also more prone to heart attacks. The 36 people involved were assigned to one of two 12-week exercise programs. The first program was a series of standard aerobic warm-up exercises followed by walking or jogging and cool-down movements, lasting 55 minutes in all, performed three to four times a week. The other group

The psychological benefits

■ Studies have shown that regular exercise increases:
  academic performance
  mental agility
  self-control
  emotional stability
  independence
  coordination
  sexual satisfaction
  energy levels
  work efficiency
  sense of well-being
■ It decreases:
  absenteeism
  alcoholism
  anxiety
  depression
  dysmenorrhea (period pains)
  phobias
  psychotic behavior
  tension
  work errors
  a general sense of being
    unwell

90

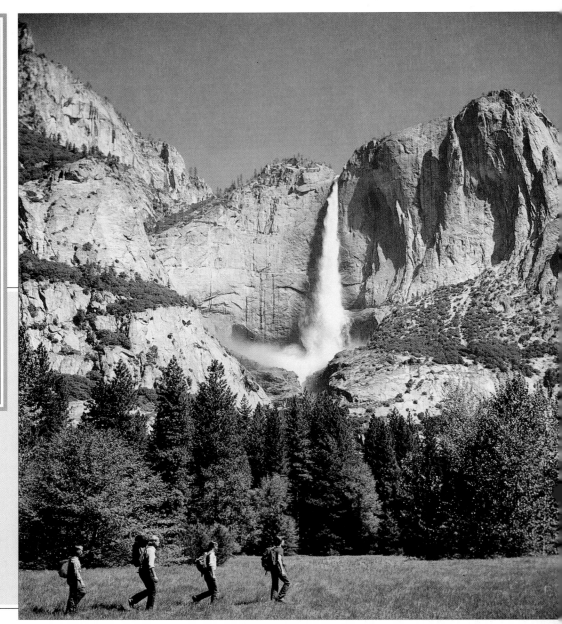

▶ **The wilderness experience** *is highly sought after by stressed city dwellers, particularly in the United States. The combination of physical exertion, fresh air, beautiful scenery and running water can have a profound effect on the mind and body. Many people seek insight or solace through a walking holiday in one of the world's more exotic destinations.*

was assigned a nonaerobic pattern of warm-up exercises, training on a circuit of exercise machines and cool-down exercises lasting 70 minutes and done two to three times a week.

Both before and after the exercise program the participants were tested for cholesterol level, blood pressure, heart and lung fitness and Type A behavior. In addition, a two-hour mental stress test was administered. Heart rate and blood pressure were monitored and a blood exfusion pump slowly withdrew blood to assess stress hormone levels while the participants completed a series of mental arithmetic problems.

The results were striking. Although both forms of exercise were beneficial, the aerobic exercisers produced a different and better pattern of results. Not surprisingly, they showed a greater aerobic capacity (averaging a 15 percent improvement), but also experienced an increase in HDL ("good") cholesterol. Both groups showed a significant reduction in Type A characteristics: they were less likely to interrupt and were judged to be less hostile and aggressive during their tests and interviews.

The results of the mental-stress test produced a unique and potentially important set of findings. The aerobic exercisers showed a significant reduction of heart-rate and blood-pressure responses to mental stress, much greater than that shown by the anaerobic exercisers. They also recovered more promptly from stress. Aerobic exercise appears not only to make people feel better, but to reduce the physical and mental agitation produced by stress.

Guidelines for exercising

Developing a safe, effective, health-enhancing exercise program that suits you means looking at a number of factors. Age, current health status, personal interests, personality type, finances, the climate you live in and the availability of exercise facilities all need to be taken into account. What are you hoping to achieve by exercise? Are you looking for overall fitness, weight reduction, improvement of a specific body part or simply relaxation? You will have to consider all these things in order to devise a program that you will enjoy, that you can stick to and that will do you good.

Most physicians agree that people over 35 should have a complete checkup before starting a vigorous exercise program. Exercise stress testing is often done on people who are already at risk from heart disease. Talk to your doctor about your plans, especially if you are very inactive, overweight or elderly. You may need to start off slowly, but even the most frail or unfit person can develop some sort of useful regular exercise plan. **MW-R JAB**

Physical benefits of regular exercise

■ Studies have shown that regular aerobic exercise increases:
    the efficiency of the cardiovascular system
    aerobic capacity (the efficiency with which the body uses oxygen)
    muscle mass
    HDL cholesterol ("good" cholesterol that helps to clear fats from the blood stream)

■ Regular aerobic exercise decreases:
    LDL cholesterol ("bad" cholesterol that carries fats into the blood stream)
    body-fat
    blood pressure
    heart rate
    the risk of heart disease

■ Regular anaerobic exercise increases:
    strength
    flexibility
    muscle and bone mass

■ Regular anaerobic exercise decreases:
    joint stiffness
    body-fat
    the risk of osteoporosis (brittle bone disease)

Tennis player Arthur Ashe, despite his extreme fitness, had a massive heart attack. Fitness in this case did not prevent heart disease but did reduce its impact. Ashe's doctors claimed his heart attack would have killed an ordinary man, but Ashe survived and recovered rapidly.

The guru of jogging, Jim Fixx, died of a major heart attack at a relatively young age, but he came from a family with a dismal history of serious heart disease and had already suffered a heart attack as a young man. His doctors calculated that his jogging may have increased his natural lifespan by as much as 15 years.

How often should I exercise?

■ Exercise should be undertaken at least three times a week and not more than five times for maximum benefit. If you exercise less than three times a week you will lose in the periods of inactivity whatever benefits you gain from the periods of activity.

The body does need to rest from the strain of exercise, and it is best to give yourself a break; otherwise wear and tear on the muscles and injuries such as stress fractures or shin splints will undo most of the good work. Most people work up to exercising every other day.

How quickly should I improve?

■ As you become more fit, what was a tough workout will become easy. To improve and maintain your body you will probably want to increase the length, repetition and frequency of your exercise, up to 45 minutes to an hour in length and as much as five times a week.

Anaerobic exercises that you once did 10 times you may increase to 20 or 25. In exercise involving weights you can increase the repetitions (for endurance and muscle tone) or increase the weight (for muscle strength and bulk); in time you may do both. It is important not to increase duration, repetition and frequency too rapidly.

If you do too much too soon you may injure or overtire yourself — or even bring on the heart attack you are trying to avoid. Exercising every day is not recommended, as your muscles and joints need time to recover from the strain you have put on them.

91

12

Making Exercise Part of Your Life

Is your spirit willing but your flesh weak when it comes to exercise? ● *It can be a worthwhile exercise in itself to think consciously about what would make you start and keep up a get-fit program* ● *It may save your life.*

MANY PEOPLE find it quite easy to plan out an exercise program. Actually getting started, however, and sticking to it, are other matters. Motivation is essential for both beginning and maintaining an exercise program. You must feel that the activity is worthwhile, and that it is within your capabilities. If you know that your lifestyle is unhealthy and could be improved by exercise, it is worth asking yourself why this knowledge has not resulted in action.

Having the motivation to change

There are four stages in making an exercise routine a part of your life. First is the process of thinking about the need to exercise. From this there may arise, second, the motivation. Third, is the act of starting an exercise program, and, fourth, the task of maintaining it.

When you experience problems with any particular stage, the source of the difficulty can often be traced to the previous step. If you do not feel sufficiently motivated, your reasons for starting may be poorly defined; or if you are having problems maintaining your program, it may be that the plan you initiated was too strenuous or not enjoyable enough to sustain your motivation.

If you have thought vaguely about exercising but have never actually begun, think about specific reasons for undertaking a regular workout strategy. Are you at risk from

Too late to start?

■ John is a 47-year-old business executive. Both his parents suffer from heart disease. When he decided to start an exercise program he weighed 88kg (194lb). A checkup revealed that his cholesterol level was higher than was desirable, as was his blood pressure (140/85). On a treadmill test, John was able to exercise for six minutes at a heart rate of 175 beats per minute (as high as it was safe for him to go). The following recommendations were made:

Type of exercise: walking and jogging.
Intensity: to maintain 138-144 heartbeats per minute.
Duration: 35 minutes.
Frequency: three times a week.

After 16 weeks on this program, John had a second checkup. His weight had dropped to 83kg (182lb). His cholesterol level had dropped and his percentage of HDL cholesterol was better. His blood pressure was now 135/80. During a treadmill test he exercised for 8.5 minutes at a heart rate of 175 beats per minute, and his aerobic capacity (his oxygen uptake) had increased by 15 percent.

These improvements are not unusual. They show a significant improvement in overall health and a reduced risk of heart disease.

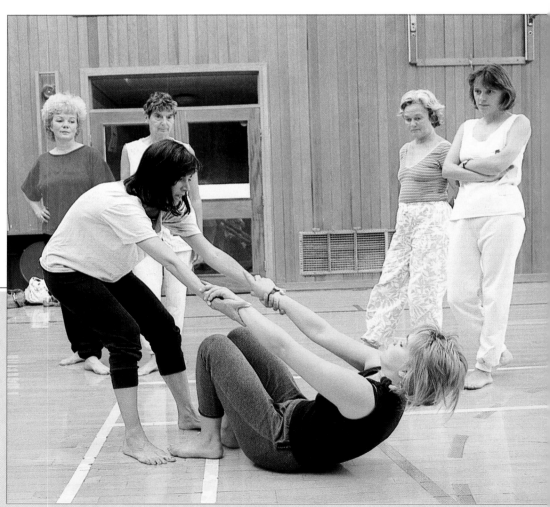

▲ **Make an investment**. *Many people find that making a cash commitment by joining a health club, or signing up for dance classes, especially one like this aimed at beginners, encourages them to start and continue a program. Buying exercise equipment can also help to keep your motivation alive. It does not involve the added social investment that joining a club or class does, however, and equipment may simply accumulate in a corner of the basement.*

heart disease? Do you get winded easily if you run up a flight of stairs? Do you want to improve your cardiovascular fitness? Do you need to lose weight? Do you want to increase your energy level?

Even if you are already exercising, you will find that the things which motivate you change over time. They should be reassessed periodically in order to maintain a commitment to exercise.

Choosing your activity

You will probably want to develop an exercise plan that involves aerobic exercise (for cardiovascular fitness), anaerobic exercise (for strength) and stretching (for flexibility). It should also be of an intensity, duration and frequency that will result in the improvements in your health that you hope to see, fits your schedule and is best for you

(see *Ch 11*). Given these considerations, you will find that there is a wide range of activities available and it is a matter of finding one that you enjoy and can stick to. If you hate getting wet and choose swimming as an exercise because it is convenient, you will not keep to your exercise program for very long.

Is there any activity that you enjoyed as a child and would like to go back to? Perhaps you loved ballet classes and would benefit from jazz dancing or other dance activities. Are you happiest in a social situation? Joining a gym, exercise class or jogging club might be helpful. Do you crave time for yourself?

Cyclers, joggers and swimmers often find their exercise gives them plenty of time to relax and unwind by themselves. All of these activities are examples of aerobic exercise adapted to the needs of individuals.

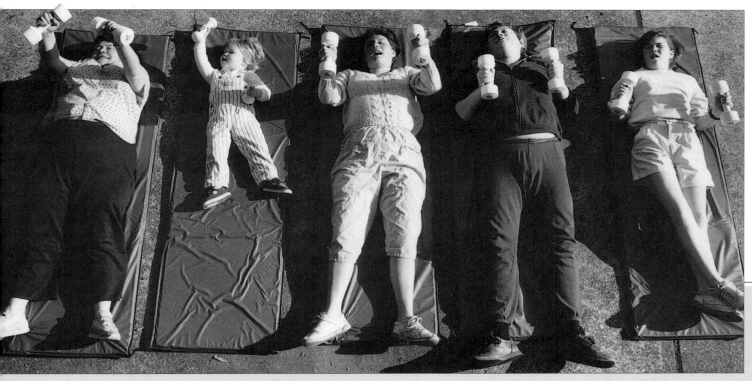

▲ **Every bit of exercise helps**, *but can a family sustain for long a program like this? The health benefits of exercise may be enough motivation to get you started, but eventually you need to make the transition to exercising for pleasure. Choosing an activity you enjoy and that fits into your lifestyle makes for a lifetime of exercise motivation. Children below the age of 12 should not lift weights.*

"No pain, no gain?"

■ Exercise should not be an activity that causes you real discomfort. The popular catch phrases "No pain, no gain" and "Go for the burn" are part of an exercise myth that health professionals think is unnecessary and dangerous. Exercising at a comfortable level of intensity is less likely to damage the body

(joints being particularly vulnerable to overstressing) and is just as effective.

You do have to push your body a little to work hard, and if you have been very inactive you might find it difficult to judge the difference between useful stretching of your body's resources and the warning

signs of pain. You can test for this by keeping track of your heart rate and making sure you are staying within your training range, or by using the "Rating of Perceived Exertion" chart (see *Ch 11*). If you exercise regularly you will soon get to know the difference between pain and healthy exertion.

Whatever program you choose, exercise is hard work. Many beginners discourage themselves with an over-ambitious program that never really allows them to get started. It takes a little time to feel the benefits of exercise, and if you push yourself too hard you will never keep up a regular pace. Learn to determine your optimum heart rate and find out how to take your pulse, and use this as a measure of how hard to exercise (see *Ch11*). You will get more health benefits and will be less likely to injure yourself if you choose activities and intensities appropriate to you as an individual.

Once your exercise plan is in full swing, it is not too soon to begin thinking about how to keep it going. Exercise has to be maintained in order for its benefits to be realized. Unfortunately, most exercisers do not think about this until it is too late, after they have begun to backslide on their exercise commitments. Most people who begin a program of activities drop out within the first few weeks.

The exercise dropout

Research into common patterns of exercise has paid considerable attention to the problems and characteristics of the typical exercise dropout. By identifying the factors that contribute to dropping out, strategies can be developed beforehand to counter or minimize the risks. Several important elements have been associated with the risk of dropping out. Poor motivation is a primary factor. Lack of support from the spouse or family, or no social support during or after exercise, puts off many people from continuing.

Any vigorous or overambitious activity is also likely to deter beginners. The program may be too strenuous for them, but even if it is suitable, the dropout rate from high-intensity programs is always higher than that from low-intensity ones. It is always better to start slowly. Small

inconveniences or a choice of exercise that is not enjoyable for the individual involved may also contribute to poor maintenance of an exercise program.

Lapse, relapse and collapse

Any single lapse can snowball into total collapse of a program designed to change your behavior in the long run. The person's interpretation of and reaction to this episode

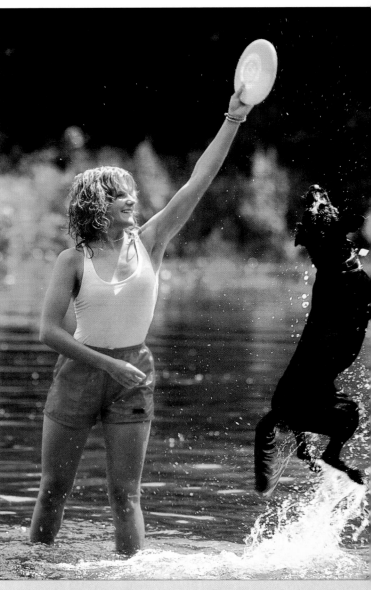

▲ **Owning a pet that needs exercise** *can be good for your health. Your dog will insist on a routine that benefits both of you. Having a friend who needs an exercise partner can be just as good. A partner can make exercise more enjoyable by giving it a social element. You* *should be able to talk comfortably without becoming breathless; if you cannot talk, you are pushing yourself too hard.*

94

Exercising through the seasons

■ Many people start exercising enthusiastically in spring, but become discouraged by the unpleasantness of exercising in very hot or very cold weather. Dressing to suit the elements and choosing the right time of day can go a long way toward minimizing discomfort and maximizing adherence to a program. Avoid really extreme temperatures and exercise indoors on these days.

In hot weather, decrease your exercise intensity and duration as your system is already under some strain. Drink lots of fluid, ideally two cups 20 minutes before exercising and half a cup every 15 minutes during a

workout. Avoid caffeine as this causes dehydration. Wear light-colored, lightweight, loose clothing and try to exercise in the early morning or the evening when the temperature is lowest.

In cold weather, try to exercise at noon, when the day is warmest. Dress in warm, loose layers. The layer next to your skin should still be cotton to absorb perspiration quickly. Include progressively heavier materials and one layer resistant to wind and rain. Remember to wear gloves and warm socks, as body extremities lose heat rapidly; 80 percent of body heat is lost through the head – be sure to wear a hat.

will determine whether a relapse occurs or is prevented. This rule of thumb, known as the relapse prevention model, has been applied to exercise by many health professionals and researchers. The key terms are lapse, relapse and collapse.

A lapse is a single slip in carrying out an exercise program. Perhaps a session is cut short, or skipped altogether. Relapse is a string of several such slips. Maybe a week of exercise is missed, or only four sessions in the course of a month.

In a state of relapse, the person is repeatedly falling short of exercise goals – falling back into their sedentary, pre-exercise-program state. Collapse is the total abandonment of an exercise plan. This entire process, from lapse to collapse, can occur in only four days.

Preventing a relapse

Even though the average dropout rate is high, there are many steps you can take to prevent a relapse. The first rule is easy: be aware. Keep a record of your exercise plans and achievements so that you can see easily if you are falling behind. Exercise needs to become a habit, but until it does you need to remind yourself of the importance of doing it regularly. This can be done by means of a graph or diary; you can even write your exercise sessions in your appointment book and tick them off. The act of recording itself makes you feel more accountable, and a record of improvements – say, a daily graph of time or distance or weights or heart rate – can encourage and reinforce exercise motivation.

Identify risk situations, times and places. If you have a lapse in exercising, when does it tend to occur, and why? Do you falter in your resolve when you are on vacation, or when it is cold and wet? Do you tend to forget your workout gear? Do you go out to lunch instead of the gym? Change your exercise times or develop alternative strategies to prevent further lapses. If you normally jog but hate to go out when it is cold, choose another activity that you can do indoors on cold days. Keep an extra set of exercise clothing at work or join a gym that provides them. Stop trying to exercise at lunchtime – schedule it for another part of the day – or arrange to go out to lunch after your exercise session.

Keeping on your toes

Perhaps your exercise prescription needs to be re-examined. It may be too difficult, or perhaps you are getting bored and need to step up the pace. Or it may be that the exercise you have chosen is simply not that much fun for you. Experiment with different types of activity, slow down your pace, or try a more difficult stage of exercise. Use your heart rate as a guide and stay within your training range to assess the level of challenge your program is giving you.

Above all, do not despair. Just as eating one piece of cake is not the end of a sensible diet, one slip or even a series of slips is not the end of an exercise program. **SLP JAB**

95

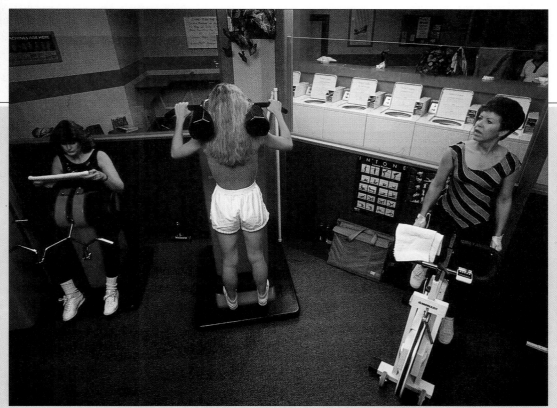

◄ **Finding the time**. *Your own neighborhood laundromat may not double as a gym, but there are probably other opportunities in your life to double your value for time spent. You can do other things you have to or want to do while still fitting in about three half-hour exercise sessions each week. If you pay a little more for a quiet rowing or cycling machine, for example, you can use it without drowning out your favorite radio or television program.*

13

Are Sports Good For You?

Sport may help you get fit, but it is not necessarily good for your health ● *Injury and physical strain are often the results of overenthusiasm* ● *Handling competition and aggression may prove to be more difficult than you think.*

SPORTS should be as beneficial to health as any exercise activity. We tend to think of top athletes as people in the peak of physical condition. But sports are not automatically good for either psychological or physical health. Understanding the ways that sports can help or impair well-being is the first step to a healthy sporting life. To promote health effectively, sports should be organized so that they are available to people of all levels of competence and fitness, and should be both enjoyable and rewarding.

Why are sports different from exercise?

Although many aspects of sports are very similar to exercise, there is one extremely important difference. When you are playing sports, your performance is rated or scored and there are winners and losers. Unlike exercise, competition with others is a central element and the main goal is not physical benefit but winning. There are forms of exercise that can be treated competitively, but instructors of exercise tend to discourage this and urge exercisers to challenge only their own achievements. The effect of competition on your overall health can be either positive or negative depending very much on how it is handled and on how well the competitors are matched.

Sports do require physical effort, but this is not the point of the activity, and many games do not even require the participants to be physically fit. Stop/start activities such as squash, fencing and tennis call for short bursts of energy that do not fully condition the players aerobically. On the other hand, sports demanding high levels of strength like weightlifting and wrestling may not involve enough continuous endurance to provide a full aerobic workout. In fact, most athletes gain any physical or medical benefits more from training than from the game itself.

If you want your health to benefit from sports, you should take these factors into account by choosing an activity that will help you to become fit in training and playing. You should also think carefully about the competitive aspect of the game you have chosen. Will you enjoy it, or will you find

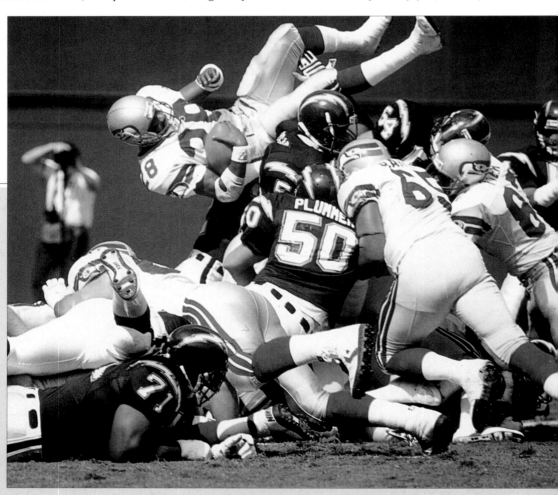

▶ **Joining in the rough and tumble** *will not always leave players in the peak of condition. Sports involving high levels of risk and physical contact will inevitably lead to injury sooner or later. High-contact sports are really only suitable for young adults who are already very fit. Even for them, the risk of injury poses a serious threat and should be a major consideration if you want to take up a sport chiefly for health reasons. Professional players of high-contact sports like football and rugby may, in fact, be quite unfit (even overweight) despite being highly skilled.*

it stressful and depressing? Sports vary considerably in their physical and competitive elements, and you have to find the one that is right for you.

Choosing to suit your needs

People who choose sports as part of their physical fitness plan usually want to feel that they are having fun, not just working out. The right sport for anyone is one that is enjoyable and rewarding for the person concerned. If you do not get substantial personal gratification, your involvement will diminish to nothing in a short period of time. If your health is to benefit, the sport you choose must involve activities that you enjoy.

Sports vary in the rewards they have to offer to participants, but effective rewards are the ones that sustain your interest and participation over time. If you find that you are lapsing in your training, review what it is that you enjoy about the sport and what it is that you do not like. Then look for a compromise that includes more of the enjoyable elements and fewer of those you dislike. If you respond quickly to social interactions and support, these are greater during play in a team sport such as volleyball than in a one-on-one sport such as tennis.

Access for all

The competitive nature of sports can encourage feelings of inadequacy and failure even in purely amateur players. There is no reason, however, why the most unskilled and unpracticed people cannot learn and develop in competition with people at their own level of ability. Many poor golfers and tennis players get enormous rewards from their sport and even enjoy competition as long as they play with people of a similar ability.

Sports need not be expensive, either; there is a sport available for every income as well as every level of skill. The popularity of basketball and soccer in inner-city areas is no accident. Little equipment is needed, you can improvise within the space available, and a player can even practice certain parts of the game alone. By contrast, the organizational demands of a marathon or fun-run are great and need some committee work. Golf and skiing equipment costs a great deal and restricted or expensive access to facilities place these sports beyond the reach of many people. They also require an investment of time, and you may prefer to choose a sport like racquetball, for example, in which you can play a competitive (and physically beneficial) game in less than an hour.

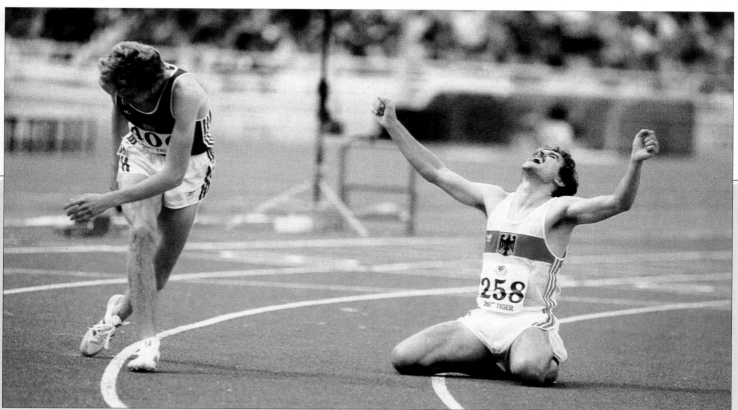

▲ Pushing yourself to the limit in front of an audience often gives athletes a surge of adrenaline allowing them to produce record-breaking performances. When so much motivation and personal ambition hangs in the balance winning produces a feeling of pure elation, and losing is all the more bitter. Successful performance in directly competitive sports includes learning how to deal successfully with losing as well as winning.

Am I too old?

Your age and the possibility of long-term participation are also important factors in choosing the right sport. Games requiring speed, balance, power and coordination favor the young. Cardiovascular endurance, muscle strength and flexibility can be maintained by anyone regardless of age, and sports that focus on them, such as cycling, will provide health benefits throughout a lifetime. Football and basketball may be less attractive to the older person.

The range of ages thought appropriate for any given sport is often based on factors unrelated to health and more strongly related to concepts of aging. Fortunately such barriers are beginning to fall, and men and women now run marathons into their eighties, because this sport focuses on abilities that last. Sports can be fun and good for you at any age, as long as you find the right one.

Children do not have to be sports stars

■ Children are easily made to feel that they have no role in sports. It can take years to learn to ignore this message and participate with enjoyment.

Coaching techniques emphasizing rewards for the best and punishment for a poor performance are particularly damaging. Parental pressure to win can also be counterproductive. It may even drive a child out of sports altogether.

Studies confirm that children who most enjoy playing sports experience little of this sense of pressure. Children nevertheless derive a good deal of their satisfaction from the attention and support of parents. If sports participation and achievement is ignored, they can feel uncared-for, just as when parents ignore other aspects of their lives.

■ **The price of success.** Children who do aspire to high levels of competition however, may develop problems if their parents and coaches do not raise them with care. The American researcher B J Brandemeir and her colleagues have shown that children who are involved in high-contact sports may have less well-developed moral reasoning and can justify intentional acts of violence in competition.

Such children may also suffer physically through stress on developing limbs and joints or through effects on the endocrine system that can delay puberty and menstruation.

Children involved in top-level sports may find almost all of their waking hours devoted to practice, travel and competition, isolating them from the normal social and educational experiences that will equip them for adulthood. This is especially tragic when a retiring athlete's self-image is tied up in the performance of sports skills that he or she can no longer perform well, and has no other avenue of gaining self-fulfillment and respect.

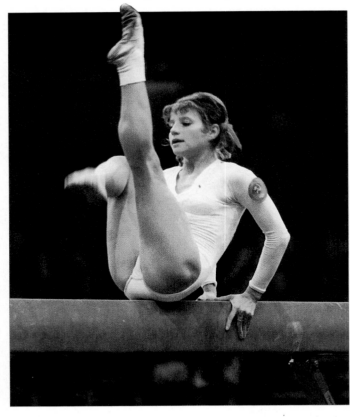

▲ **World-class gymnasts,** *displaying extraordinary stamina and flexibility, can reach their peak in their early teens or before. The physical consequences of this level of training may be crippling, even before the emotional toll can be reckoned.*

▶ **Are sports "character building" for children?** *Many parents think so. Aggressive group sports are often thought to combine physical exercise with risk, excitement and learning about teamwork. Children who perform badly can feel very inferior.*

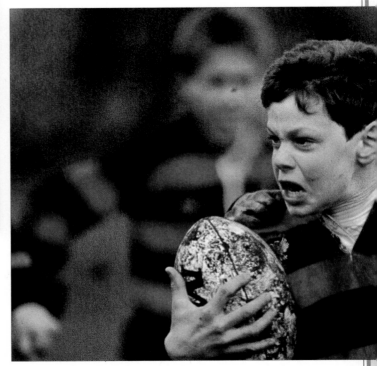

Making sure sports are good for you

Preparation for sports has two components: being physically fit enough to participate and having the basic skills and knowledge of the sport. Physical fitness is the result of exercise and diet, and it provides the basic physical capability to carry out the skills of the sport. But achieving a high level of physical fitness before you start to participate in a sport is often overemphasized. Enjoying a sport at a level of low physical demand can provide immediate rewards that will be the basis of motivation for becoming more physically fit in order to enjoy the sport at a higher level of involvement. Setting high initial fitness standards can stop many people from even considering taking up a new sport.

Some sports do demand high initial fitness, especially those with a high injury level, such as skiing, or those involving spurts of intense activity, such as squash and racquetball. People at risk from cardiac disease sometimes take up these sports to improve their health, push themselves too hard too soon, and can end up having a heart attack on court. If you take up this sort of activity you will need to maintain your fitness between games. Serious injury and illness usually occur in those who try to play a fast, hard game after a long interval with no regular exercise.

Combining exercise and sport

All sports enjoyment can be improved by proper training. Most team games have formal training sessions to improve general fitness and promote expertise in certain areas. Training can be as much fun as actually playing the game, and the increase in skills it brings will also raise your level of play and probably encourage you to be more energetic. If your sport involves no formal training, however, it might be a good idea to combine it with other forms of exercise that will benefit your playing or make up for the fitness gaps in your sport.

For example, marathon runners might not be getting enough anaerobic exercise to maintain their strength and flexibility, which are useful to long-distance running but which marathons themselves do not actually promote. Shot putters, javelin throwers and jumpers might be strong and flexible, yet have poor cardiovascular fitness. They might want to take up running, swimming or cycling to increase their aerobic capacity; this will ultimately improve their performance as well. If you want to take up more than one sport, think about combining an aerobic and an anaerobic one to provide yourself with the greatest physical benefits.

Keeping up the momentum

Just like exercise, if a sport is to do you any good you need to do it frequently – probably at least three times a week. The more you play, the better you will get. If yours is

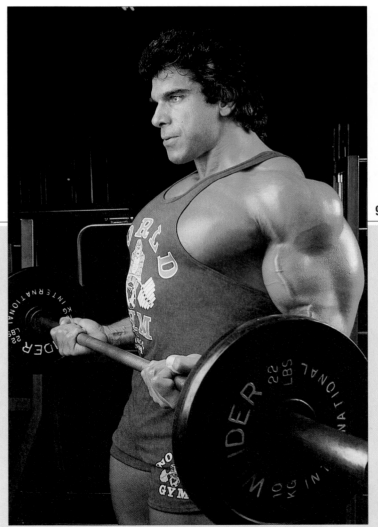

99

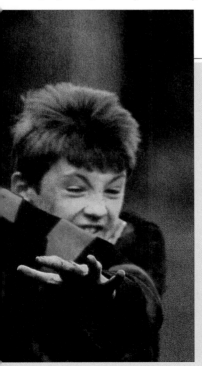

▶ **Professional bodybuilders** *often use extreme measures to achieve competition results which are not, in fact, good for their health. This exercise, known as a barbell curl, is specifically intended to develop well-rounded biceps. Pumping iron to build muscle can be exhilarating, but it is too often done to the total neglect of cardiovascular fitness. Competitors fear that running or cycling will burn off the pounds that they have carefully acquired. As contests draw near competitors follow a diet very low in fat, and may even dehydrate themselves so that their skin becomes paper-thin, showing their muscle definition to its maximum advantage.*

a team sport that is only played once a week, try to attend training sessions several times during the week and avoid missing them carelessly. If you are not playing very frequently and are missing games, re-evaluate your motivation. Is the sport not as enjoyable as you thought at first? Perhaps you need a change of activity to something that suits you better. It may be that the sport does not fit your timetable very well. Or it may be that your skills and physical fitness have improved to such an extent that you are bored with the level of play that was once exciting and challenging.

Fortunately, it is possible to change the level of challenge or difficulty as your abilities change. Look for partners or teams that match your level, and do not be afraid to try new things – it will benefit everybody to play with people at their own level. Play more frequently, for longer periods of time and with greater intensity. Use your heart rate to measure your needs. If you are not playing at 70-85 percent of your maximum heart rate at the height of the game, it is not doing you much good and you need to increase your level of play. Raise your ambitions to match your skills and you will continue to get the most out of your sport.

Coping with injury

Most people who play sports suffer from the occasional injury. Usually it is quite minor but the effects can be minimized by using proper equipment and care. Serious injuries include damage to limbs and joints, and also to the head

Psychological benefits of sports

■ A study based on interviews with a group of figure skaters showed that they could divide the rewards of their sport into four major categories:
● better interpersonal relationships – including closer bonds with friends and family
● feelings of competence – including the satisfaction of performing well and the joy of winning
● social recognition – including attention from others for doing well
● the actual performance of the sport – including enjoyment of the physical action and of the sense of exuberance and well-being this aroused.

All of these rewards are available to participants in any sport, regardless of skill level.

Participation teaches social skills

■ Sports throw participants into difficult situations that test goodwill, tact and stamina. Typical situations include not giving up when things are going badly, handling negative as well as positive outcomes gracefully, effectively directing others, accepting criticism and direction positively and coping with the stress of competition.

In team sports, participants learn to work as part of a group, taking responsibility for their actions and providing support and assistance to others. In one-to-one sports they learn courtesy and fairness.

Your experience with sports may not always be positive. Negative coaching can communicate feelings of incompetence and failure, and your own unrealistically high standards can make you feel discouraged and upset. In the heat of the moment you may not always behave in socially acceptable ways, and some sports figures will even use tantrums to boost their own adrenaline levels and distress other players. Such tactics are a sign of poor social skills and may be an attempt to mask the insecurity of the player.

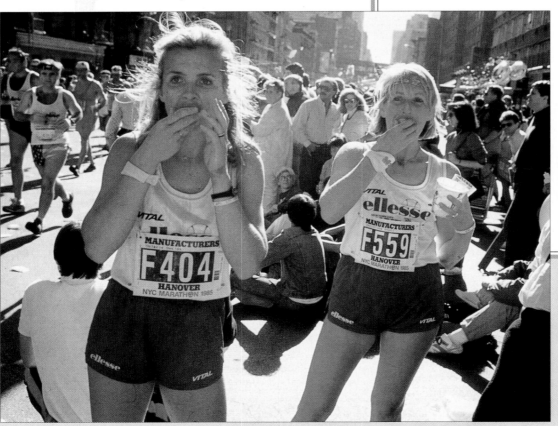

◄ **Sport is for everyone.** *The maxim that it is not winning that is important but "how you played the game" is particularly relevant to marathons where participation is all. The success of this event is measured in the range of participants, representing every degree of attractiveness, overweight and aerobic fitness.*

and spinal-cord due to collision and impact. Some sports are more dangerous than others: football, skiing, boxing and motorcycle racing all have a much higher level of injury than do golfing and tennis.

Injured players, particularly in team games, are not always treated well. They may be encouraged to continue in spite of pain, and they are often isolated and made to feel weak if they stop to receive medical treatment. Pain is a warning and without treatment the result can be a more serious or even permanent physical injury.

Researchers have long wondered if one personality type is more likely to experience injury than others, but have found no evidence for this. What has been discovered, however, is that people are more likely to be injured if they lack social support and the skills needed to deal with change and stressful life events. Competitors who have

close friends and family and who have learned to handle stressors are less likely to be injured, and a friendly environment in which coaches and players are supportive of each other can prevent or minimize injury.

Striking the balance

Sports can be enormously enjoyable, physically beneficial and psychologically helpful as long as the balance is right. Picking the game that fits your individual abilities, age, free time, finances and interests is crucial. Enjoying sport as part of an all-round physical health strategy can make staying fit easier and more pleasurable. If we maintain the right attitude and do not become bogged down in the pursuit of winning, sports can relieve many of the stresses and strains of our lives and teach us valuable lessons about getting along with others. **M G**

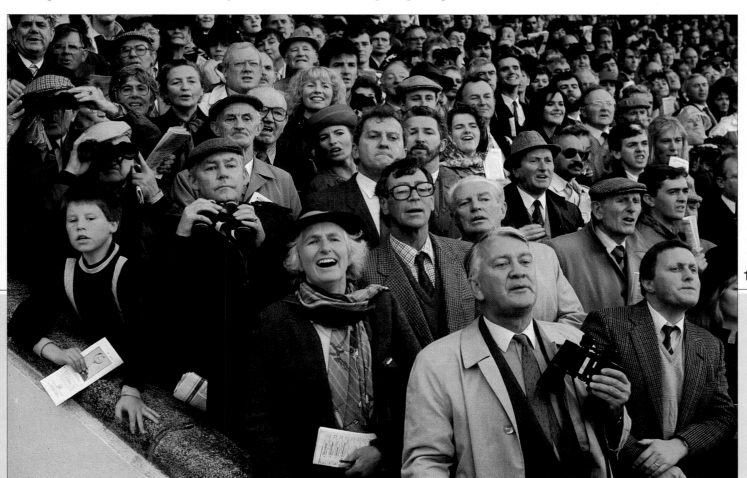

▲ **Spectators are the most numerous participants** *in major sporting events. Many of them simply enjoy the sights and sounds of a day out; others feel the "second-hand" thrill of exertion and competition. Of course, watching others will not*

improve your level of fitness. Spectator sports can still be good for your personal well-being simply because they involve social activity and may provide you with the motivation to make new friends and take up new interests. Particularly

when play becomes aggressive, spectators can sometimes present a serious danger to themselves and to players or officials if they become too involved in the conflict or the outcome of the game. Often team games invite enormous

loyalty from followers who become overdependent on the result for their own sense of confidence and self-worth. These race-goers in Dublin, Ireland, however, look tranquil at the moment.

101

14

Smoking

Avoiding tobacco smoke is one of the best preventive health measures you can take
● *Quitting is not easy, but the rewards include many that are immediate and others that can save your life in the long term.*

CIGARETTE SMOKING is the single most important preventable cause of death in almost every developed country. In the United States, more than one in every six deaths can be attributed to it. In addition, millions of people who have not yet died from the effects of smoking suffer poor health because of them. Included among these statistics are thousands of nonsmokers who have inhaled air contaminated by smoking parents, friends, marriage partners and fellow workers.

For the last three decades, there have been vigorous anti-smoking campaigns – and one smoker in three has quit. Nevertheless, 25-30 percent of adults still smoke and more and more teenagers are experimenting with cigarettes; of these, about 80 percent will become addicts in adulthood. Information about why and how to avoid starting – and, if addicted, why and how to quit – is as important as it was 30 years ago. There is also much more of it.

How dangerous is smoking?

More than 90 percent of all deaths from lung cancer (representing 30 percent of all deaths from any form of cancer) are due to smoking or to breathing other people's smoke. Lung cancer usually starts in cells of the bronchi, the main air-passage tubes into the lungs, when tars carried in cigarette smoke interfere with the cells' genetic systems for controlling cell division. Cells divide out of control and a

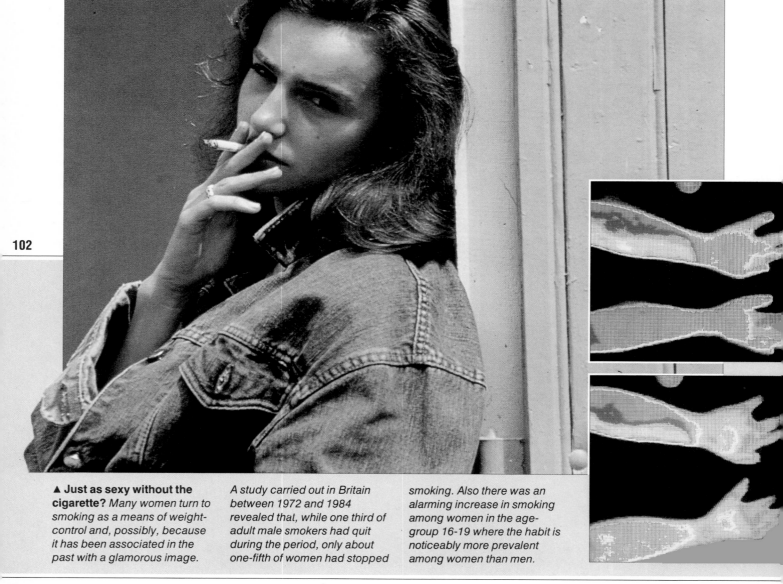

▲ **Just as sexy without the cigarette?** *Many women turn to smoking as a means of weight-control and, possibly, because it has been associated in the past with a glamorous image.*

A study carried out in Britain between 1972 and 1984 revealed that, while one third of adult male smokers had quit during the period, only about one-fifth of women had stopped

smoking. Also there was an alarming increase in smoking among women in the age-group 16-19 where the habit is noticeably more prevalent among women than men.

tumor develops. Within one to five years it may spread to the rest of the lungs where cancerous cells are picked up by the bloodstream and carried to other parts of the body to establish secondary tumors in the brain, the liver, bone marrow or the skin.

Smoking (and passively inhaling other people's smoke) causes deaths from heart disease and strokes. By stimulating blood vessels to constrict, the nicotine that the blood picks up in your lungs increases the resistance of your entire arterial system to the pumping action of the heart. This drives up blood pressure, and while pressure is high, arterial walls are susceptible to damage. Fatty deposits form at sites of damage, narrowing the arteries and further contributing to high blood pressure.

Peripheral vascular disease (hampering circulation in the legs and arms) is a risk for long-term smokers. A more serious risk is any narrowing of the arteries of the heart and the brain. When these narrowed arteries are blocked, heart attacks and strokes may result – about 38 percent are attributable to smoking.

Smoker's cough can become chronic bronchitis: damaged linings of the bronchial passages become susceptible to recurrent inflammation. Apart from the constant discomfort of bronchial inflammation and coughing, bronchitis victims are at risk of serious complications. Many bronchitis sufferers become dangerously or fatally ill with pneumonia.

Another risk is emphysema, with chronic shortness of breath. Bronchitis makes you breathe forcefully, subjecting the tiny air sacs in the lungs to above-normal pressure. This weakens their elasticity – they become stretched and less efficient, or they burst and blister. It can lead to respiratory failure, if infections such as pneumonia do not kill the victim first.

In addition, smoking may contribute to cancer of the lips, tongue, salivary glands, floor of the mouth, throat, cervix, larynx and bladder, and probably to cancer of the stomach, pancreas and kidney. All forms of cancer are more likely to occur if you combine smoking with even moderate drinking of alcohol. Smoking a pipe or cigars instead of cigarettes may reduce your risk a little, but is still seriously detrimental to health. Chewing-tobacco irritates the mouth and throat, and can cause mouth cancer. It is also damaging because of the high nicotine intake.

Smoking is also a factor in a number of health problems that are not so directly life-threatening – for example, periodontal (gum) disease. Gastric diseases (including ulcers) are at least partly caused by swallowing the irritants in tobacco smoke. Retardation of fetal growth and development (leading in some cases to miscarriage or stillbirth) is an effect of regularly inhaling tobacco smoke or smoking during pregnancy.

Osteoporosis (brittle bones) can result partly from smoking. The underlying reason may be nothing more than the fact that smokers have less energy and so take less of the exercise that stimulates bone cells to produce osteoid – the material that gives mass and strength to our bones.

Premature aging of the skin is one consequence of the poorer circulation of blood from which smokers suffer.

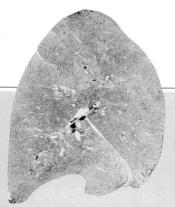

◄ **Smoking affects blood-flow to the hands**. *The top picture shows a pair of warm hands before smoking; the lower picture shows the same hands, now much cooler, after smoking. Within seconds of lighting up, the capillary blood vessels – especially those in the hands and feet – contract, significantly reducing the local blood supply.*

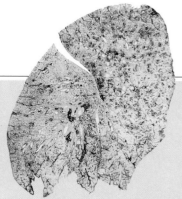

▲ **Smoking affects the lungs**. *TOP LEFT A section of normal healthy lung tissue. TOP RIGHT A section of tissue from the lung of a smoker, showing the distribution of tar deposits. These cause congestion and physical damage, and are likely to trigger lung cancer, a major killer. The most effective prevention is simply not to smoke.*

Getting ready to quit

■ **Focus on the immediate benefits of quitting**. All smokers know that their habit is damaging their health – but heart disease and cancer seem a long way in the future. Why worry, in the short term?

With reasoning like this, you will probably never break the habit. It is helpful to think as well of all the immediate benefits.

● You will breathe more easily and physical exertion will be more enjoyable.
● You will have few chest and throat infections.
● Your hair, breath and clothes will smell better, and people will like being with you more.
● You will be a better role model for your children.
● Your friends and family will breathe cleaner air.

■ **Have faith in yourself**. Do not be discouraged if you have made unsuccessful attempts to quit in the past. Most permanent quitters report that they had a number of failures first.

But such attempts should not be thought of as failures. Every time you give up smoking – even for only a few days or weeks – should be regarded as a partial success.

Believe in your willpower. The fact that you have been able to kick the habit temporarily shows that, the next time, there is a good chance that you will be able to give it up for good. And, if nothing else, quitting for even a few days will contribute something toward your general health.

Why do people go on smoking?

Tobacco contains nicotine, which is a substance as addictive as heroin or cocaine. Stopping nicotine-use leads to withdrawal symptoms including increased irritability, headaches, insomnia, poor concentration, decreased heart rate, gastrointestinal upset and a general feeling of being unwell. These withdrawal symptoms are at their most acute during the first few days or weeks after quitting. The practice of smoking is first and foremost a physical addiction.

Depending on the amount taken, nicotine can act either as a stimulant or as a tranquilizer. Smokers learn, usually unconsciously, to regulate their nicotine-intake levels to obtain these different effects. Nicotine is absorbed rapidly from the lungs, reaching the brain in seconds. One effect of

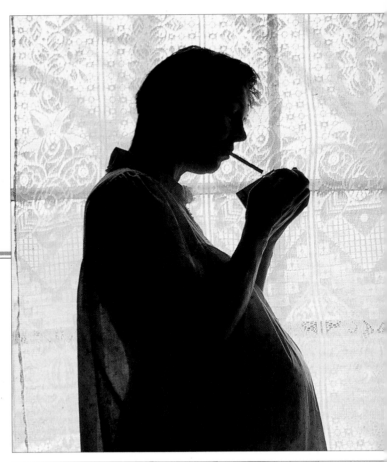

A program of action

■ **Make a commitment**. Set a firm date to quit, and tell all your friends about it. Write down your plans for quitting: this can strengthen your resolution.

At the same time you can build up unpleasurable feelings associated with smoking – try chain-smoking three packets of cigarettes: you will probably feel sick. You can keep around you visual reminders of the more repulsive aspects of smoking – for example, collect all your butts in a big glass jar: whenever you look at it or smell it, you will be reminded of how unpleasant your habit is.

■ **Identify the high-risk situations**. Each time you crave a cigarette, note down the time and the circumstances; soon you should be able to identify high-risk situations. These might include wanting something to help you concentrate when you are working; wanting something to help you relax when you complete a task; wanting to share the ritual of smoking in social situations.

Once you know what those situations are, you can plan how to cope with them using means other than a cigarette.

■ **Easing off nicotine**. To lessen the impact of withdrawal symptoms, try "nicotine fading" – tapering off your daily nicotine intake. Switch to a lower-nicotine brand or reduce the number of cigarettes you smoke each day. It is best to do both: a major drawback to switching to a lower-nicotine brand is that you tend simply to smoke more cigarettes, so that your nicotine intake remains the same.

■ **Getting through the first stages**. The first few days and weeks without cigarettes will be ones of discomfort and temptation. How can these be minimized? Nicotine gum can be used at first to give you your ration of nicotine, plus the pleasant oral sensation of chewing, while your dependence on cigarettes, in particular, is reduced.

You may prefer nicotine-free substitutions for smoking: chewing gum, a raw carrot or anything else that appeals to you.

Tell yourself to relax for a few minutes in times of stress – until your urge to smoke has passed. Avoid high-risk situations. For example, if you have a strong craving for a cigarette after dining out, choose to go to a restaurant with a no-smoking policy. Avoid passive smoking – this often is associated with alcohol too. Instead of going to a smoky bar for a drink after work, do something else. Go for a stroll or a drive, see a movie – anything you find relaxing. Ask your friends not to offer you cigarettes, or let you "borrow" one in a moment of weakness.
● Put all your ashtrays some-

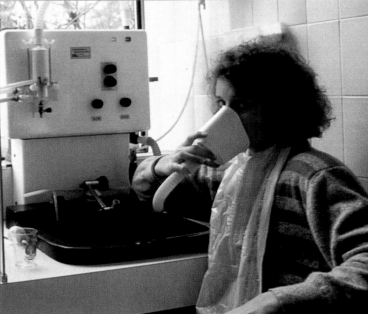

where inconvenient, or even throw them away: often the trouble of having to find an ashtray will give you enough time to change your mind.
● Avoid buying cigarettes yourself.

● Give yourself small treats, or save up some of the money you would have spent on cigarettes, then buy something you really want.
● Be proud of every day you go without a cigarette.

the drug (at least among addicts) is to improve alertness, so that they find it easier to concentrate. Nicotine has some effect as a mood elevator, and can help reduce feelings of stress (smokers use more cigarettes when put under stress). The body develops tolerance to nicotine, so that progressively more of it is required to produce the same effect: today's "moderate" smoker is likely to be the heavy smoker of tomorrow.

How is smoking a habit?

Physically, smoking is an addiction; psychologically, it is a habit and this is another reason why people go on smoking. Social, environmental and emotional factors are responsible for the habit aspect of continued smoking. The association of pleasurable activities with smoking should not be underrated. A person who enjoys smoking while relaxing after work will find that the pleasant feeling evoked by the situation becomes linked to having a cigarette. Similarly, people who have become accustomed to smoking in order to counteract mild stress in one situation – like speaking to a stranger on the telephone – will find that they turn to cigarettes at other times of mild stress.

Some people have personalities or lifestyles that make it much more difficult for them to quit. Someone with a Type A behavior pattern (see *Ch 4*) may, under stress, smoke more heavily and inhale more deeply for a longer time. A person like this will find it hard to stop. Heavy drinkers have more difficulty giving up smoking. **ACK**

◄ **Pregnant women who smoke** *are risking not only their own health: they are endangering the survival of their unborn child. The worst damage smoking can do to human beings is before they are born. Nicotine and carbon monoxide are easily passed on to the fetus. The result can be miscarriage (spontaneous abortion), stunted growth, deformity, mental retardation or stillbirth. Even if only the father smokes, the mother's passive smoking can damage the unborn child.*

◄ **When you want to stop** *it may be an investment to pay for a course of intensive treatment at a health spa. The residential patient LEFT is having a sonic aerosol treatment to clear the sinuses. This institute at Aix-Les-Bains in France offers an anti-stress program including drinking the local waters which are rich in calcium, sodium and sulfur. Patients report that the waters do reduce their desire to smoke.*

► **Making it through the high-risk situations**. *Socializing with friends who smoke will be one of the biggest challenges you will face after quitting. You can keep calm and confident by telling yourself how good it makes you feel to be in control of your urges.*

■ **Quitting for good**. The vast majority of smokers would like to be able to quit. The fact that almost 75 percent of them have made at least one serious attempt shows that most of them can at least sometimes summon the fortitude to tolerate withdrawal symptoms.

Unfortunately, after a few days or weeks of abstinence, when, ironically, withdrawal symptoms are quickly becoming much more tolerable, they start thinking that "one cigarette will not matter," and soon they are smoking as heavily as ever.

For a successful investment of the effort you put into quitting, it is crucial not to become overconfident after your initial victories. Regard yourself as a nicotine addict for life – an addict who happens not to smoke. Over the months and years, the temptation to have that "one cigarette" will decrease, until eventually you may find the very idea revolting.

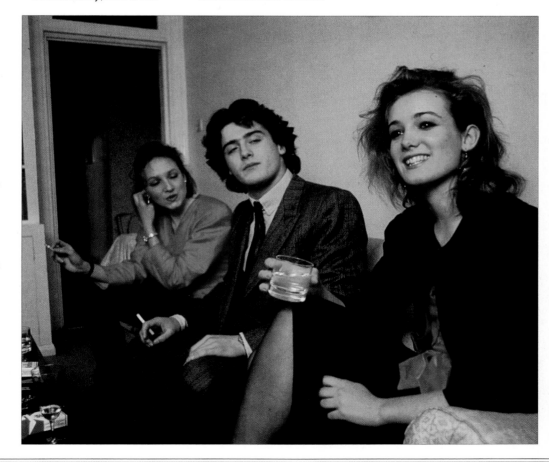

105

15

The Effects of Alcohol

Alcohol may produce a "relaxed" feeling because it is a depressant, but it is physically addictive, and emotionally dependence easily develops ● Wine and beer can be just as harmful as hard liquor ● How much is too much for you?

DRINKING is a major part of any social event; weddings, parties, business meetings, dinner with friends and dates are all occasions for alcohol. We drink because we enjoy the taste, because drinks are for celebrating and because of the pleasant feeling that alcohol gives us. But alcohol is a drug, and drugs can be dangerous if we take them for granted. If we want to combine alcohol with a healthy and moderate lifestyle, we need to understand the physical and psychological effects of drinking.

A depressing substance

Alcohol is a chemical substance that alters body and brain functions. Specifically, alcohol affects mood, because it is a depressant. This may surprise you. Most people think that drinking has a stimulating effect – it makes us feel less inhibited and more daring or enthusiastic. In fact, alcohol slows down our normal responses so that we act on our primary emotional impulses. Someone who is normally rather shy may, under the influence of a drink, become less anxious and self-conscious. But the more we drink, the more deeply the depressant effect of alcohol works. That is why a person who drinks throughout the course of an evening out may go from cheerfulness to ebullience to self-pitying tears to a complete stupor.

In the short term, a few drinks may alleviate sadness or anxiety, but when someone stops drinking their sadness or anxiety rebounds. Removing any mood-changing drug – alcohol or tranquilizers – produces a rebound effect where the nervous system returns to its former state suddenly like a coiled spring snapping back. All the effects masked by the drugs reappear and may seem worse than before. If we want to enjoy alcohol safely, we must remember that the "lift" is temporary and the long-term effect is depression.

The physical effects

The depressant effect of alcohol works on us physically as well as emotionally. Even a small drink slows down reaction times. It also makes us hold our bodies less rigidly.

Spot the danger signs

■ Do you drink alone? Do you *need* a drink to perform a task or to cope with a particular person?

Do you find it extremely hard to be in a social situation unless you have a few drinks? Do you rationalize about your drinking?

Do you pretend – to yourself or to others – that you drink less than you do?

These are signs of a serious drinking problem. You may need help from a professional treatment center or a self-help group such as Alcoholics Anonymous. It is important to overcome not only the physical addiction but psychological dependence as well.

If you come from a family with a history of alcohol or drug abuse, you may want to look for a program or group that specializes in that area. There are also organizations that provide counseling and support for families and friends.

Your doctor may be able to advise you.

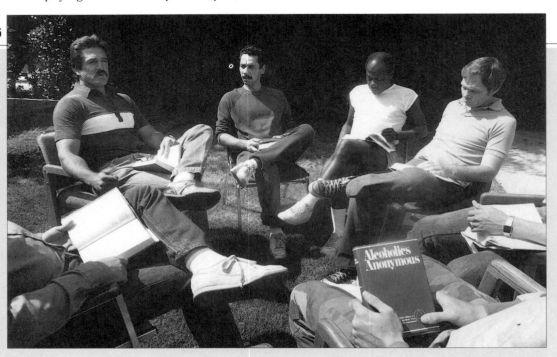

▶ **Which of these party-goers is going to drive home?** *Alcohol interferes with our control over emotional and physical reactions. If you have been drinking, you should not drive.*

◀ **Alcoholics Anonymous** *has the best-known program for sobriety, founded over 50 years ago; many treatment centers incorporate it into their own programs. Alcohol can cause physical addiction and a range of life-threatening illnesses. Psychological addiction, unlike physical addiction, is not related to amounts of alcohol consumed.*

Many people find they can dance better after a drink because of this muscular relaxation – but if you drink too much you will not be able to control your movements at all.

Alcohol can affect your body in many more extensive ways. These can range from the merely inconvenient, such as headaches and sleep disturbance, to the life-threatening, such as heart disease, cancer and brain damage. Some of these effects come about with moderate consumption, but most only with prolonged abuse. Even occasional excessive drinking can result in memory blackouts – being unable to remember what happened the night before. On any occasion, one or two drinks will affect the time we need to think and react. In particular, routine decisions become slower and judgment is poorer. After eight drinks we are ten times more likely to have a car accident. Tragedies that result from drinking and driving are among the most common, but also the most avoidable, effects of overindulgence.

Getting the balance right

Alcohol influences our relationships at home, at work and with our friends. Excessive drinking may lead to family difficulties – arguments with other members of the family or the failure to look after children properly. Because alcohol reduces inhibitions, we may do things that we would not do otherwise, becoming aggressive or breaking the law. At work, even a few drinks at lunchtime can reduce effectiveness. Our social lives may become narrow – focused on nightclubs or bars to the exclusion of other, healthier pursuits. Heavy drinking quickly affects other parts of our lives too. We may not lose our jobs, homes or friends, but we may miss chances of promotion and cause unnecessary pain to those who care for us.

Nevertheless alcohol remains an integral part of the social lives of many adults – and there is no denying that we enjoy it. People are drinking more than ever before. Alcohol is becoming cheaper and more readily available. In 1950 it took 10.6 hours for the average worker to earn enough to buy a bottle of whiskey – in 1980 it only took 2.1 hours. Alcohol clearly poses dangers to our health. Should we avoid it altogether or are there safe limits? Most of us can safely take a moderate amount of alcohol without danger, as long as we are aware of and can control our intake.

Are you drinking too much? Are you suffering some of the

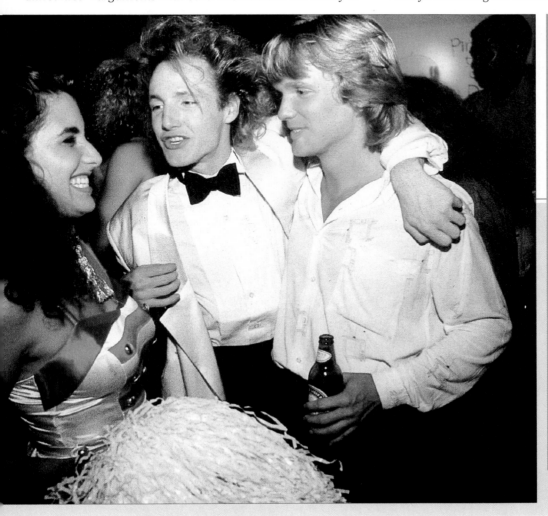

Are teetotalers more healthy?

■ Compared with abstainers and light drinkers, heavy drinkers are twice as likely to die of a heart attack, three times more likely to die in a car crash, six times more likely to commit suicide and twelve times more likely to get cirrhosis of the liver.

But research shows that moderate drinkers – who consume a unit or two a day, say a glass of wine with dinner – are slightly less likely to have a heart attack than teetotalers.

Perhaps moderate drinkers handle stress better – however, this may be a benefit of their moderate personalities, not the alcohol. Teetotalers in such studies usually do not exclude those who have stopped drinking because of poor health, and are more at risk than those who have always been teetotal.

A glass of beer a day may not actually improve your health, but it is possible to drink moderately and stay fit as well.

effects of moderate drinking – putting on weight, the occasional hangover? You can cut down on alcohol by changing how you think and what you do.

First, assess your drinking habits to determine what you should change. Start by keeping a diary of how much you drink, where you drink and why you drink. Work out how many units of alcohol you have consumed – this gives you a baseline to judge your progress against. Do you want a drink because you are tense, because everyone else is having a drink, because you are bored or because you are lonely? Ask yourself whether these are good reasons for drinking or whether there are other ways of reducing tension, curing boredom or loneliness.

Use your diary to identify risky situations. Are there times of the day when you should try to avoid drinking – perhaps straight after work? Are there people who you should avoid drinking with, do you drink too much after an argument at home or work? Work out your own danger situations. Then

you will be in a position to make the changes that will lead to a moderate, healthy lifestyle with alcohol.

When you try to change a habit, it is easier if you have a target. Your target must be realistic; there is no point aiming for a level that you cannot achieve since you will just give up. If you are a man, your upper limit on one day should be between four and eight units, and if you are a woman, between three and five units. Most days you should drink less than your limit. You should aim to have at least two days of rest each week. This allows your body to recover and you learn to enjoy things without the help of alcohol.

What is alcoholism?

For some people, trying to modify their drinking may be surprisingly difficult. Often, when we suspect we have a problem, we try to rationalize it: "It will pass. It can't be serious." It is difficult to admit that our drinking is out of control. "I know I have been drinking a lot recently but I only

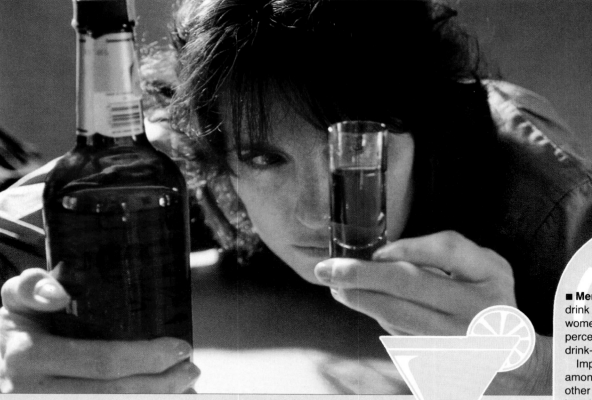

■ **Women and alcohol.** Women are drinking more now than ever before. Ten years ago the ratio of people asking for help with alcohol problems was one woman to every eight men; it is now one woman to every three men.

The safe physical limit of drinking for women is lower than that for men. Not only do women have a lower body weight than men, but a lower proportion of their bodies is water. The same amount of alcohol has a greater effect on the level of alcohol in their blood and physical damage such as cirrhosis of the liver occurs earlier in a woman and at lower levels of drinking intake.

There is no safe psychological limit, and one sex is not more prone to developing drinking problems. Women's increasing drinking may reflect the fact that many women now have the stress of coping with dual career and family responsibilities, but women are more likely than men to seek help.

■ **Men and alcohol.** Men can drink more alcohol safely than women, but on average a higher percentage still suffer from drink-related problems.

Impotence is more common among heavy drinkers than other men. Men who drink heavily often have a beer belly. This is not only unsightly but it is also unhealthy. It is possible to be overweight and undernourished at the same time. Alcohol provides the calories to generate the fat, but does not provide the proteins, vitamins or other nutrients that are necessary for a healthy body.

It can be particularly hard for men to give up heavy drinking – "a real man likes a drink" is still a common stereotype.

Practice refusing drinks

■ If you are out with friends taking turns to buy each other drinks, do you drink more? There are ways of dealing with this kind of social pressure.

You can simply say that you do not want to drink much and that you will buy your own drinks, or when it is your turn you can leave yourself out. You could still enjoy the company of friends but have nonalcoholic drinks instead of your usual order. If this is too difficult, perhaps you should avoid drinking

with these people in future and make arrangements to see them in some other situation.

There is often great social pressure to drink when you do not want to, especially at parties and celebrations. If you are going to be put under pressure, practice ways of refusing drinks. Before you get into an awkward situation, rehearse statements such as "No thanks, my doctor says I'm drinking too much" or "I've got a lot to do later and I need to stay alert."

do it on the weekend – it's under control." People who drink heavily or regularly may deny that there is a problem, or admit to the problem but blame it on a high-pressure job, financial worries or a family crisis – or even on one specific person. Rationalizing, illusions of control, denial and blame are common in alcoholics and in their families.

The word "alcoholic" to many people implies someone who is regularly drunk or extremely belligerent, and whose overall appearance, including poor personal hygiene, suggests serious problems. In fact, there are many alcoholics who are not noticeably out of control in their behavior after a few drinks, and whose lives appear to be normal – even models of perfection.

The frequency of someone's drinking may be an indicator, not just the amount consumed. The stereotype of the alcoholic drinking straight whiskey or gin is another myth. It is perfectly possible to be alcoholic and only drink wine or beer. **DJC**

Units of alcohol

■ The physical damage caused by alcohol is firmly linked to how much is consumed. It is the amount of alcohol that matters, not how much liquid is drunk, or whether it is consumed as wine, whiskey or beer.

Alcohol is measured in units and varies considerably from one kind of drink to another. There are safe limits; if you go above these limits you increase your chances of physical damage to a significant degree and run the risk of becoming

physically addicted to alcohol.

Alcohol may also be psychologically addictive. The key to psychological dependence is not how much is consumed, but when and why.

If someone habitually responds to stress, for instance, by taking a drink, this may be a sign of alcoholism.

People who have a family history of alcohol or drug abuse are particularly at risk of becoming addicted to alcohol and to other drugs as well.

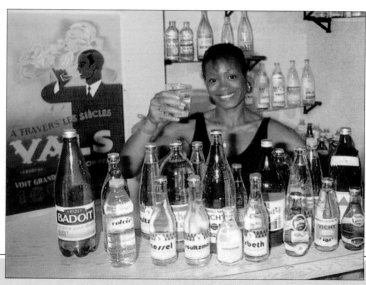

109

▲ **Cheers!** *This Paris water bar offers an array of mineral and spring water as an alternative to alcohol. In addition to the health benefits of substituting water or fruit juice for alcohol, there are also social benefits: there is no need to restrict underage drinkers.*

■ **Keeping a drinking diary.** Work out how much you have had to drink in the last seven days. Think back over each day. Try to remember what you did, where you went, whom you spent time with and how much you drank. Use the figures RIGHT to work out how many units of alcohol you consumed over the last seven days. Was this a normal week or did you consume more or rather less than usual? Was this excessive?

■ **Number of units in common drinks**

1 glass of table wine	1-2
1 measure of liquor (vodka, whiskey, gin)	1
1 can (440ml – 12oz) of beer	1.5
1 can of strong beer	4

Some drinks vary considerably in their strength. Cocktails usually contain a mixture of liquors – allow a unit for each type of liquor contained.

■ **What are the weekly limits?**

Men	Women	
35 or more units	20 or more units	too much – your health may be affected
21 to 34 units	14-19 units	you should cut down
20 or less	13 or less	within safety limits

Time of day	What did I drink?	Amount drunk	What was the social situation?	How did I feel?	What should I drink next time?
6.30pm	5 glasses of beer	7.5 units	Drinks with friends after work	Thirsty and tired. I drank what everyone else had	2 glasses and then fruit juice
8pm	3 glasses of wine	4.5 units	Dinner with a date	A little nervous – I felt we should finish the bottle	A spritzer (wine and mineral water) or order a half bottle

16

Drugs, Pills and Painkillers

Coffee, cigarettes, aspirin and cocaine are all drugs ● *Laws distinguish legal and illegal, prescription and nonprescription drugs, but even aspirin can harm us if taken carelessly* ● *Many legal drugs can be addictive.*

HOW OFTEN do you take drugs? If your answer is never, then it is very likely that you are thinking about illegal drugs. But tea, coffee, cigarettes and alcohol are all drugs; so are painkillers, cold remedies, antidepressants and tranquilizers. Nearly everyone takes drugs but in different degrees. It is a long way from the habitual coffee drinker to the heroin addict, but it is important for you to know what kind of drug you are using and why.

Some people treat almost everything themselves and only call the doctor when all else has failed. Others will go to the pharmacist – many are known as "Doc" even though they are not medically qualified. Some people will pick up the telephone and ask to see the doctor immediately. There are those who see illness as a sign of weakness to be denied; some see it as a chance to get plenty of attention; others accept illness as part of a healthy life and attempt to minimize its effect with the help of simple remedies. People who deny symptoms of illness or use prolonged self-medication to avoid taking time off to get well are putting their long-term health at risk.

Before attempting to cure your symptoms, ask yourself, "Are they telling me something important?" There are times when it could be dangerous to take medicines to feel better; an extreme example might be the athlete who kills himself by taking stimulants that in the short term enable him to ignore the pain of fatigue.

On the other hand, you may have commitments vital to your career and be willing to pay for relief in order to go on functioning for a specific period of time. Each of us needs to make a decision about how far we are prepared to go in

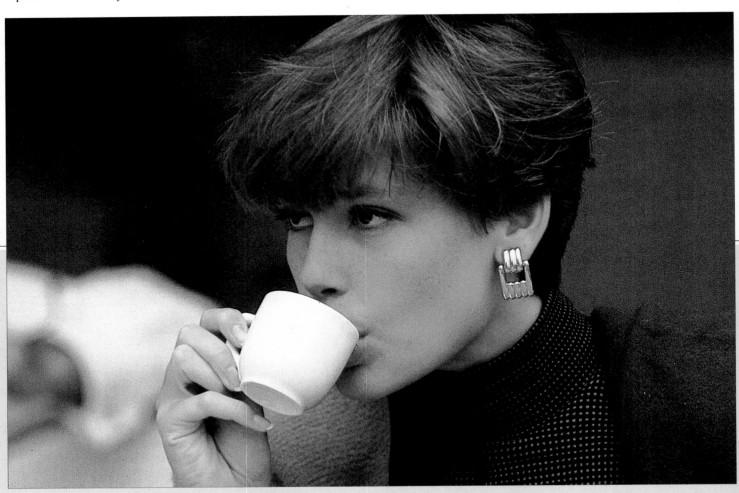

▲ **Caffeine is a drug.** *Like cigarettes, it is a legal drug, and the conditions associated with using it are far removed from those that occur with many other drugs. Unlike cigarettes, caffeine will not kill you – or the people around you. Six cups of coffee a day is probably not good for you, but researchers have been consistently unable to link moderate consumption to any specific illness. The most serious side effects of using caffeine seem to be insomnia and stained teeth.*

putting our health at risk in order to achieve the things we want. Your place on this scale will depend on a number of things. For example, it is likely that the younger you are, the more willing you will be to take risks.

Risks and side effects

There are risks and side effects with all drugs. You may develop an allergy, you may have an idiosyncrasy that makes you react to a drug in a particular way, or you may damage yourself by long-term use of a drug with dangers you are unaware of. You will not know you are going to react badly until it happens. For example, aspirin can be the cause of severe and sometimes fatal hypersensitivity, severe hemorrhage from the stomach, stomach ulcers and other reactions that make it dangerous for 12-year-olds and younger children to take. Acetaminophen (Paracetamol) causes chronic kidney damage if used in large doses over a period of years. These are the two most commonly used pain relievers.

What to ask for

Most countries limit drugs available over the counter by legislation. In the United States this dates from the Pure Food and Drug Act passed in 1906. The Food and Drug Administration decides which formulations are classified as "prescription" and "nonprescription."

These kinds of drugs are identifiable in three ways: by their chemical name, normally only used by scientists and research workers; by their generic name – the official name by which they are known once they have been approved for use; and by the trade name of the drug company that manufactures them. The list can be confusing when the same drug is manufactured by different companies. Some companies supply mixtures of nonprescription drugs offering a . range of treatments, judged to relieve a cluster of symptoms, that are known by their trade names only.

Asking for drugs by their trade names can be considerably more expensive. If you use the generic name it can cost you a fraction of what it would cost if you asked for the drug by

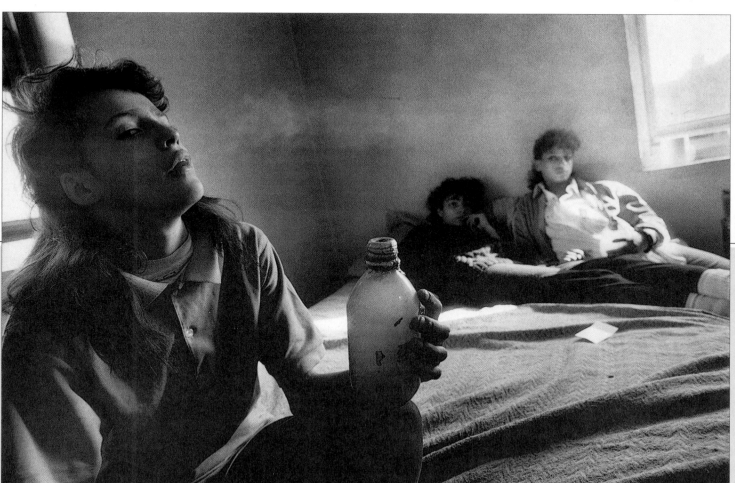

▲ **Crack,** *derived from cocaine, began to appear in the late 1980s along with "crack dens." Most crack users are teenagers* *and young adults who live in the inner cities, where daily life is dominated by the drug. The violence of the drug trade has* *left few people untouched in sections of cities like New York. The epidemic has become an international concern. In* *Colombia, the world's leading producer and exporter of cocaine, the drug trade has provoked civil war.*

111

its trade name. A powder or capsule containing a mixture of drugs is even more expensive. It is a good idea to ask your doctor or pharmacist for recommendations and then ask for drugs by their generic names. If you are recommended a mixture or trade preparation, ask what advantages it has over the generic alternative.

Treating minor illnesses

The most common complaints for which we seek medication tend to be aches and pains, colds and fevers, indigestion, constipation, diarrhea and allergies.

How often do you reach for nonprescription painkillers? They can be very effective if used with caution but it is worth remembering that an overdose can be lethal. Long-term use of any of the apparently mild pain relievers is also unwise and should not be carried out without a doctor's supervision. Aspirin, for example, can cause internal bleeding, although prescribed doses are valuable in the treatment of certain conditions. Evidence has shown that long-term use of aspirin in low doses can prevent miscarriage and help to control heart disease. It is frequently prescribed for the care of heart patients because it acts as a blood thinner. This would also help to minimize the most common type of stroke, caused by blocked arteries to the brain, but it would not be helpful at all for the less common type of stroke, in which an artery in the brain bursts. Most companies produce combinations of painkillers containing caffeine for use in the morning and the sedative antihistamine for evening use. Others add a stimulant which helps to dry up mucus in cold-sufferers, but this stimulates the nervous system and heart and probably should not be taken by people with a coronary condition.

Legal psychoactive drugs

The medicines that you can buy over the counter or that have been prescribed by your doctor are not far removed from certain kinds of illegal drugs. There are a number of drugs that can be prescribed by your doctor and are perfectly legal, yet they fall into the category of psychoactive or mood-altering drugs. Tranquilizers, antidepressants and sleeping pills are taken by millions of people who are not physically ill but who, for various reasons, are experiencing problems such as depression or anxiety. These drugs are addictive or habit-forming.

How do they differ from each other? The effects of tranquilizers and sleeping pills can be very similar and in some cases their use is interchangeable. The main difference is the length of time they need to take effect. This depends on how quickly they are absorbed into the body and enter the brain. Another difference is the length of time they continue to be effective after they have begun working.

Tranquilizers offer relief from anxiety during the first six weeks of treatment. Most sleeping pills cease to take effect after 3-14 days of continuous use. The longer these drugs are taken on a continuous basis, the less effective they become. They can be effective over a longer period if not taken continuously; otherwise, they are merely serving to increase the addiction.

The placebo effect

■ One of the ways in which medical drugs and over-the-counter pain relievers succeed in making us feel better is through the "placebo effect." This is the ability we all have within us to ease pain and escape the symptoms of illness simply by believing that what we have taken is going to do what we are told it will. Medical research has conducted innumerable experiments to prove the power of this effect. It has been established that if you give a group of patients a completely inert drug, referred to as a "placebo," leading them to believe it is a powerful medicine, usually about one-third of them will show reduced symptoms.

Another factor in the effectiveness of the placebo is our internal production of endorphins ("morphine within"), the body's natural painkillers. They affect the body very much like opiates do and we can learn to control their release with imagery. In a study at the University of California, 23 dental patients who were recovering from extractions were given a placebo and told that it was a painkiller. Over one-third reported pain relief, but when they were later given another substance that blocks endorphin activity, pain returned to them. Their belief in the placebo had triggered the release of their own natural painkillers.

Addiction to tranquilizers

■ The classic sequence of addiction is that a person must take increasingly large doses to achieve the same effect, and will go to any lengths to obtain supplies. This is true of drugs like cocaine and heroin and has to do with their chemical make-up. With drugs such as caffeine and nicotine, consumption usually remains at a steady level once the habit is established.

With tranquilizers, however, most dependents remain on the prescribed dose and sometimes even manage to reduce it. This is probably because dependence on tranquilizers is mostly psychological and results from the doctor continuing to prescribe them.

Nevertheless, people do become dependent on these drugs, and very often those who become addicted cannot recognize the fact. The drugs are extremely easy to get hold of, and repeat prescriptions are often given without question. Withdrawal symptoms can include anxiety and insomnia, which might be one reason why addiction is so difficult to spot — the symptoms of addiction look remarkably like the original symptoms that tranquilizers were prescribed to relieve.

Drugs do not provide a solution. It is important to find other ways of coping that might involve a change of lifestyle.

"Beta-blockers" are occasionally prescribed to calm a patient down. These are not tranquilizers but can diminish physical symptoms of anxiety like shaking and palpitations.

Antidepressants are not generally thought to be addictive but there is increasing concern that people do seem to have trouble cutting down once they begin to take them. They are effective in relieving depression in 70 percent of the people who take them. They are thought to be more effective for people who exhibit physical symptoms of depression such as insomnia and loss of appetite and for people who seem to be depressed for no apparent reason, rather than those who are reacting to a specific event such as a bereavement.

They only work if the correct dose is taken, and initially people may feel worse, causing some to give them up altogether or to reduce the dose to a level that has no effect.

When they are effective, the first things that occur are improved sleep and appetite and eventually the feelings of depression begin to lift.

Common problems and some remedies

■ For minor illnesses, most people go straight to their medicine cabinet. No one likes to be uncomfortable, but ask yourself if your symptoms might be trying to tell you about a chronic condition. If you get frequent headaches, you should see your doctor rather than consume steady quantities of painkillers. The chart below lists some common complaints, the usual over-the-counter remedy and possible side effects.

Salicylic acid is a chemical that forms in aspirin that has been stored on the shelf for too long. If the aspirin has a sharp sour smell like vinegar, you should throw it away; it is too old and will almost certainly upset your stomach.

Problem	Drug (trade name(s))	Effect on body	Side effects/risks
High temperature, fever	Paracetamol, Acetaminophen (Panadol, Hedex, Tempra, Tylenol) Aspirin (see below)	Lowers temperature Relieves mild pain	Allergic skin rash Kidney damage in long-term use Severe liver damage with overdosage
Muscular aches Headaches Mild arthritic pain	Paracetamol, Acetaminophen Aspirin type drugs: Aspirin, Sodium salicylate, Methyl salicylate	Lowers temperature Relieves pain Stops blood clotting	Allergic skin rash, sun sensitivity Stomach upset and hemorrhage Severe brain and liver damage in children under 12
Arthritic pain	Ibuprofen (Brufen, Motrin, Nurofen)	Suppresses inflammation Reduces pain in arthritis Promotes fluid retention	Stomach ulceration and bleeding Rashes, dizziness, blurred vision, Heart failure in those with heart disease
Indigestion	Magnesium trisilicate tablets, Aluminium hydroxide mixture	Neutralizes stomach acid Neutralizes stomach acid	Loose bowel movements, constipation Possible risk of aluminum absorption if used for long periods
	Sodium bicarbonate	Neutralizes stomach acid	Too much sodium is bad for blood pressure and prolonged use can cause bone and kidney disease
	Numerous preparations available; find the one that suits you best; if you have recurrent or prolonged symptoms, consult your doctor		
Diarrhea	Rehydration fluids (Rehydrate, Diorylate), Loperamide (Imodium, Lomotil)	Replaces body fluid and salts Slows the rate of bowel movement	Disturbed body chemistry if fluid not made up correctly Abdominal cramps Constipation
Constipation	Senna (Sennakot, Glysennid) Bisacodyl (Dulcola)	Stimulates bowel movement in 6 hours Stimulates bowel movement in 6 to 12 hours	Griping abdominal pain, dependence in long-term use Rectal burning if given as suppository
Allergies, Hay fever, Itching, Conjunctivitis	Chlorpheniramine (Piriton, Chlor-trimeton) Terfenadine (Triludan)	Blocks the action of histamine in skin nose and eye membranes Blocks the action of histamine in skin nose and eye membranes	Drowsiness, fatigue, slows reaction time Do not drive or operate machines within 8 hours Causes less drowsiness, less effective for itch; possible side effects not yet identified

113

Taking drugs for the experience

In his study on the effects of mescaline, *The Doors of Perception*, Aldous Huxley said: "That humanity at large will ever be able to dispense with artificial paradises seems very unlikely. Most men and women lead lives at worst so painful, at best so monotonous, poor and limited, that the urge to escape, the longing to transcend themselves if only for a few moments, is, and always has been, one of the principal appetites of the soul."

Huxley's view is a bleak one, and there is some truth in it. Laborers in the Third World often use naturally-available drugs such as betel or coca leaves to alleviate the pain and exhaustion of their daily lives. In Western society the use of a "fashionable" drug may start with a small, elite group and then filter down, while remaining too expensive for the very poor. But people of all income groups may use drugs for pleasure or as an escape and the reasons why may depend on a complex interplay of factors which will vary with each individual.

A person might choose to take drugs out of curiosity, because of peer group pressure, or simply because the drugs are freely available. Once they have found the experience a pleasant one, however, they are very likely to want to repeat it. At this point, although it is by no means a foregone conclusion, it is important to be aware of the dangers of dependency.

Dependency can be either physical or psychological. From a medical point of view, physical dependency is characterized by two things: the first is the physical tolerance that can be built up over continued use, so that

Commonly used illicit drugs

■ The drugs that cause the greatest social and medical problems, tobacco and alcohol, are restricted very little by law. Neither are tea and coffee – together perhaps the most commonly used drugs worldwide.

Most countries do have laws against:

Cannabis – available in three forms: herbal cannabis, which is the dried leaves and flowering tops of the plant; cannabis resin obtained by scraping the leaves; and cannabis oil.

"Dope" is usually smoked but can be eaten, for example, baked in a cake.

It induces relaxation, talkativeness, hilarity, sometimes distortions of time and space, heightening of the senses, hunger. It is not physically addictive, but mild psychological dependence occurs. Chronic use can produce apathy, and may cause lung and respiratory problems.

Opiates – opium, morphine and heroin, all derived from the milk of the opium poppy.

Heroin, commonly known as "smack," comes in powder form and may be white, brown, beige or gray. It may be sniffed, smoked, taken orally or injected. Similar substances, such as methadone, are produced synthetically.

Opiates provide relief from anxiety, physical pain, discomfort and hunger. They produce feelings of well-being. Nausea and vomiting may accompany first-time use. Larger doses can cause stupor, coma and death.

Repeated use will cause both physical and psychological dependence. Withdrawal can be extremely unpleasant: physical effects compare with flu and depression; psychological dependence is harder to break and longer-lasting than physical addiction.

Cocaine – "coke" or "snow," is a powerful stimulant. It is a white powder extracted from the coca leaf by a chemical process and is normally sniffed, although it may also be taken orally or injected. Coca leaf is chewed.

Cocaine produces a sense of energy, strength, confidence and euphoria. It enhances enjoyment of most activities but effects are short-lived. Large doses can cause irritability, anxiety and agitation.

Chronic use can produce insomnia, loss of appetite, anxiety, irritability, even paranoia. Physical addiction is a possibility, but psychological dependence is much more likely.

Crack, a derivative of cocaine, has found popularity on the streets and in the poorer areas of American cities.

Amphetamines – usually referred to as "speed." They are synthetic stimulants available in a white powder or in tablets.

The powder is usually sniffed, but the drug may also be taken orally or injected. They induce excitement, energy and confidence, with talkativeness and a high level of activity. Exhaustion, depression and hunger may follow. Psychological dependency is more likely than physical addiction. Chronic use can cause anxiety, irritability, restlessness and paranoia. Nausea, weight loss and insomnia are also common.

Ecstasy, a variety first produced in 1914, reappeared in

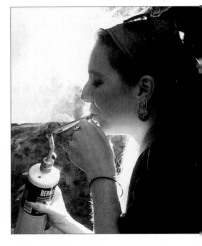

▲ **In addition to the chemical effect** *of crack, people who use it may enjoy collecting "paraphernalia" associated with their method of consumption.*

the 1980s associated with the phenomenon of "acid house" music.

Hallucinogens – their name suggests, have a powerful effect on the mind. The best-known is Lysergic acid (LSD), commonly referred to as "acid."

Some naturally-occurring hallucinogens are mescaline and "magic mushrooms" which contain such substances as psilocybin, and which are not illegal in their natural state.

LSD is normally swallowed in blotters (squares of paper

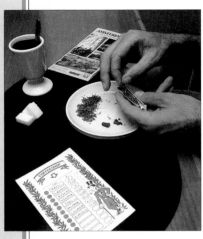

▲ **Marijuana** *(cannabis) is usually smoked in the form of a homemade "cigarette." It has a mild effect and is not physically addictive.*

the user needs to increase the dose of the drug in order to achieve the same effects; the second is the physical process of withdrawal that takes place when the user stops taking the drug.

Psychological dependency is more complex. In a sense, it is possible to become psychologically dependent on any-thing – people, television, coffee, gambling – even routine itself can provide a sense of security. Drugs offer a tempo-rary escape from boredom, anxiety or other emotions or situations that a person may want to avoid. Sometimes, for the length of time that the effects last, they also offer some-thing extra: a feeling of excitement, a sense of well-being, a belief that we are better, more successful people than we really are. Unfortunately, this belief does not usually stand up to the cold light of reality. Nor does it do any good to

ignore things that you may be unhappy about; on the con-trary, this can be very harmful.

Physical dependence can be treated medically. Psycho-logical dependence can be more difficult to treat because it is not only the person's lifestyle that is involved, but fre-quently family background as well. Children who grow up with drug- or alcohol-dependent parents are much more likely to become dependent. Even those who do not become dependent on drugs or alcohol are likely to have "addictive personalities" and to become addicted to a wide range of habits from smoking and overeating to compulsive shopping and working. It is much more difficult for such people to conquer psychological dependency. Often they successfully break one habit (such as dependence on tran-quilizers) but may find it impossible to break a second (such as smoking) – or may even acquire a new one (over-eating) to compensate for the loss of an old habit.

These factors may sound overwhelming, but it is possible even for people with "multiple addictions" to overcome both physical and psychological dependency. Although the field is relatively new, the study of addiction has developed rapidly in the USA in the last 10 years and much "self-help" literature is now available in addition to professional treat-ment. There are also support groups such as Alcoholics Anonymous, Narcotics Anonymous, Overeaters Anonymous and Gamblers Anonymous, which are now spreading throughout the world.

The first step in conquering dependency is to recognize it. Once this has happened, the process of change must start from within. Especially for people who are psychologically dependent, recovery means not only changing your lifestyle but also changing the negative self-concepts that may have contributed to or resulted from the dependency. This will take time. SL

115

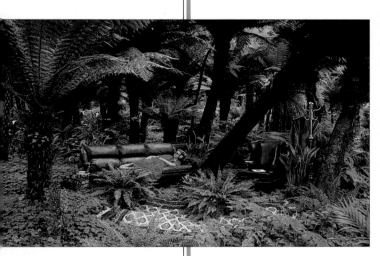

▲ **Altered states produced by hallucinogens** *will vary according to the person taking the drug, and the mood they are in when they take it.*

treated with the drug) or micro-dots (tiny tablets incorporating the drug with an inert base).

The powerful psychological effect depends on the user's personality and environment. Reactions range from euphoria to terror. There is distortion of the senses, and some users report mystical experiences.

There is no physical addiction but a danger of psychological disturbance. Regular use may encourage detachment from reality. "Flashbacks" can occur long afterward, in which parts of a "trip" may recur.

Are drugs going out of fashion?

■ The late Norman E Zinberg, a Harvard psychiatrist who had studied national patterns of drug use since 1963, identified four major waves in the USA which began with LSD in the early 1960s, marijuana in the mid to late 1960s, heroin from the late 1960s to the early 1970s, and cocaine in the late 1970s and 1980s.

He saw the shifting patterns as signs of the times: "Cocaine became the drug of the eighties because it's a stimulant," he said. "People were looking for action. It fitted the mood, just like psychedelics fitted the mood of the early sixties."

Other researchers have found these patterns influenced by regional variations and the movement of drugs through the class structure. Traditionally, the use of a particular drug starts within a small, elite group and filters down through the social classes until it permeates the ghetto or the city streets. David F Musto, the Yale medical historian who wrote "The American Disease: Origins of Narcotic Control," tells us: "The first people to go on a drug are the avant garde and the wealthy, and they are the first to go off it too. But in the inner city, drugs become a source of

status and money, at least for the dealers."

Musto believes that the most important trend is the dimin-ishing use of illegal drugs by the middle classes, a trend that has cut through all of the other cycles since 1979. He has pre-dicted that by about 2010 or 2020 drug use will reach an all-time low.

Overcoming a drug dependency

■ Drug addiction is often much easier to overcome than drug dependency. Addiction means that your body has adjusted chemically to the drug and that a painful physical readjustment will take place if the drug is stopped. Overcoming the addiction may simply involve putting up with the short-term discomfort of withdrawal.

However, physical withdrawal is usually complicated by dependency. The victim derives emotional satisfactions – eg relaxation – from taking the drug. The challenge of achieving these satisfactions in new ways – or doing without them – can be a long-term crisis of psychological readjustment.

Do drugs alter mood?

Research suggests that many of the effects that are attributed to recreational drugs are largely products of the users' own minds. This is not to say that any dependency they have on their drug is imagined or exaggerated; but the root cause of the dependency may lie more within the user than is realized – and likewise the power to overcome it.

Chemicals often magnify the existing emotions of a drug user. Research has shown that people will adjust to the mood of the setting they are in or of the people they are with, regardless of the pharmacological properties of the drug they are taking.

Volunteers who have taken heroin in laboratory conditions found it boring or unpleasant, whereas regular users usually describe their first experience as an amazing "high."

Conversely, studies in large cities have shown that the "placebo" effect applies to recreational drugs too. People will become dependent on "heroin" that consists mainly of talcum powder, and exhibit all the signs of addiction. People have become drunk on water they believed was gin, have swal-

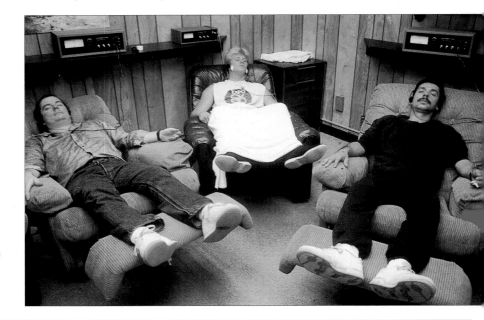

▼ **Treating drug addiction** *on an individual level addresses not only physical addiction but also psychological dependency, which is harder to overcome. A combination of group therapy, individual counseling and relaxation practice through biofeedback (shown here) all encourage patients to overcome dependency from within.*

Does someone close to you have a drug problem?

■ If you suspect that someone you love has a problem with drugs or alcohol, the first thing to do is to examine your own feelings. Ask yourself how well-founded your suspicions are and how far you are prepared to go in offering your support.

Should you decide to confront the other person, forearm yourself with as much information as you can. Remember, also, that confrontation need not be unpleasant or angry; handled with tact and diplomacy, it can be the most constructive way to deal with a situation.

Choose your moment carefully. It should be a time when

you are both relaxed, perhaps after sharing a joke or a confidence. But do not expect it to be easy; the other person is likely to feel vulnerable, isolated, guilty and defensive.

Be careful not to make accusations but concentrate on showing concern and offering your support. If the reaction is denial, mention things that have happened as a result of the problem and make it clear that you would like to understand. Re-emphasize your love and concern. Be willing to listen. But do not expect too much the first time – be prepared to take things in stages.

Codependency. Remember though, that ultimately the other person must take responsibility for his or her own recovery. You can offer support, love and understanding, but you cannot do it for them. If you feel that you are too involved with the issue of someone else's dependency – "Everything in my life will be all right when they get help" – then you may need help too. This syndrome, where someone who has a relationship with a drug- or alcohol-dependent person feels that the other person's problem controls their life as well, is called codependency. People who grow up in

families with a history of drug or alcohol abuse are particularly affected. An increasing amount of research has been done on this subject in the USA since the 1970s and the number of therapists who specialize in treating codependency is growing, as is the number of support groups. ACOA ("Adult Children of Alcoholics") and Al-Anon were originally founded by and for family members of alcoholics, but alcoholism and drug dependency have much in common, and meetings are usually attended by (and welcome) a wide range of people trying to cope with diverse situations.

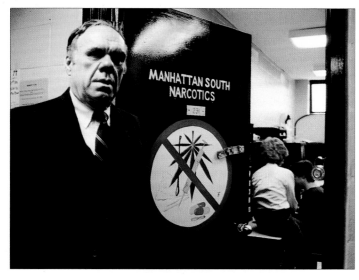

► **Controlling the supply of drugs** *is one government response to solving social problems associated with drug use. Most major cities now have special narcotics units working independently and in conjunction with larger national organizations and Interpol. Social services, drug clinics and therapists take the opposite approach: eliminating the desire for drugs instead of the supply.*

lowed salt tablets and shown clear signs of sedation, and become "stoned" on inert material they were told was cannabis.

Losing a dependency

Weaning yourself away from a drug to which you attribute, rightly or wrongly, some of your nicest experiences, or even your ability to cope day-to-day, is a cycle of psychological change. Some people complete the cycle. Others drop out and then have to go through the process again. Some try only once and give up trying, but most make a series of repeated attempts.

A crucial factor in successful change appears to be the expectation of a good outcome. People who do go through the whole cycle find that their belief in their ability to change improves as they go. This is very valuable in counteracting temptation which is at its peak at the beginning of the process and gradually diminishes.

Coping with lapses

People do lapse, and in this situation it is important both to learn to deal with the lapse and to try to prevent it happening again. The key to coping with a return to old behavior is not to expect to manage the situation without problems: *coping* rather than *mastery* is the thing to aim for. If we give ourselves credit for small successes, we are more likely to continue trying and,

ultimately, to succeed. Any major adjustment in your life needs to be accomplished gradually, bit by bit. The danger of an all-or-nothing approach is that the inevitable failure can bring with it a dramatic loss in confidence and a return to old behavior patterns.

In trying to prevent lapses it can be useful for us to think of our lives as a road map. American drug researcher Alan Mavlatt uses this analogy to illustrate how parts of our journey will be easy to cope with and others will be tortuous and difficult. High-risk times will be moments of choice, when we can develop alternative responses or return to a habit.

In looking at the roads we might take, we are preparing ourselves for possibilities; looking at those we have taken in the past can help to identify the most dangerous routes. The routes that are likely to be the most successful are not necessarily the easiest ones. The hardest places to get to can be the most enjoyable and personally satisfying.

Often, a very effective way of changing an old habit is to replace it with a new one. Life-enhancing activities such as exercise, deep relaxation, meditation, learning new skills, tackling personal problems with counseling, or simply meeting a new set of people, can all be valuable.

Habit-breaking strategies

■ Here are some strategies for breaking the habit of using any drug. Look too at the advice given in Chapter 14 about quitting smoking.

● During withdrawal, try to spend more time doing the things you want to do instead of things you have to do.
● Begin replacing old bad habits with good new ones such as exercise, meditation, a new interest, new friends.
● Avoid situations (or people) that might encourage you to return to drug use.
● Learn to "ride through" your cravings – they will subside.
● Watch out for apparently irrelevant decisions – just happening to choose a route to work that would lead you past a convenient supply, for example, could be an early sign of a craving.
● If you lapse, try to limit the damage it may do – the less it affects the other areas of your life, the easier it is to stop again.
● Do not use negative techniques – eg, telling yourself, "You're a loser if you do not succeed." Use positive statements to boost your sense of confidence and self-worth: "I'm OK," "I'm strong enough to do this."
● Share your problems with others – there are many sources of support available, both professional and self-help, most of which can be found through the telephone directory or your local doctor's office.
● Remember that change is a gradual process – do not expect too much at once.

117

17

Illness and Disability

When we are enjoying good health, we can suffer from the illusion of invulnerability ● *Now is the time to think what it would be like to have an infirmity* ● *Eight out of ten people develop a disabling illness in their lifetime.*

CHRONIC health problems range from those as minor and common as shortsightedness to more serious but manageable conditions like asthma or diabetes, as well as major permanent problems such as paralysis or loss of a limb. It may seem odd to group together the shortsighted with amputees, but both have a physical problem that will not go away, and that requires adaptations to lessen its effect. Most people will be affected during their lives by a major or minor health disability, either in themselves or in someone in their family. Understanding the disability, how it might affect you, and what you can do about it is the first step to coping well with a chronic health problem.

What is disability?

The World Health Organization defines three main elements of a chronic condition. Impairment refers to the parts or systems of the body that are faulty. Disability encompasses the things that a person with an impairment cannot do as a result. Handicap is a disadvantage of a social, personal, or economic nature resulting from a disability. In general, the term "disability" is used to refer to the whole range of consequences of a chronic health problem.

If you are shortsighted, your poor vision is an impairment, your inability to navigate safely out of doors is a disability, and not being able to get a driver's license is a handicap. Fortunately there is an easy solution to this problem: you can get a pair of glasses. Not all disabilities are so easily or completely managed as poor vision, but the basic aim of any disability management is the same. The impairment itself is examined and aids are developed to correct, eliminate, or at least soften the consequences of its negative effects. Some people with disabilities go on a step further than this by insisting that as society creates handicaps and discrimination, society – rather than the person with a disability – should change. The effect of this logic can be seen on public buildings and transport which are often "wheelchair accessible" – and also accessible to those who push baby buggies.

Why should I be concerned?

The more serious a disability is, the more complex and extensive is the network of problems that arise. People with disabilities are not a uniform group that can be treated as a single entity. There are as many differences between people with disabilities as there are between people of the same sex, race or religion. What people with disabilities want and need is to be treated as individuals in their own right with their own talents, skills and problems, rather than as a unit in a disadvantaged group. That treatment needs to come from family, friends, health carers and the general public if discrimination is to be eventually eliminated and people with severe disabilities are to have the same rights as others.

While we are enjoying good health, we often suffer from the illusion of invulnerability. We find it difficult to believe that we will ever become seriously ill or develop a chronic

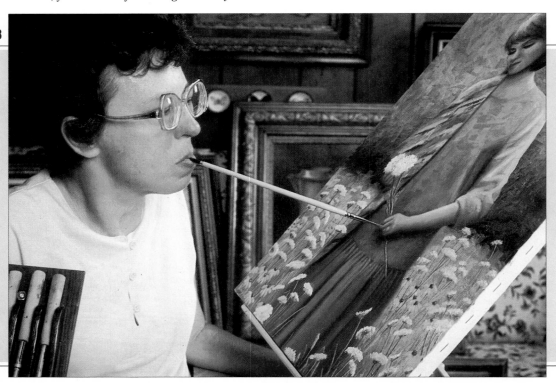

◄ **Living a purposeful life**, *Nancy Litteral finishes another painting. Psychologists have found repeatedly that people have an enormous capacity to adapt to disability, both emotionally and practically. A healthy lifestyle is a crucial factor in coping with personal disability. This involves not just physical health but the mental stimulation of finding a goal and developing ways of reaching it.*

Setting the pace

▶ **"Disabled" does not mean "unhealthy."** *To raise money for the National Institute for Neural Injury, and to prove that people in wheelchairs can be fit and mobile, Peter Werner, at 43, made a sponsored trek of 10,000 miles in his chair, first from New York to Los Angeles, then from Dallas to Washington. Backed by Dutch and German helpers, Werner was also expressing gratitude to the American people for the Berlin airlift of the late 1940s, when he was growing up in the blockaded city.*

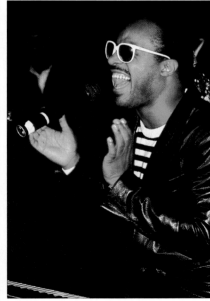

▲ **"The people I feel sorry for are those who have sight but still don't see,"** *says Stevie Wonder, who dismisses his own blindness from birth as no real handicap to him. In a professional musical career that started at the age of 10, and has included mastery of several instruments, he has created such highly acclaimed works as "Songs in the Key of Life." One of his most popular collections is the long-playing album "Inner Visions."*

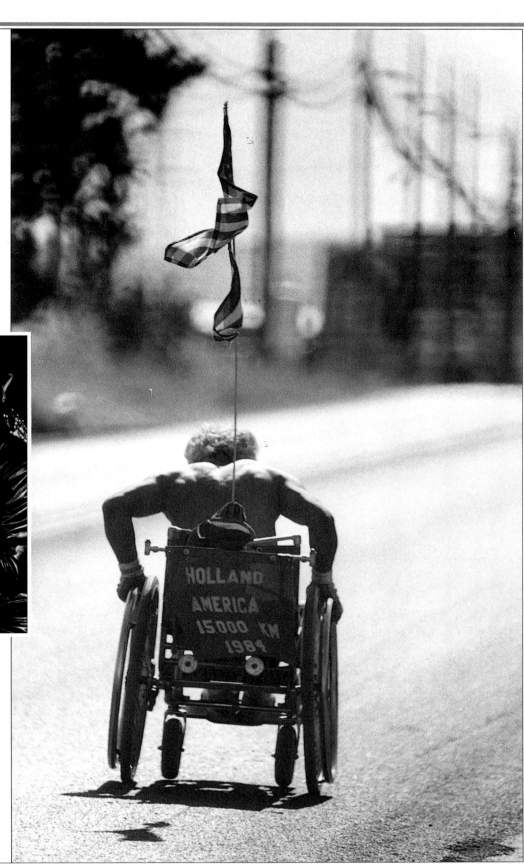

119

health problem. As a result, we often find the presence of people with disabilities hard to deal with and do not know how to treat them. People in wheelchairs often find that others act as if they were invisible. Even if they are noticed, others seem unable to figure out why a set of steps or a narrow doorway creates special difficulties for them. Many people are simply unaware of the potential problems of others until they themselves or someone close to them suffers a disability.

For your own sake, as well as for the sake of the people with disabilities you meet, it is now, at your present age and in your present state of health, that you should think about what might happen and what could be done if you or a family member acquires a disabling condition. Eight out of ten people will develop a potentially chronic disabling illness in their lifetime.

How does it happen?

There are three broad categories of disability. Genetic diseases are passed down through families, like hemophilia and Huntingdon's disease (a nervous disorder that often does not develop until after victims have passed on the disease to their children without knowing they are carriers), or are the result of faulty chromosome pairing and splitting in the developing ovum, like Down's Syndrome. Other illnesses are the result of accidents or damage at birth (especially complex brain damage leading to conditions such as cerebral palsy) or damage later in life, mainly from traffic accidents. A third category of impairments are acquired over time as the result of diseases such as multiple sclerosis and diabetes. It is possible that some of these diseases also have a genetic component.

Different sorts of disability affect different age groups. Cystic fibrosis, juvenile-onset diabetes, and spina bifida are regarded chiefly as diseases of children, because although the problems they cause persist throughout life, methods of coping have to be developed in childhood. Multiple sclerosis and Huntingdon's disease do not usually appear until adulthood and their management is complicated by the need to make major changes in lifestyle. Conditions such as heart disease, arthritis and chronic respiratory disorders account for 25-50 percent of the disabled conditions and are usually diseases of the elderly, so treating them requires careful consideration for the needs of an aging patient.

Medical screening – catching problems early

■ Screening aims to detect the symptoms of disease at an early, readily treatable stage. It is aimed at risk groups – people whose age, sex, medical or family history or lifestyle makes it more likely for them to develop a particular illness or disability.

■ **Before birth**. Prepregnancy screening helps those who have not yet been conceived. The mother-to-be will have a thorough medical examination to determine her basic fitness and freedom from disease. The doctor should be told about any regular medication either of the prospective parents takes. This needs to be changed if it might affect a fetus.

A careful doctor will ask questions about the lifestyles of both prospective parents. Heavy drinking or smoking by either the mother or father can damage a baby's health, and you may be advised to give up or cut back for as much as three months before pregnancy.

You will also be asked about the history of genetic disease in your family, and if necessary you will be offered genetic counseling to help you decide how to respond to the risks of having a child with a disability.

Regular checkups during pregnancy ensure that the baby is growing normally and that the mother's health is stable. Blood tests make sure that the mother does not have anemia and that there is no blood group incompatibility (the Rh factor) between mother and child. Problems such as genetic disease, spina bifida and Down's syndrome can be picked up early in pregnancy through chorionic sampling (early examination for chromosome irregularities in a sample of cells taken from the membrane surrounding the embryo) or by amniocentesis (later examination for chromosome irregularities in a sample of cells taken from the amniotic fluid surrounding the baby in the womb).

Chorionic sampling and amniocentesis are usually only offered if there is a known risk of

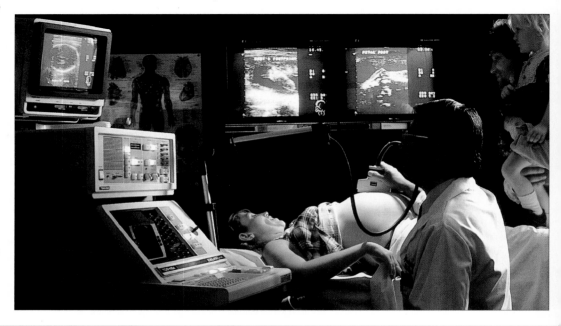

What can I do to avoid the risk of handicap?

In many instances, the way you lead your life contributes to health problems which may result in some form of disability. You can prevent or delay the onset of many disabling diseases by taking exercise, not smoking, drinking only in moderation and watching your weight. Even if you do get a disabling disease, a healthy lifestyle will make it easier for you to cope and may make the illness less damaging. Adult-onset diabetes can cause blindness and damage to the circulation resulting in the amputation of a limb, but people with diabetes who keep themselves fit, control their weight, and follow a sensible diet are less likely to be affected by such severe results. Even if your lifestyle is not directly connected to the cause or progress of a disease, it can influence the way you cope. People with multiple sclerosis and Parkinson's disease lose mobility regardless of lifestyle, but if they are overweight and underexercised they may find it even more difficult to manage their symptoms.

Many people see increasing age as a major cause of disability in its own right, and there is no doubt that disability overall increases with age. This is not inevitable, however, and healthy practices in youth, middle age and even old age will mitigate the wear and tear on the body that is a natural part of growing old. Healthy living is particularly important for reducing the incidence of conditions such as heart disease and respiratory problems that are the major causes of disablement in the elderly.

Reading the symptoms

Many people find their quality of life deteriorating before they realize that they are actually ill. For these people the diagnosis of a disabling illness can come as a relief. Some conditions such as multiple sclerosis are marked by insidious, vague symptoms including numbness and tingling in the arms and legs, clumsiness and extreme fatigue which may be dismissed as "all in the mind," the result of laziness or an emotional problem. Once the illness is diagnosed at least these symptoms have a name and a cause which can be understood.

For other people diagnosis can bring on depression; it can seem like a sentence of death. Information on the nature of their condition, and help with understanding and coming to terms with natural feelings of anxiety or depression, can be of immense value.

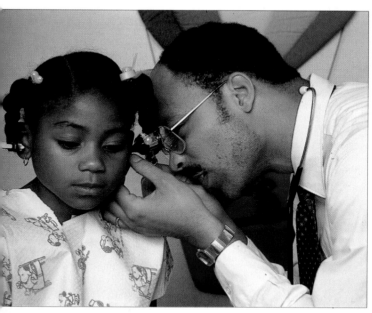

◄ **"Healthy and alert"** *is the news from the womb, as ultrasound screenings provide this expectant mother with an image of her child. Screening usually finds nothing wrong. This combats anxiety, which can itself be a risk to health (see Ch 5).*

▲ **Preventing loss of hearing** *through medical checking. Untreated middle ear infections can permanently damage hearing, which should be checked regularly throughout childhood. Some children become adept at lipreading in order to disguise their problem.*

Down's Syndrome or another chromosome irregularity. You should think carefully about taking these tests if you are not prepared to consider a termination in the event of an abnormal result.

Regular urine and blood-pressure testing will ensure that the mother is not developing toxemia (also called eclampsia), a condition which can be fatal for both mother and child. Fortunately it is not common and can be treated successfully if caught early enough. Most pregnancies proceed uneventfully, and regular checkups can catch many problems that arise before they become serious.

■ **Infancy and childhood.** Within the first minute of birth babies are given an "Apgar test," named after the doctor who invented it, rating their color, heart rate, respiration, muscle tone and response to stimuli. This test is given to all babies to identify any immediate distress which might threaten the infant's life. Further checks follow at 30 minutes to look for abnormalities such as dislocation of the hip, abnormal head size, undescended testicles, hernias, cataracts and heart irregularities which may need further treatment.

Normal checkups between the ages of 6 weeks and 18 months will concentrate on assessing the child's rate of development. They aim to detect delay in reaching certain milestones of development such as walking, talking and continence so that preventable causes of delay in development may be treated and steps can be taken to enable the child to catch up.

Inoculations against serious childhood diseases begin at eight weeks. Children begin to respond reliably to tests for vision and hearing from about 2 years, and these will be checked regularly throughout the time they are at school. Adolescents will be checked for normal sexual development and also for distortions in the growth of the spine which may only become obvious during the growth spurts of puberty. **KW**

121

Symptoms are important in many disabling conditions because they provide a readily available source of information for monitoring the progress of the disease and assessing the impact of the person's environment on his or her condition. Some people may notice that extremes of temperature consistently make them feel worse, and use this knowledge to ensure that their house and working environment maintain a comfortable temperature, planning outings for times of the day and year when the climate is mild.

Many conditions such as arthritis and Parkinson's disease follow an unpredictable course, and paying attention to symptoms allows the person to respond depending upon how they feel. Since medications for disabling diseases may have adverse side effects, it is best to keep them to a minimum. People with disabilities also need to be flexible in choosing when to do certain daily tasks. If you need to go shopping, for example, you should tackle it when you feel at your best rather than sticking to a fixed schedule which may not fit in with the state of your health. People with disabilities have to think ahead and prepare a number of flexible plans of action in order to live well within the physical limitations of their condition.

Getting up steps

People with health problems may not be able to dictate all their own terms and surroundings, however. Public facilities are often not geared to anyone but the able-bodied. Getting through doorways, up steps, and onto trains and buses can be difficult for people with a mobility problem, whether they are in a wheelchair or have mild arthritis. Campaigning for disabled access to buildings and transport systems has resulted in some improvement, but many public places are difficult for the disabled to use even though they pay taxes like everyone else to help maintain public services.

The public health and social services in your area have a responsibility to raise public awareness of disability problems, and in many countries these services will act as consultants to planners, advising where to widen an entrance, what sort of door is easiest to open, or where a ramp or an elevator is needed. They can also offer help and advice on how to adapt the disabled person's home, providing information and sometimes financial assistance to modify bathrooms, stairways, beds and kitchens, so enabling the person with a disability to live a full and independent life where at all possible. Hospital and community services

Adult screening

■ Women who are sexually active should have a screening for cervical cancer at least every five years. This involves a painless pelvic examination and the removal of a tissue sample swabbed from the neck of the womb which can be examined for irregularities.

Women using oral contraceptives should have their blood pressure checked regularly, and those with an IUD or coil need an examination at least once a year to check that it is still properly in place. Those using a diaphragm should have its fit and size checked every six months and whenever they gain or lose 10lbs.

Breast X-ray (mammography) is useful in detecting tumors in the dense breast tissue of older women. Although breast cancer is relatively rare in those under 45, self-screening for lumps is recommended for all women (see Ch2).

Everyone should also keep a check on moles and other spots. Skin cancer is on the increase, particularly in hot sunny climates among those who do not use a sunscreen. If a mole changes shape, size or color, tell your doctor – it can be treated easily if caught early.

Males are four times more likely to suffer from coronary heart disease in early life than women are. Men should have a regular checkup every five years, especially after 35, to look at coronary risk factors, including cholesterol levels.

Men should also examine their testicles for any unusual lumps, hardness, or tenderness (see Ch2).

■ **Later life**. From the age of 45 in men, and after the menopause in women, coronary artery disease is the major preventable cause of ill-health and death, and the risk factors are well known (see Ch2). Living a sensible life with proper diet, good exercise, no smoking and alcohol in moderation is your best safeguard. Regular screening for cardiac disease and cholesterol levels will identify those individuals who need to take special care.

Women in sexual relationships should continue to have cervical screening until at least 65. Mammography in women over 50 can detect breast cancer at an early stage and regular X-rays are advised.

In retirement, regular vision and hearing tests should be taken and difficulties in walking and moving monitored regularly before serious problems develop. Many disabilities which people put down to age are in fact treatable. **KW**

Psychological strains

■ Disablement can lead to depression and sometimes serious psychological disturbance. Stress and depression are most common in the early stages of a disability and can be alleviated by individual or group counseling, where discussion about different ways of solving problems and the psychological effect of these problems will help to prepare for difficulties to come.

Severe psychological problems generally occur only with advancing stages of serious disabling conditions such as multiple sclerosis and Parkinson's disease. It is the severity rather than the kind of disability which is associated with psychological distress.

Family and friends can often help by being willing to listen and by trying to understand. Ignoring the condition will only increase their isolation and frustration. Many counseling groups welcome family and friends, and these can be a great help in understanding the disease and the variety of ways that people respond to their disability.

You are more likely to notice and feel affected by the symptoms of an illness if you are bored or anxious. Also, you tend to notice symptoms that fit in with what you expect to find, and ignore those that you do not know to be significant. Being told you have a disabling condition appears initially to increase the symptoms you experience.

122

such as physiotherapy, speech therapy, occupational therapy, counseling, dietetics and clinical psychology provide a valuable source of advice on how to achieve a lifestyle that the person with a disability and his or her family can adapt to successfully.

It helps, though, if the person with a disability knows what to ask for. The health services in any area are often busy and understaffed. If you or someone in your family becomes disabled, severely or mildly, it helps if the person with a disability is able to state what they want from the health care system and what lifestyle they want to achieve. If you can approach your health service with positive ideas and suggestions you are more likely to get the help you need. There are an increasing number of well-organized and effective self-help groups that can advise you. Many people with disabilities live full, happy and, despite their disabilities, healthy lives. Some people with disabilities feel that their condition has changed their life for the better, giving them a clearer idea of their values and perspectives on life. It has made their relationships more meaningful and helped them to appreciate the spiritual rather than the material aspects of their lives. Just like the healthy person, the disabled person wants to improve the quality of their life. Living a healthy lifestyle, learning to interpret and act on symptoms, planning a flexible schedule, and making the most of the available services can help the person with a disability to achieve and maintain an enjoyable and worthwhile life. **LE**

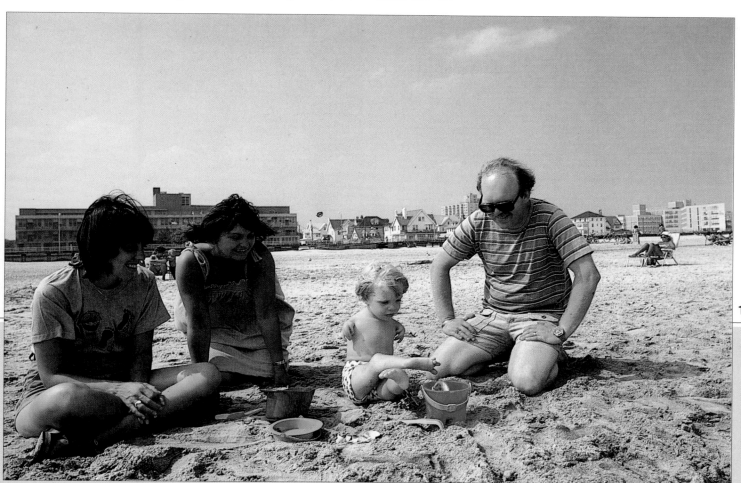

▲ **Making maximum use of malformed limbs** is child's play for this boy, at the beach with his physiotherapist and his parents. Disabling conditions have very different consequences depending upon the stage of life when they occur. Children born even with a severe impairment may cope better than those who are disabled due to injury or illness in late adulthood, so long as they have experienced loving care which has not hidden or ignored the consequences of their condition. They grow up developing coping resources and strategies, are less inclined to think of their condition as something that marks them out, and are more likely to think of themselves as individuals with their own abilities (a positive approach) rather than as people primarily characterized by a lack of ability (a negative approach). Adults may have to make major changes to their careers, leisure pursuits and personal ambitions, even their plans for a family, which can be very hard to cope with, particularly if the person had been physically very active.

18

Hospital Care

A hospital stay need not be an unpleasant experience ● *Modern medical practice allows patients to be more informed and involved* ● *This improves their sense of control and minimizes feelings of anxiety and helplessness.*

GOING into hospital for any length of time is stressful to some degree for everyone. Normal routines are disrupted, hospital routine rather than personal control determines activities, and there is little privacy. For those undergoing surgery, some pain and a period of recovery are to be expected. Not surprisingly, some people will do anything to avoid going into hospital for treatment, even if this means ignoring a serious ailment. But hospital treatment is intended to increase the quality of your life. It is there to reduce problems, not to create them.

Good surgery can transform your state of health and even save your life. People who have delayed surgery for years are sometimes surprised, once they have had treatment, to find how restricted their lives had become under the weight of their illness without their even realizing it. But all surgery involves cutting or removing tissue, and most involves some kind of anesthesia, so there are always some side effects to take into account. These must be weighed carefully against the possible gains.

The stressful and negative aspects of surgery and hospitalization can be reduced by your own efforts. Knowledge about your illness, and the purpose, effects and the probable outcomes of the treatment you will undergo, will enable you to decide how much you can help yourself and when it is better to let others help you. The more you are

able to participate in a partnership of care, the more likely you are to recover quickly, uneventfully and with the minimum amount of pain.

How do you decide to go into hospital?

Your family doctor or the medical specialist that you have been referred to will usually be the first to suggest the need for tests, treatment or surgery which must take place in hospital. But the decision is yours – the doctor who performs the procedure is required by law to have your written and informed consent about any treatment of this kind. Even so, as many as one third of patients do not even know the name of the treatment they are expecting

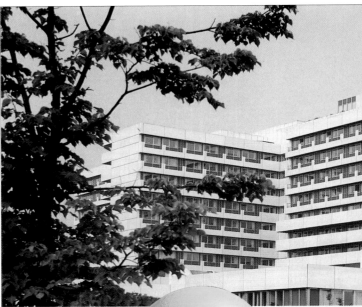

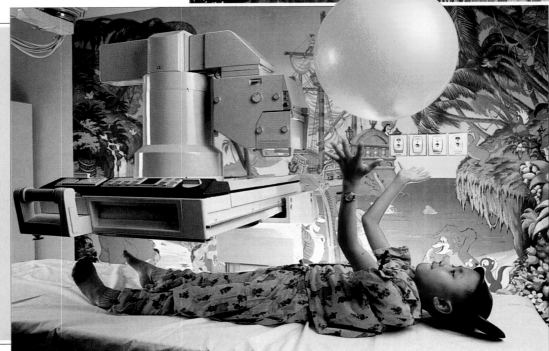

■ **Hospitals are intimidating** *to many people who may feel uncomfortable even going to visit a sick friend or relative. The most modern attempt to be attractive but the design of any hospital must give priority to practical needs, and the effect may be uninviting. Inside, effort is usually made to brighten up the patients' surroundings, especially in children's wards* RIGHT. *However, the most important aspect of a hospital is not its appearance but its equipment and qualified personnel* FAR RIGHT.

or have any clear idea of what the doctor intends to do.

Ask your doctor for a detailed explanation of what could be done. Medical staff are often busy and overworked, but they do understand the need for you to know what is happening. If you fail to get a satisfactory answer, do not be afraid to ask for a second opinion. It is, after all, your body that is being treated, and you have a right to know what the experts intend to do.

Preparing to be admitted

Just going into hospital will disrupt your routine. You can prepare for this in the same way as you would for a business or holiday trip, by canceling commitments (and home deliveries if you live alone) and informing those who need to know that you will be away, telling them for approximately how long, and where you can be reached.

Practical arrangements depend on the length of time you will be in the hospital and how serious the treatment is. Ask your doctor for some idea of how long recovery usually takes – when will you be able to leave hospital, and how long after that will you be able to resume everyday tasks. You will also need to know how long you are likely to be away from work. Doctors can never give precise answers to these questions because so much depends upon how the operation goes and how you as an individual respond to treatment, but they can give you some guidelines. This will allow you to be prepared, and will give your relatives, friends and colleagues some idea of what to expect.

If you have children they may need special attention, particularly if you have not been away from them before. Talk about things you will share when you return; with older children you can explain something about your need to go into hospital and what will be done to make you better. If your children will be able to visit you in the hospital, there are many widely available story books to help a child understand what a hospital looks like and the kinds of things that happen there.

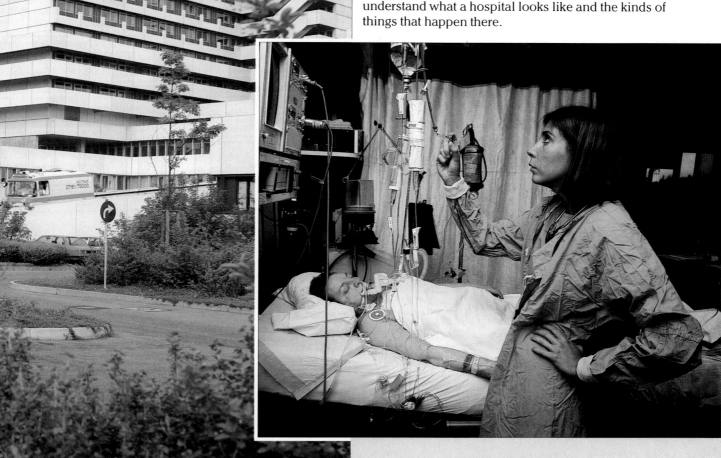

125

What to expect with an operation

■ The routine of preparing for surgery under a general anesthetic is similar for many sorts of operations. The doctor will check to see if your chest and breathing passage are clear, your heart rate is strong and your blood pressure is normal. The stress of surgery will be easier for you if these basic bodily functions are working well. If you have a cold or flu, for instance, a doctor may decide to postpone the operation until a later date.

You may have some blood taken to check for abnormalities and to have your blood group identified. Body hair near the surgical area may be shaved. You may be given an enema to empty your bowels, and you will probably be given no food or water for 8 to 12 hours before the operation. This is to prevent choking during the operation or loosening or emptying of the bladder and bowels under anesthesia. General anesthesia makes

many people feel sick, so an empty digestive system prevents distress.

You may be sent for extra tests such as X-rays and scans before the operation, in order to determine the proper surgical procedure more accurately. Shortly before surgery you may be given a pre-operative medication or "pre-med" to relax your muscles and reduce anxiety, although you may prefer to relax yourself in your own way. Once you are

wheeled to the operating room the full anesthetic is given, and a pain-relieving drug is sometimes injected during surgery so that it will take effect before you wake up. After surgery you are taken to the recovery room, and once you regain consciousness there you will be taken back to your bed. Within 4 to 8 hours, depending on the seriousness of your surgery and your reaction to it, you will be allowed to sit up and take some food and drink.

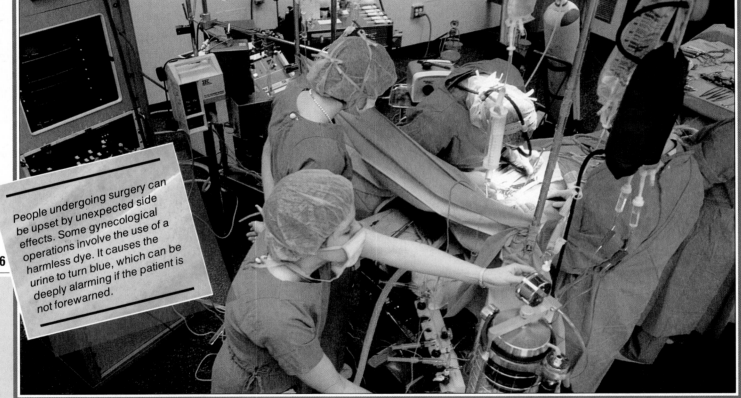

People undergoing surgery can be upset by unexpected side effects. Some gynecological operations involve the use of a harmless dye. It causes the urine to turn blue, which can be deeply alarming if the patient is not forewarned.

126

The importance of mental preparation

■ Recovery time and the general level of anxiety after surgery can be greatly reduced by knowing what to expect.

A study compared women undergoing laparoscopy (a minor surgical technique used to diagnose causes of pelvic pain and infertility) with women having the same surgical

procedures for sterilization.

The gynecologists in charge of these patients were surprised to hear the study's results: that women undergoing laparoscopy were more anxious than those having sterilization, even though cutting or clipping to close the fallopian tubes causes more pain than simply probing to dis-

cover the possible causes of infertility.

This was because the women having laparoscopy for infertility were less well informed. As many as 25 percent thought the examination would not require an incision and were upset to discover only hours beforehand that the procedure involved

being put to sleep with a general anesthetic.

The women having hysterectomies knew that it was minor and very common surgery and were both less anxious before the operation and less upset by their recovery from the anesthetic afterward.

The results of surgical treatment

The recovery rate of all patients is heavily influenced by their fears and expectations about what is wrong with them and to what extent they will be able to recover from it. The patient's expectations matter particularly as they approach each of the major "hurdles" of recovery, such as that painful and woozy first walk after surgery.

Physical stress is caused by the physical shock of the surgeon's knife and removal of tissue, and by the drugs used to relax muscles, control consciousness, reduce pain and prevent or encourage blood clotting. People vary enormously in how well they recover from that stress. A great deal depends on how much they can control tension and fear. Anxiety is natural but it stimulates stress hormones such as adrenaline which hamper the body's natural clotting mechanisms designed to heal wounds. Stress hormones also cause muscle tension which can increase our awareness of pain.

Stress can cause other problems too. A tense person who does not really understand the cause or probable duration of discomfort can be the prey of unnecessary fears. Chest pain, tiredness, poor concentration and shortness of breath are common after heart surgery, but patients who do not know this may fear they are having a heart attack, especially if they have never had chest pain before. Patients who know what to expect, especially those who have had a heart attack or angina and know the difference between this and pain after surgery, are more likely to feel calm. They report less

pain, begin to move about more easily and often feel more optimistic about recovery than those who find chest pain a new, unexpected and frightening experience.

Knowledge reduces stress

Since so much stress arises from being ill-informed, having accurate information improves the way people experience surgery and hospitalization. Many hospitals now provide booklets about common medical treatments. These contain information about what surgery is designed to do. The better ones include details about the sights, sounds and smells to expect in the anesthetic room and recovery area, the physical sensations to expect, and how long these may last after the operation. If you know you are going to have to go into hospital you can collect and read this literature well in advance.

An important part of hospital information is concerned with people's management of their own illness. Self-help techniques can encourage patients to make the best use of the information that they have been given. These include relaxation exercises which replace or supplement pain control through drugs, advice about when to ask a nurse for help and how to cope with post-anesthetic nausea and dizziness.

Researchers have found that people provided with such detailed information are less anxious before the operation, have less pain afterward and are able to get up and be ready to leave hospital sooner. They are able to return to normal

Being informed is healthy

■ If you are able to opt for a choice between treatments on the basis of all the facts, you are likely to be more satisfied with your decision. In Liverpool, England, a group of women with breast cancer were offered two surgical treatments which the doctor believed were equally effective in controlling cancer – removal of the lump of cancerous tissue alone (lumpectomy), or the removal of the whole breast (mastectomy). Some women prefer lumpectomy because it is less disfiguring and recovery time is faster; others feel safer with more radical surgery like mastectomy. Since between one third and two thirds of women suffer from anxiety or depression after breast cancer surgery, it was hoped that the offer of a choice would help women cope better with their surgery.

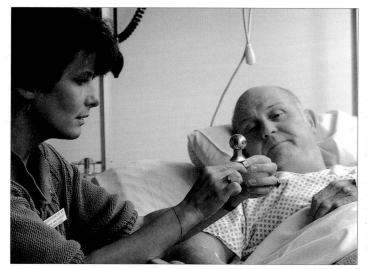

◄ **Patients who know what to expect** *are better prepared to cope with the physical and psychological stress of surgery. Surprisingly, the amount of tissue damage is not the only indication of how long it will take someone to recover. Another is the patient's level of anxiety. Information about how a procedure will affect the body may allay fear and usually tends to reduce the overall stress of the patient.*

At first many of the women felt unable to decide, given the basic facts about each treatment. The women then saw a psychologist who counseled them carefully about the pros

and cons of each method and how this would fit in with their lifestyle and body image. All of them ended up deciding for themselves and feeling happy about having made a choice.

Very few experienced serious distress after the operation. They knew what to expect and felt in control of their bodies and their treatment because they were kept informed.

activities up to twice as fast as poorly-informed patients. When well-prepared people are surveyed as to how advance information helped them to cope, they reply that inform-ation has given them a sense of control. It let them know when they could passively accept advice and help, such as letting the nurse escort them to the toilet when they were still drowsy from the anesthetic, and when they could do something for themselves, such as deep regular breathing to reduce nausea and discomfort. The management of their recovery was consequently more straightforward and much less stressful.

When to withhold information

Some people do panic when they are given too much specific information about what is likely to happen. Young children, the confused elderly and people of a naturally timid or anxious disposition may become distressed if they are told too many details or are given too long a time before an operation to think about what might happen. It used to be common practice to hide the full knowledge of a potentially fatal illness from a patient; cancer victims in particular often never knew how ill they were. Relatives often beg doctors not to tell a patient the full extent of an illness. They do this with the best of motives; they want to prevent distress and help the patient remain cheerful for as long as possible. But medical staff now tend to resist this way of dealing with sickness even in the case of very young children or the very old and confused, because they have seen that ignorance is, in fact, much more distressing than useful knowledge.

People who are sick are usually in full possession of their mental faculties and are perfectly well aware that something is wrong. Not only do they feel unwell; they are surrounded with medical equipment and are subjected to a barrage of

tests. They know that most people only go to the hospital when they are ill. Hiding information can be counter-productive as it may convince patients that things are much worse than they actually are. Even if you feel that a relative would not handle distressing information very well, it is almost always better to give the patient some idea of what the illness is, its implications, how surgery might help and how the patient is likely to feel afterwards, even if all the "gory details" are withheld.

Combating pain

It is only natural for people waiting for surgery to worry "Will it hurt?" Advice about how to manage pain is one of the most reassuring things that medicine can offer a patient. Surgery always involves cutting, which causes damage to nerve endings. This prompts the nerves to send messages to the brain which we feel as pain. Cutting into tissue also releases a chemical called histamine into the blood, which further stimulates the nerve endings to send pain messages to the brain. Because pain is the body's way of warning us that something is wrong, stress hormones intended for use

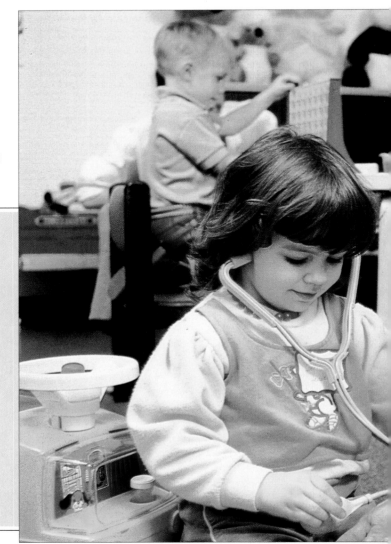

When the patient is a child

■ When children need to go into the hospital parents are often distressed about how to explain the need for treatment. Hospitals can be very frightening for children, but if they know beforehand what will happen and what to expect, their fears can be reduced.

One of the best ways is at school or playgroup. Pretend hospitals can be set up in classrooms, and the children encouraged to investigate the toy medical equipment and learn about different proce-dures. Some hospitals organize tours and produce videos which show children the inside of the building and what goes on there.

Most hospitals now encour-age parents to stay with their young children if at all possible, and may provide "play therapy" for the seriously ill and those undergoing distressing treat-ment. This involves using miniature toys and hospital equipment RIGHT to describe treatments to children and allow them to act out fears.

Children need this informa-tion, but it is not a good idea to tell a child about going into the hospital too far in advance. A day or two beforehand enables a child to organize books and toys and to ask questions, but this is not enough time for anxiety to build up.

in defense and attack are also produced, which stimulate damaged nerve endings even more and cause tension.

The brain has its own chemicals which reduce the perception of pain, including endorphins and other opiate-like substances. The actual perception of pain in the thinking part of the brain, the cortex, seems to be able to activate these endorphins. The cortex can also send messages closing off "gates" in the spinal cord which conducts nerve messages, in order to stop pain signals getting through in the first place. People who have broken a limb often say they do not feel any pain until long afterward, and this "gating" effect caused by the shock of the accident may be why. Pain relief from more minor injuries often comes from rubbing small bruises or scrapes. When we do this we are stimulating nerve fibers in the skin, and these messages interfere with the pain signals going to the brain.

The effects of drugs

The mind can reduce pain reception, but most postoperative shock is severe enough to require drugs. Anesthesia, whether general (causing loss of consciousness and the lack of all sensation) or local (removing pain sensation by numbing a selected group of nerves), allows surgery to take place without our feeling any pain at the time. The cut nerve endings will continue to send pain messages to the brain for some time, so other drugs may be given to lessen the after effects.

Strong morphine-based drugs act on the same part of our brain as natural opiates, but they do have disadvantages. Used over a long period or in large doses, they become addictive (we need more and more to get the desired effect and experience pain or withdrawal symptoms when they are removed). They may also make us drowsy and constipated,

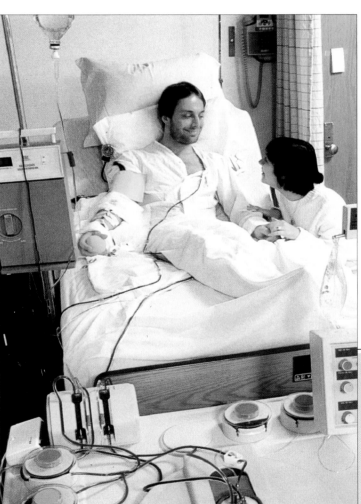

▲ **Keeping the patient cheerful** *has always been important to recovery. It is no longer normal medical practice to withhold information from severely ill patients but in some cases it is necessary to assess whether this information will upset them. It is never desirable to pretend that nothing is wrong; the person will suspect the worst if others refuse to discuss their condition. But in the case of children, the confused elderly or people of a naturally nervous disposition, it may be best not to give too many alarming details.*

129

and can even cause death by inducing too slow a rate of breathing or by straining the heart.

Particularly in the case of serious injury, which is likely to need long-term treatment and which increases the chance of heart and lung failure, alternative methods of pain management can be very useful.

For patients facing less serious surgery, drugs tend to cause slower recovery if used extensively because the drowsiness they induce prevents the person from getting up going to the toilet alone, eating properly or carrying out any of the other self-care tasks that are part of the recovery process. This slow recovery can lead to complications like bed sores, constipation, bladder infection and general debilitation from poor nutrition.

Extended drug treatment also requires a longer hospital stay. People undergoing minor surgery who can manage without extra pain-killing injections after the operation, or accept local instead of general anesthesia, can often go home the same day.

Pain management without drugs

You may recover faster without drug use, but what about pain? Hospitals are reluctant to overdo drug treatment, but if you feel your pain is severe you are the best judge. Tell the

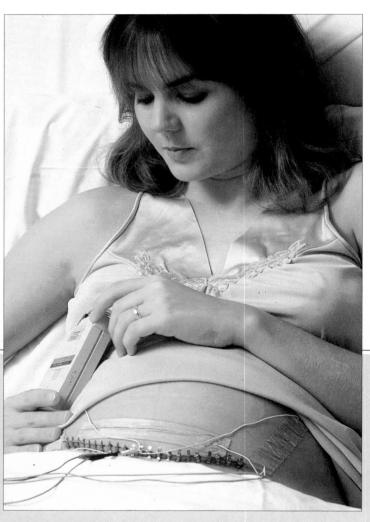

▲ **Recovering from a Caesarean birth**. *The pain of surgery as well as childbirth used to be relieved by drugs. An alternative technique now widely in use is TENS (transcutaneous electrical nerve stimulation). A small device, easily held in one hand, delivers electrical impulses to the nervous system via small electrodes on the skin. The sensation of pain is blocked from reaching the brain, where pain is felt.*

Self-hypnosis to combat pain

■ Burn injury involves the destruction of layers of skin. The outer layers contain many nerve endings which become damaged and exposed to the air. As a wound heals, nerves regrow, so even where a wound was so deep as to destroy nerve endings and be painless at the center of the burned area, it can become painful as the nerve endings regrow around the edges of the wound.

Burn patients face weeks or months of healing and many painful procedures such as surgery, wound-cleaning, changes of dressing and skin grafts. Because of the dangers of long-term drug use, particularly in such critically ill people, alternative methods of pain relief have enormous value. Methods of distraction (using music, for example) or relaxation are helpful, but self-hypnosis has proved to be extremely useful.

The technique of self-hypnosis involves a process of autosuggestion, using relaxation methods to calm and relax the mind and then suggesting positive images and feelings

Self-dosing and pain management

■ The drugs you take in hospital are usually brought round at intervals of 2-3 hours, or at longer intervals during the night. Patients do not necessarily get medication when they need it. If drugs are not given until the patient's pain is severe this may require more medication than usual; other patients may get more drugs than they really need. Hospitals have begun to experiment with self-dosing based on the recommendation of psychologists. The principle is that if patients know how and when to dose themselves, they will be able to gauge what they need themselves.

Self-dosing patients are usually given pills and a chart with instructions about dose levels and minimum intervals between doses, and allowed to skip a dose if they feel able to cope. Research on patients in Seattle, Washington, suffering from burns, heart-bypass surgery, and other operations were given this option, and actually took fewer drugs than those being dosed by nurses. They reported less pain and were able to get up earlier. So long as an illness is not interfering with the patient's thinking processes, self-dosing appears to be a valuable way to decrease dependence on drugs and improve recovery time.

doctor or nurse and they will give you additional medication. There is no need for you to feel ashamed or a failure because you are in pain. Hospital staff are now beginning to encourage alternative methods of pain management, and it may be worth trying these before turning to drugs. They will also give you greater control over your own illness. Techniques include relaxation methods (see *Ch 5*), hypnosis by a professional or self-hypnosis which involves visualizing the good results of surgery, breathing deeply and imagining relaxing or distracting scenarios. These methods will not control severe pain but they can be a great help in managing post-operative discomfort.

hich will continue during dis-essing procedures. It is taught y a psychologist or hypnosis pecialist and can be learned by hildren and adults. Hypnosis lies on the power of the nagination and motivation; in urn patients, pain control is ften to the fore of their minds.

Researchers in an army hos-ital in Houston, Texas com-ared the experience of burn atients using self-hypnosis rith those who were assisted nly by regular counseling from psychologist. All the patients rere on a self-dosing drug

regime as well. Patients of all ages, 6 to 70, regardless of the extent of their injuries, did better with self-hypnosis.

They gave themselves significantly fewer drugs, felt more relaxed, and in some cases had a sense of being divorced from or "not bothered" by their pain, almost as if it were happening to someone else. They were also discharged from hospital sooner.

This is perhaps one of the strongest proofs of the power of the mind to influence the body in a positive way.

Coming out of hospital

Most people do not spend a long time in the hospital any more, even after major surgery. Convalescence happens mainly at home, and emphasis is much less on rest and more on active rehabilitation. Even a couple of days of bed rest can lead to a rapid loss of fitness, and over a prolonged period of rest muscle tissue weakens and aerobic capacity decreases – you will find you have less strength and will tire more easily. Once your doctor gives you the go-ahead to start moving the damaged parts, however, you can begin to help lessen this deconditioning by undertaking a gentle exercise program.

No matter how fast you begin to get moving again, you will be tired and less strong. Even a light general anesthetic leaves chemicals in the blood for several days, and your body is using energy to rebuild damaged tissue. You should expect to move more slowly than usual and do not push yourself too hard. You may feel stronger and more capable than you really are. You must also avoid pulling on the scar area, particularly in the first few days when the healing process has just begun and the stitches are still in place.

The speed with which people recover varies enormously. The nature of the operation and the general health of the patient will determine the rate of recovery, but so does the patient's own state of mind. An ill-informed person may worry about trivial symptoms and make fewer efforts to regain a full activity level. A person who knows what to look out for and who knows that it is important to get going as soon as possible will recover faster. You can control your hospital experience and recovery much more effectively if you understand what to expect and take the trouble to learn what you can do to help yourself. **LMW**

131

▶ **The better the hospital experience, the sooner the patient can go home.** *The patient's experience in the hospital depends both on the quality of care they receive and their ability to approach their own treatment positively – as an opportunity for better health instead of something to be dreaded. People who are not anxious about hospital procedures will experience less pain, are less likely to have an infection, and will have a shorter recovery time – leading to an earlier release.*

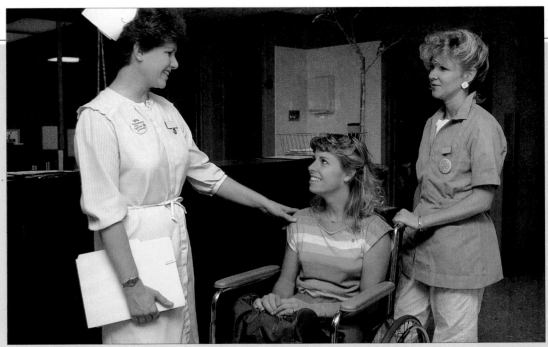

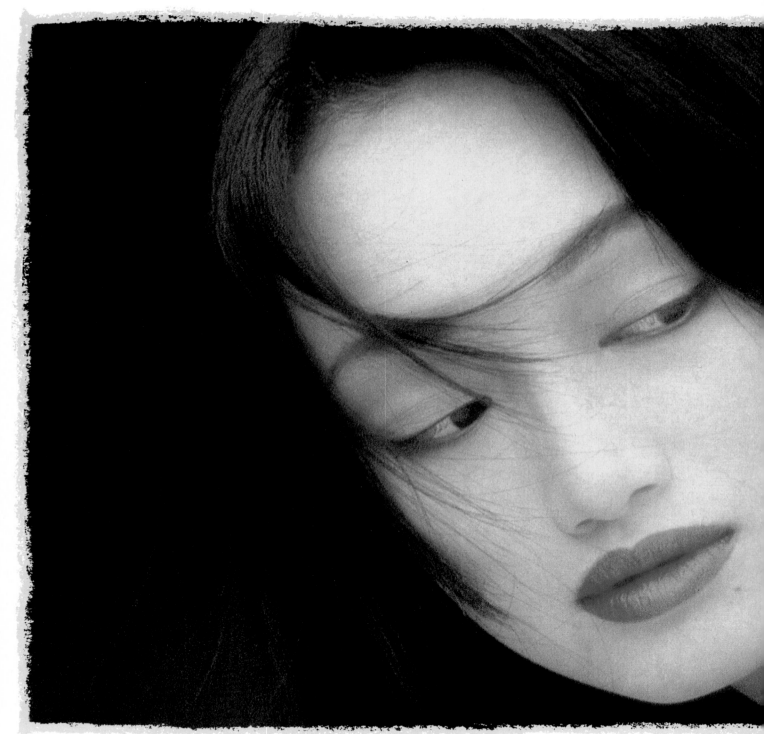

Your Appearance

PART

2

19

Do Looks Matter?

"Beauty is only skin deep, but ugly goes right to the bone" ● *Those who are either very good-looking or very bad-looking may be judged, as people, by different standards than those who are average* ● *But what are good looks?*

IN FAIRY TALES the prince is always handsome and the witch is always ugly. In cowboy movies, underneath their white hats "the good guys" have firm chins and clear blue eyes; "the bad guys" are shifty and sinister looking, perhaps with scars or other disfigurements. In the real world we know that this sort of simple equation is unfair, but psychological research shows that we still tend to judge people by their appearance. There is clear evidence that looks matter enormously to us, and that even when we think we are using objective criteria to describe people or to assess their abilities, we may unconsciously allow their physical appearance to influence our thinking.

At the same time, people tend to live up – or down – to what is expected of them, and as a consequence people's personalities and characters are shaped, in part, by their looks. If you expect someone to be a sour, disagreeable person, you tend to act in ways that help to cause their disagreeable behavior. If you expect someone to be charming and delightful, your actions tend to encourage them to show such positive personality traits. People who are regarded as attractive, consequently, are likely to be more successful in their personal and public lives. But if you are not, there is no need to despair. First, what makes a person attractive is a complex web of talents and traits, of which physical beauty is only one. Second, we can all improve our appearance and the impression we make.

The good, the bad and the ugly

Do we really treat people differently according to how they look? Most people feel that making discriminations on the basis of looks is wrong, but privately most of us seem to assume that attractive and unattractive people are different. Most often we perceive that attractive people have the more desirable traits. Research has shown that most people assume that the good-looking are far more socially appealing and socially skilled and somewhat more intelligent, effective and well-adjusted than the homely. Consequently the good-looking get better treatment. Over time, a sort of self-fulfilling prophecy occurs. The way we treat people

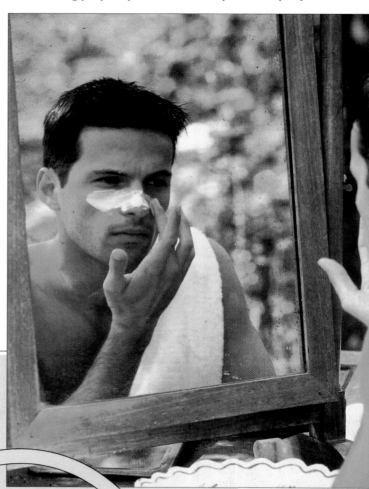

Caring about appearance

■ *Is this vanity? While looks should not be emphasized at the expense of all other qualities, everyone can benefit from taking care of their appearance. When we look in a mirror, we are checking how we look, and often the result is that we do something to make ourselves look better. The act of making improvements may itself increase our confidence, increasing the likelihood that others will find us attractive. What do you see when you look in the mirror? Is the person you see there good-looking, average, plain? Research shows that the cycle of expect-* ation RIGHT *depends mostly on how attractive people think they are, not necessarily on how attractive they really are.*

Good-looking people are expected to be more intelligent and socially adept. This influences the way they are treated.

With such favorable treatment, they respond more positively and confidently, confirming and reinforcing positive expectations.

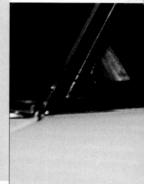

shapes the way they think about themselves and, as a result, the kind of people they become. Studies show that this sort of cause and effect occurs in many areas of our lives.

Good looks at work

Time and again studies have shown that personnel managers and employers are more likely to hire good-looking men and women, to pay them more and to promote them more readily. In three national surveys, conducted by the University of Michigan's Survey Research Center, researchers interviewed more than 1,270 men and women, aged 16 and up, who were working full time. First, interviewers rated the employees' physical appearance. (Were they strikingly handsome or beautiful, good-looking, average-looking, quite plain, or homely?) Then, the interviewers asked them exactly what their jobs were and how much they were paid. They found that for both men and women, good looks were closely linked with salary and occupational prestige. The income of handsome men was as much as $1,869 higher than that of plain men. The income of beautiful women was on average $1,227 higher than that of their plain counterparts. Height and weight also play a part – tall men tend to get on better than short ones, and slim women better than their plumper equivalents.

The researchers assessed employees' occupational prestige according to *Duncan's Socioeconomic Status Scale*, which lists the prestige of almost every conceivable job on a scale of 1 to 100. The prestige rating for good-looking men's and women's jobs was around 49-50. (The jobs in this range included clergymen, music teachers, floor manager, bookkeepers, photographers, student nurses and managers of food stores.) Homely looking men and women had jobs of lower prestige rating, in the 31-34 range. (These jobs included housekeepers, building superintendents and managers, boilermakers, machinists, and managers of service-stations.) Obviously good looks pay – both in money and in prestige.

Fitting the looks to the job

Physical attractiveness is only one factor that helps determine how quickly men and women are hired, how much they are paid, and how quickly they are promoted, but other things count too. A person's appearance must be appropriate for the job they want to do. Some jobs seem more suitable for men, others for women. For a traditional man's job such as a mechanic, delicate beauty might be a disadvantage. And different jobs might have different physical qualifications. The same rough good looks that we would regard as ideal in a sports personality might work against someone looking for a desk-bound job. Professional

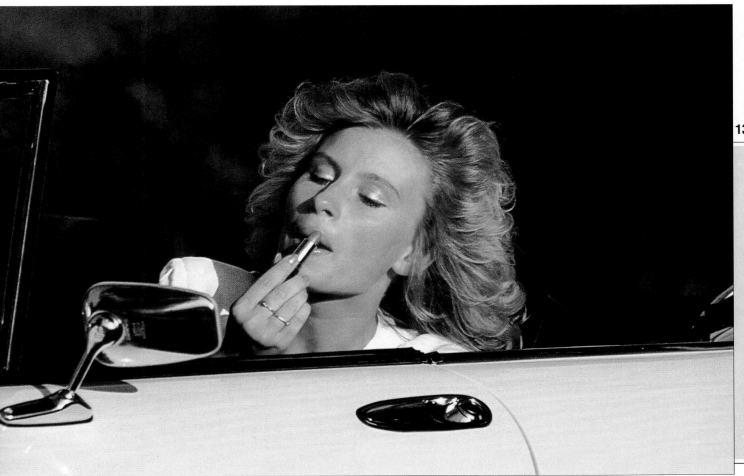

demeanor, intelligence, education and experience are critically important too. Although appearance is clearly important in the business world, it is probably more important to look appropriate and to seem intelligent, well qualified for the job and hardworking.

Living up to expectations

How do our looks affect our social interactions? Do homely people have restricted social lives? Do they get along with people differently as a consequence? Often expectations are a sort of self-fulfilling prophecy.

The fact that people often act just as we expect them to was demonstrated in an intriguing study by Mark Snyder, Edward Tanke and Ellen Berscheid. Men and women at the University of Minnesota, who were strangers, were recruited and paired off for a study on "the processes by which people become acquainted with each other." As the men and women arrived, they were sent to different rooms without meeting each other and they had to use the telephone to become acquainted.

Before the conversation began, each man was given a snapshot of his partner, along with some biographical information. They were not allowed to see their partner in person, however. In truth, the snapshot was not of their partner, but was of either a good-looking or a homely woman. Men were asked their initial impressions of the women before the telephone conversations began. Men who thought they would be talking to an attractive woman expected her to be sociable, poised, humorous, and socially adept. Men who had been led to believe that their telephone partner was homely, expected her to be unsociable, awkward, serious, and socially inept. Those were the men's *expectations* and they do not surprise us. We already know that good-looking women make a more positive first

impression than homely ones. What is startling is that the men's expectations had a dramatic impact on the women's responses in the short space of a telephone call. Some men talked to a partner they thought was beautiful. Others talked to someone they thought was quite unattractive. In fact, the women on the other end of the line had no resemblance to the photos shown to their male partners. Some were attractive, some average, some extremely plain. Nonetheless, the women became what the men expected them to be. What the men and women said on the telephone was recorded separately.

The researchers then asked judges to listen to the women's voices and to estimate what they might be like. If a man thought he was talking to a beautiful woman, she soon sensed that, and began acting that way, too.

Women who had been presented as attractive became more animated, confident, and socially skilled. Women who had been presented as homely acted exactly that way. As the organizers put it: "What had initially been reality in

Good looks on trial

▶ Special treatment is given to all people who are extremely attractive, not just to well-known personalities and movie stars. However, there are disadvantages. Very good-looking people stand accused, by common assumption, of being selfish and vain. Confirmation of the assumption may be seized upon, whenever it seems to appear. RIGHT Good-looking celebrities are constantly on trial in the public eye. If their livelihood depends on their looks, they may find their lives falling apart when they begin to age. Famous people may be criticized in the media if they

gain weight, begin to wrinkle or otherwise let themselves go; stars are supposed to be beautiful forever.

■ **Appearance influences the perceptions of judges and jurors** in courtroom trials. Good-looking defendants who engage in illegal activities are less likely to get caught in the first place. If caught, their crimes are less likely to be reported; if they do go to court, they are likely to receive more lenient treatment – except attractive women who have used their looks to commit a crime.

Consulting about your image

■ Politicians, actors, and some people not so much in the public eye, employ image consultants to advise them how to dress, style their hair, apply makeup, even how to walk and talk, to convey the desired image of authority, confidence or sensuality.

An image consultant will go through your wardrobe and advise you what to keep, what to throw out, and what to have altered. They will take you on a shopping trip to buy new and more suitable clothes.

You will also learn *how* to shop and what your weak-nesses are in this area – do you buy on impulse and then regret your purchase? Are you too cautious? Image consultants will help you build up a set of clothing and accessories that will suit you, your job, and your lifestyle.

They will also make recommendations about how you might change your hair and makeup, either in ways that will suit your face or that are more in keeping with what you do. A woman lawyer, for instance, might be persuaded to tame attractive but girlish long hair into a neater style which is still attractive but gives her more authority.

Politicians and film stars often take elocution lessons. You may feel this is unnecessary, but image consultants can give tips for self-presentation which make enormous differences – trying not to raise your voice at the end of a sentence, but lowering it instead makes your speech sound more confident.

Some people who employ an image consultant have their instincts about clothes, hair-styles and self-presentation confirmed; others can be radic-ally transformed. In either case you have the assurance that you are doing the right thing about your appearance, and that in itself builds confidence.

It can be expensive, as you will have to pay a consultant's fee and commit yourself to pur-chasing new clothing; but the consultants argue that you actually save money by equip-ping yourself with a good work-ing wardrobe, and that your improved image will reap divi-dends in new work and social opportunities. Certainly improved self-confidence is worth a great deal.

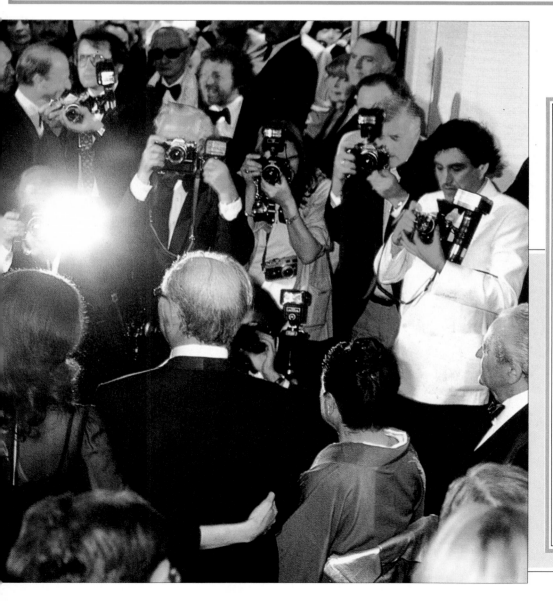

The attractive child

■ Teachers expect a cute child to do well in school, and looks do seem to play some part in the evaluation and grading of children.

In a typical study, two psy-chologists asked 400 teachers to take a look at a few children's academic files, which included false photographs.

Some teachers saw a picture of a boy or girl who was quite attractive in a file. For others, the same file included a photo-graph of an exceedingly plain child. In spite of the abundance of more objective information, when files included attractive photographs, teachers assessed boys and girls as more intelligent. They thought that their parents were more interested in education, and that they would be more likely to get advanced degrees than other students. The teachers in the experiment expected good-looking students to be popular as well as academic.

the minds of the men had now become reality in the behavior of the women they interacted with." The men expected beautiful women to be more sociable so anyone that they perceived as beautiful acted in that way.

How looks influence behavior

What happened to transfer the perceptions of confidence, humor and friendliness in the minds of the men, into reality in the behavior of the women? When the men's sides of the conversations were analyzed, it was found that those who thought they were talking to a beautiful woman were more

sociable, sexually warm, interesting, independent, sexually permissive, bold, outgoing, humorous and socially adept than were men who thought they were talking to a homely woman. The men assigned to an "attractive woman" were also judged to be more comfortable, to enjoy themselves more and to use their voices more effectively. In a nutshell, the men who thought they had an attractive partner made more effort.

If the stereotypes in these men's minds became a social reality within only ten minutes of a telephone conversation, we can imagine what happens over several years. If, year

Pairing off — like attracts like

■ Your appearance is important in almost every area of life, but nowhere does it matter more than in intimate encounters. Although most of us can describe the ideal date or partner of our dreams, what we want and what we get are two different things. We generally end up with partners whose assets and liabilities overall match our own. Studies in the United States, Canada, Germany, and Japan find that people generally end up dating and marrying someone who is similar in appearance.

In a typical study, researchers photographed and video-taped couples in a variety of natural settings — in movie theater lines, in singles bars, and at assorted social events. Next, researchers rated the daters' looks. Not surprisingly, it was found that most couples were remarkably similar in attractiveness. A handsome

man was most likely to have a beautiful woman on his arm. A homely man was likely to be spotted buying a drink for a homely woman.

It was also found that "similarity breeds content." The more similar couples were in looks, the more delighted they

seemed to be with one another, judging by the way they touched each other. Sixty percent of the couples of similar attractiveness were engaged in some type of intimate touching: they stood close to one another, engaged in horseplay, or hung on one

another's arms. In contrast, only 22 percent of those couples who were mismatched were touching.

We may be most comfortable with those who match us in levels of attractiveness because we have similar social skills and stratagems.

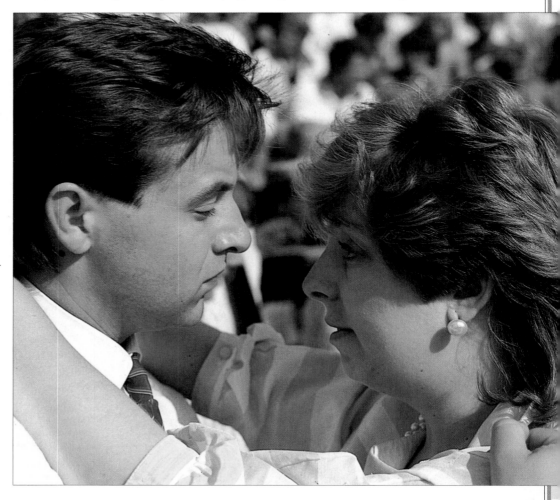

▶ **An obvious match?**
Couples are more likely to be attracted to each other when they are equally attractive. Good-looking people tend to gravitate toward others who are good-looking, while those who are plain may feel more comfortable with people of similar appearance. Studies have shown that couples who are equally attractive are more likely to touch each other and appear to be enjoying each other's company in public.

after year, attractive people are given more opportunities and more encouragement in social interaction than unattractive people, then undoubtedly, attractive and unattractive people become different social beings.

What would happen if, in a similar study, the man was not initially biased and had no idea what his partner looked like? Would the woman's real appearance shine through? In reality, do attractive men and women display more social skill over the telephone? Such a study *was* conducted and it was found that attractive men and women were judged by their telephone partners to be more socially skilled than unattractive men and women. Clearly, even when we cannot be seen, we conform to the expectations people have of us based on our appearance.

Attracting the opposite sex

In general, researchers have concluded that attractive and homely men and women have very different everyday social experiences. In one study, male and female students in their first term at the University of Rochester in New York kept records of their social encounters for 40 days. Not surprisingly, handsome men encountered more women, more frequently and for longer periods of time than homely men.

Good-looking people spent more of their time with others conversing or partying, while less attractive people spent more time engaged in tasks. Attractive men and women said they were more satisfied with their encounters with the opposite sex than less attractive people. The net result was that over time the physically attractive people became more and more satisfied with their relationships.

Other researchers support the notion that attractive men and women have the most satisfying social interactions. Some psychologists have found that attractive people tend to have more intimate and open relationships on the whole than those who are plain.

The attractive personality

Even if we did have a single ideal *physical* type in mind when we evaluate appearance, attractiveness is still not a simple issue. We all know beautiful women and handsome men who do not photograph well – and vice versa. Their laughing, talking, animated faces are more than the sum of their physical features. And we probably all remember the class clown, often an awkward, gawky child who was popular because of an attractive and confident personality. All the research on what attractiveness is shows that the ability

139

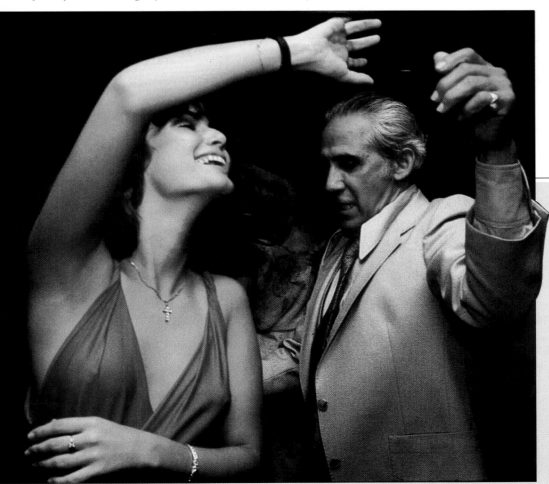

◄ **An obvious mismatch?** *Psychologist Bernard Murstein and his colleagues named the pairing of unlikely looking couples "complex matching." A couple that appear to be mismatched physically may be "compensating" in other ways. A typical example of compensatory exchange occurs when an older man with money and social status marries a young beautiful woman. He is in effect trading his prestige and power for her youth and attractiveness. Such couples appear to break the rules of pairing off because of the disparities in their levels of individual attractiveness, and bystanders may be puzzled at seeing them together.*

to put others at ease and to be amusing and interesting, is an important part of being attractive. Those who are obviously beautiful or handsome have an immoderate advantage because people expect and encourage them to be socially skilled. But the research also shows that if we project a confident and friendly personality, people will therefore expect us to be attractive.

Finding a balanced approach

The advice to be "moderate" is hard to accept. It is always appealing to see the world in simple terms. "What is beautiful is good." "More is better." But things are more complicated than that. Real life is lived in the gray areas: the realm of complexities, ambiguities and half-truths. As we

have seen, attractiveness is not a simple or a single quality, and it is easy to think that "If only I was ten pounds lighter" or "two inches taller" everything would be fine.

A variety of factors – self-esteem, intelligence, an exciting personality, vivacity, sensitivity and compassion, money, power and prestige – as well as physical characteristics, all have an impact on how good-looking we seem to others. Clinical psychologists have observed that many people focus too much on looks and neglect the things that really count. Such people may end up spiritually, personally, socially and economically impoverished and, ironically, *not* very attractive.

Becoming a more attractive person involves many different aspects of your looks and personality. If we spend too

But what *are* "good looks"?

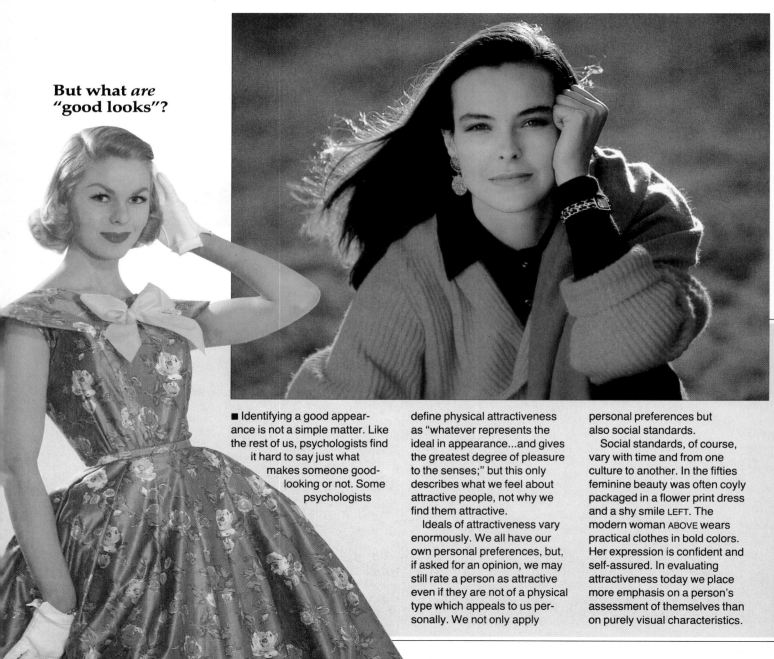

■ Identifying a good appearance is not a simple matter. Like the rest of us, psychologists find it hard to say just what makes someone good-looking or not. Some psychologists define physical attractiveness as "whatever represents the ideal in appearance...and gives the greatest degree of pleasure to the senses;" but this only describes what we feel about attractive people, not why we find them attractive.

Ideals of attractiveness vary enormously. We all have our own personal preferences, but, if asked for an opinion, we may still rate a person as attractive even if they are not of a physical type which appeals to us personally. We not only apply personal preferences but also social standards.

Social standards, of course, vary with time and from one culture to another. In the fifties feminine beauty was often coyly packaged in a flower print dress and a shy smile LEFT. The modern woman ABOVE wears practical clothes in bold colors. Her expression is confident and self-assured. In evaluating attractiveness today we place more emphasis on a person's assessment of themselves than on purely visual characteristics.

much time on our physical appearance and too little time learning about people, seeking out friends, getting an education and buckling down to work, we will not be attractive people, though we may be pleasant to look at.

Thinking positively and responsively

Balance is the key. Improving your physical appearance, for instance, is not just a matter of applying makeup correctly and dressing beautifully. Taking care of your body, eating properly and getting enough exercise and sleep are crucial to your basic appearance. Living healthily makes you look better and it makes you feel better, too. If you are confident about yourself physically you will project a more attractive image and others will respond positively in return.

Balance is also required in the other elements which go to make up attractiveness. The handicapped face special challenges and difficulties in life. Still the evidence makes it clear that even those who are the most disfigured and handicapped have a good chance of happiness if they can develop some of the other aspects of attractiveness – compassion, excitement with life and so forth. Many handicapped people are sensitive to the worries and problems of others, and have many friends who value them.

We cannot all be beautiful or handsome, but we can learn to treat other people well, to listen to them, draw them out and respond with warmth and interest. Because people tend unconsciously to associate the good and the beautiful, good listeners are often rated as popular and attractive.

Improve your personality

A good listener who has nothing to say, however, often becomes a doormat for other people. If you do not project an interesting as well as an interested personality you will not improve your overall attractiveness. Very beautiful people, for instance, may have no ability to hold a conversation. They are less attractive and successful than those who, by developing their full potential – getting an education, furthering a chosen career or pursuing a fascinating hobby – always have lots to talk about.

Your character is shaped in part by your looks. But your appearance is also affected by your personality. By developing all your strong points, you can make enormous improvements to your appearance. If you like the person you have become, you will project the confidence and zest for life which people associate with good looks – and they will respond with enthusiasm. **EH**

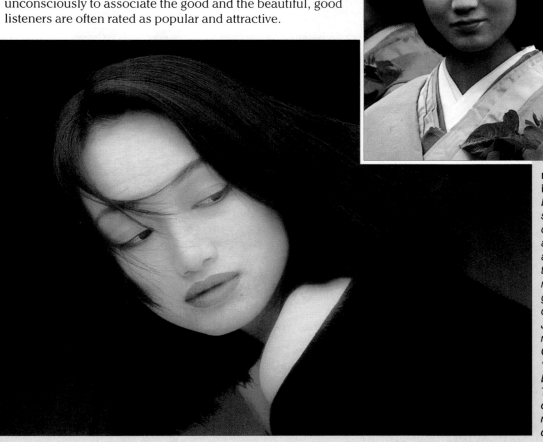

141

■ **Changing culture, changing ideals of beauty.** *As national barriers become less rigid, the standards of beauty for one culture may begin to permeate another, aided by mass media and technology. Where once the women in Japan most renowned for beauty were the geisha – ABOVE in traditional costume and makeup – many Japanese women now favor a more international look LEFT. Cosmetic surgery to create "Western" eyes and noses has become popular in Hong Kong, Taiwan, Japan and other Asian countries, where foreign models (blond Europeans) are often used in advertising.*

How much beauty is enough?

■ People generally perceive the good-looking to be special, treat them that way, and as a consequence they benefit in their education, careers and social lives. What conclusions should we draw from this? Perhaps not what you would expect. Clinicians and experimental social psychologists have come to agree that what is needed is not an even greater emphasis on beauty, but balance.

Beauty at a disadvantage

Sheer physical beauty can be a positive disadvantage in life. A famous model and actress once complained that she seldom dated at school because people found her intimidating; men felt they could not possibly be "good enough" for her. As a result she spent more time alone in the evenings than her less stunning classmates.

Good-looking people may also have trouble making friends of their own sex, and may be suspicious of approaches from the opposite sex, believing that they are "only wanted for their looks."

Research also indicates that the only thing people do not expect from good-looking people is integrity or concern for others. We expect the attractive to be selfish and self-involved. And this expectation, like the others mentioned earlier, can be a self-fulfilling prophecy.

Extraordinarily good-looking people are likely to get jobs that are dependent upon appearance and attract lovers who are very concerned about looks. This often works well so long as the person is young and beautiful. But all of us inevitably have off-days; worse still, we grow older. Being very attractive can be a difficult standard to maintain, especially on a purely physical level. We all want to improve our appearance, but in our pursuit of good looks we have to find a balanced approach in order to be truly attractive.

Average is almost as good

Men and women should certainly spend some time maintaining their appearance. Time and again research supports the notion that good-looking (or even average) men and women have a real advantage in life. But if they invest too much time in achieving and maintaining merely physical

appeal, the immediate short-term rewards may be great, but the long-term sacrifices may be even greater. We may all secretly hope to become extraordinarily good-looking, but evidence suggests that if we did, we would find, to our disappointment, that our lives would not change much.

Research reveals that good-looking people have an advantage over average-looking people who in turn, have an advantage over homely and disfigured people. But we are so obsessed with good looks that we forget that the spectrum of appearance includes "beautiful" people, average-looking ones, ugly people and people with disfiguring handicaps. If we look carefully at the relationship between appearance and a host of other variables – self-esteem, job opportunities, dating popularity, happiness – we discover that there is only a small advantage to being more beautiful or handsome than average. You would gain something if, through great creativity and sacrifice, you became a stunning person instead of an ordinary one...but not much.

Stunning people have only a slight advantage over their more ordinary peers but the average looking have a real advantage over the homely or the disfigured. **EH**

▶ **Haunted beauty**. *Marilyn Monroe, seen here with her third husband, the playwright Arthur Miller, was adored for a decade as the most beautiful woman in the world. Trends of fashion and loveliness usually do not last this long. According to cultural ideals, she should have been happy. Yet she was childless, twice divorced, suffered depression and problems with alcohol, and died in mysterious circumstances from a drug overdose before she reached middle age. The rock star Elton John paid tribute to her in "Candle in the Wind," a song describing her struggle with private demons under the glaring eye of world fame. She was hounded by the media even after her death, which is still the subject of documentaries and biographies nearly 30 years later. Ironically, had she belonged to a later generation, she would have been considered too fleshy to be the embodiment of feminine perfection.*

Good looks and self-esteem

■ Psychologists have found surprisingly little relationship between people's self-esteem and how good they actually look (as assessed by objective judges). At most there is a tendency for good-looking people to have slightly higher self-esteem than unattractive people. The tendency is extremely slight.

When reasonably attractive but ordinary-looking people sit down to complete a self-esteem questionnaire they tend to end up with scores that are surprisingly similar to those of very good-looking people.

What about the relationship between people's self-esteem and what they *think* they look like? Psychologists have found that men and women who are

satisfied with their looks also have high self-esteem – they consider themselves moral, sensitive, honest, fair, likable. Those dissatisfied with their looks are likely, on the whole, to have low self-esteem.

About 45 percent of 62,000 surveyed in a body-image questionnaire (see *Ch20*) were only "somewhat satisfied" or "somewhat dissatisfied" with their looks.

About half were *more* than somewhat satisfied. Slightly more men than women (55 percent versus 45 percent) came into this category.

A trivial 4 percent of men and 7 percent of women turned out to be quite or extremely dissatisfied with their overall appearance. **EH**

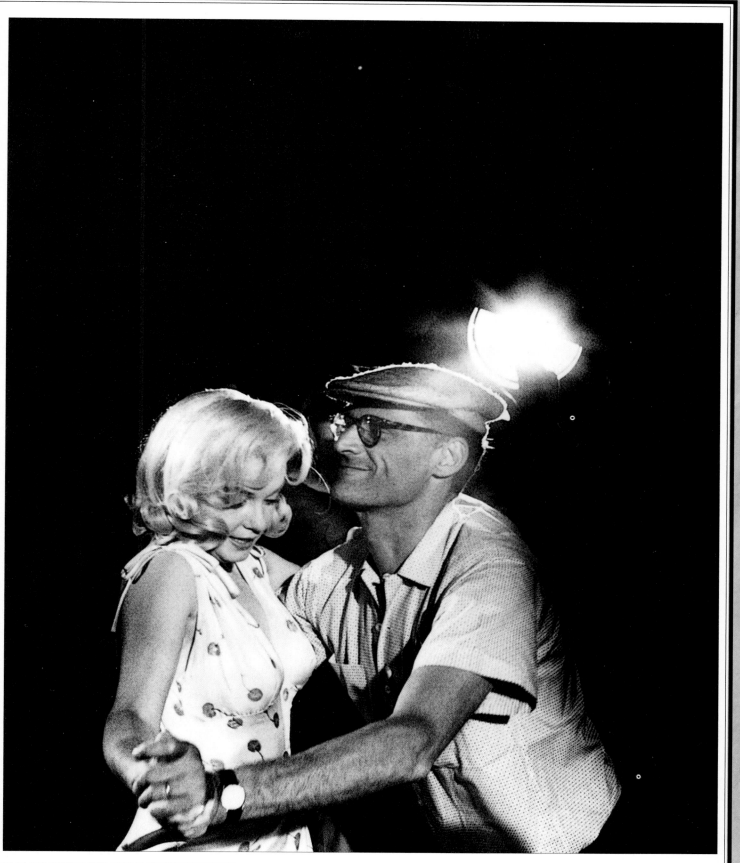

20

Your Bodyshape

How happy are you with your physique, your face, your coloring? ● *The way to a better body image starts in your own mind* ● *Often, the challenge is to change the way you look at yourself, not what you see.*

THE RELATIONSHIP between how we look and how we feel begins in childhood. Girls learn early how important it is to be "pretty," boys that it is good to be strong and tall. Research suggests that body image and self-esteem are closely linked but objective physical attractiveness and self-esteem are not; some very attractive people worry excessively about a minor flaw while other, less attractive people radiate confidence about their looks.

A healthy body image means that you accept your basic frame and body type and either feel happy about it or have realistic expectations about what you can change. A tendency to be obsessive about the way you look or the things that you feel are wrong with your appearance may signal a deep discontent with yourself and have little to do with objective reality. This lack of self-acceptance may express itself in an excessive admiration for stereotyped images of people who look "right." By contrast, people who have a positive view of themselves are often grateful *not* to conform to social stereotypes – they take satisfaction in having a strongly individual identity.

Shaping up – women looking at men

What features do men and women prefer in the opposite sex? If television commercials are to be believed, every woman wants a man with a massive upper body slimming to the waist in a classic V shape. However, some research has indicated that women find less muscular physiques more attractive. For the purpose of this study the male body was divided into four sections – arms, shoulders and chest, waist, hips and legs – and it was found that most women seemed to prefer the medium physique over others. Men with slim legs seemed to be the most favored, while those with underdeveloped chests and shoulders and broad waists and hips were liked the least.

Women seemed to prefer men whose bodyshape was similar to their own: thin women preferred thin men, and medium-sized women preferred medium-sized men. The results suggest that if you are a slim and athletic woman, then it is likely that you will prefer a man who also projects a lean and athletic image. If, on the other hand, you are heavy and do not enjoy exercise, then you may prefer a man who, by the image he projects, also seems to prefer not to exercise regularly.

Women who are traditional or conservative in outlook seem to prefer the classic male physique (the V shape) whereas more unconventional women tend to prefer male bodies that do not conform to a stereotype. The findings seem to suggest that women's preferences for male body types reflect their overall attitude toward tradition and cultural trends. The muscle-bound physique may not be currently seen as the most attractive, but the present emphasis on exercise and bodybuilding may perhaps lead to an increase in its popularity among women.

Shaping up – men looking at women

There has been a widely-held but untested belief that male preferences for the female shape were limited to the emphasis placed on individual body parts – breasts,

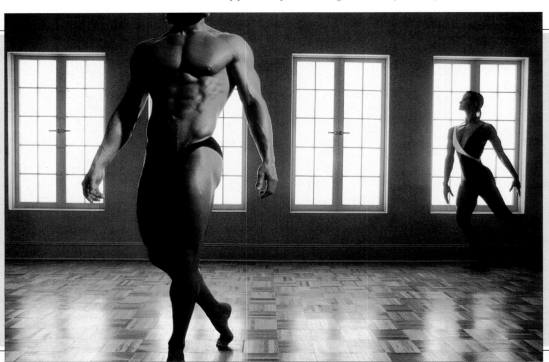

◄ **Every woman's dream man?** *The classic V-shaped male physique – massive chest and shoulders tapering to a narrow waist – has long been idealized as the way men should look. Many body building courses have based their advertising on cartoons of skinny weaklings transformed into strong men who are very successful with women. In fact, not all women prefer this body shape on a man; those who do are likely to be traditional and conservative in their attitudes toward male/female relations.*

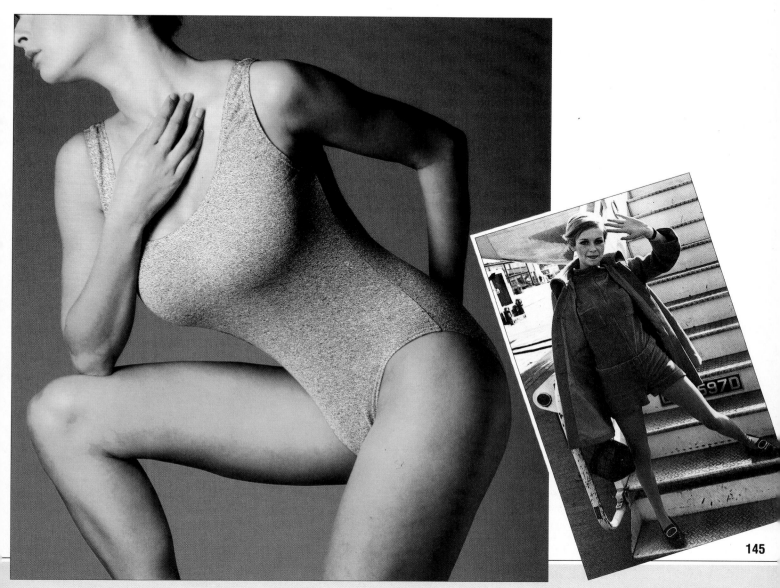

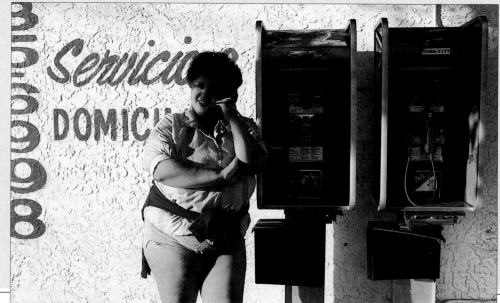

■ **Every man's dream woman?** *One study found that men's preference for female body shapes corresponds to the men's personalities. A man whose ideal woman resembles the classic full-breasted look* ABOVE *is likely to be extravagant and excessive in his behavior. A man who prefers the thin Twiggy body shape* UPPER RIGHT *is likely to be reserved, and a preference for rounded, well-padded women* RIGHT *may indicate a desire for nurturing.*

buttocks and legs. More recently, it has been found that men have a much more complex perception of what makes a woman physically attractive and that they prefer distinct body types rather than individual parts. One study found that male preferences in female bodies could be divided into five categories. Four of these revealed associations between the preferred female bodyshape and particular personality traits in the men.

The first group of men preferred the "ideal" female shape: moderately large breasts, medium to small buttocks and medium legs. These men tended to be self-confident and have a positive outlook – winning qualities usually represented in the media by glamorous people of both sexes with ideal bodies. The second group were more reserved and found women with medium breasts, small buttocks and medium legs to be most attractive. Just as they did not seem prone to excessive behavior, these men did not find excess in the female form appealing.

The third group of men selected women with Rubenesque figures – ample breasts, medium buttocks and ample legs. These men were reported as being disorganized, lacking persistence and likely to feel guilty or inferior; their choice might indicate a desire for nurturing or comfort. The fourth group clearly emphasized large breasts in their preference, which was also characterized by medium buttocks and medium legs. These proportions indicated an extravagant outlook on life where excess may be desirable.

These results suggest that men's attitudes toward female bodies are consistent with their outlook on other aspects of their lives. If you do not see yourself as excessive, in other words, you are likely to prefer a woman who also does not project an image of physical excess; if you see yourself as normal and well-adjusted, you are likely to prefer a woman who also projects a "normal" or "ideal" image.

Self-image plays a very important role for both men and women both in determining and in explaining our preferences for particular body types in the opposite sex. The findings of this research may help us to understand why we consider some people attractive and others unattractive, and why our perceptions may be different from other people's. They may also help to explain what types of people are likely to find us attractive given the image we may be projecting to others with our bodies.

146

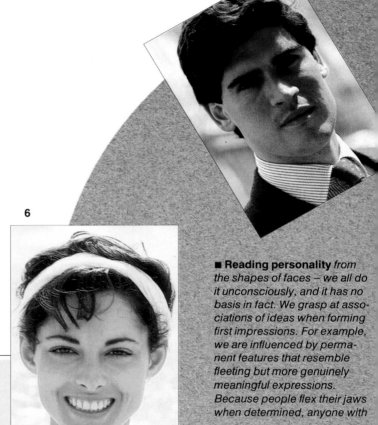

■ **Reading personality** *from the shapes of faces – we all do it unconsciously, and it has no basis in fact. We grasp at associations of ideas when forming first impressions. For example, we are influenced by permanent features that resemble fleeting but more genuinely meaningful expressions. Because people flex their jaws when determined, anyone with*

The shape of your face

■ Your face contributes more to your personal image than any other part of your body. It is to the face that we look first for information about people.

Researchers have divided facial features into general categories – rapid, slow and static:

Rapid features include facial muscles, skin tone, sweat, pupil size and direction of gaze. They play an important role in the expression of mood, emotion and attitudes.

Slow features include bags under the eyes, pouches, wrinkles, hair and skin texture, and may change over the course of a day (facial hair in men) or a lifetime (wrinkles).

The changes in slow features are usually gradual. Age, weather, nutrition and the continual repetition of a particular expression will all leave their mark over time.

Static features change imperceptibly over time and include bone structure, skin pigmentation and genetically or racially determined features.

Over these we have virtually no natural control; by and large we have to accept them.

They do seem to be the basis for our recognition of others – we are more likely to recognize other people by the shape of their faces than by facial expressions.

Forming impressions from bodyshape

Because we use other people's appearance as a source of information about them, a language of stereotypes is an unfortunate but inevitable result. For example, we sometimes unconsciously rely on the shape and weight of other people's bodies to give us an idea of their personality and temperament. According to our society's most popular stereotypes, thin people are seen as more sensitive, tense, nervous, suspicious, inhibited and apprehensive, whereas

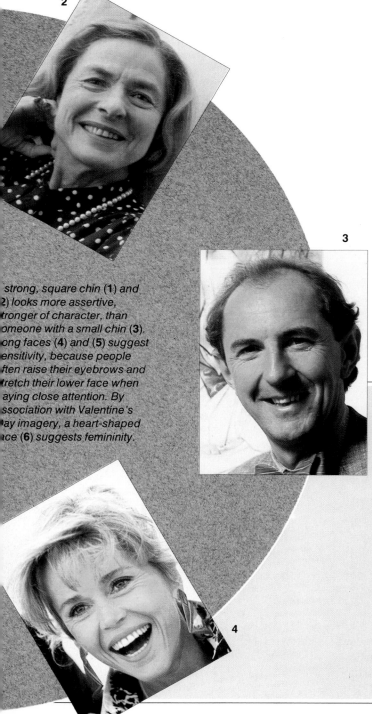

strong, square chin (**1**) and (**2**) looks more assertive, stronger of character, than someone with a small chin (**3**). Long faces (**4**) and (**5**) suggest sensitivity, because people often raise their eyebrows and stretch their lower face when paying close attention. By association with Valentine's Day imagery, a heart-shaped face (**6**) suggests femininity.

overweight people tend to be viewed as sociable, cheerful, easy going, conventional, weak-willed and perhaps even self-indulgent. People with a muscular build are often seen as being youthful in their outlook, adventurous, competitive, self-reliant, assertive, mature, bold, direct and energetic. It seems, therefore, that those people with athletic-looking bodies tend to have the most desirable personality traits attributed to them.

Few of us fit exactly into any of these extreme categories but may have characteristics of one or all of them. It is useful to be aware of stereotypes, however, because even though our basic body type is genetically predetermined to a certain extent and there is little we can do to change it, they are helpful in giving us some idea of the judgments people may be making about us.

Evidence suggests that excess weight is usually noticed and considered undesirable, and that the social stigma of obesity is understood at a very early age. It has been found that, for American women, being thin is strongly related to perceptions of higher social class. Many of them also believe that they would be more likely to win the Miss America contest if they were lighter than the average contestant rather than heavier.

Over 50 percent of American women and 30 percent of American men have reported in surveys that they wanted to lose weight, indicating widespread dissatisfaction with their bodies. But in addition to this trend toward a thinner "ideal" self, the average weight of young women has been on the increase and these opposing forces have apparently led to increases in eating disorders like anorexia nervosa and bulimia (see *Chs 9,10*).

There are other complications connected with the pursuit of the ideal figure. For example, if a woman's weight drops too dramatically, she is likely to experience problems with

147

Body parts and self-esteem

■ Research shows that certain body parts are more important for self-esteem than others. We may not care much what our toes look like, but our whole sense of worth may be precariously balanced on our face or body build.

One study found that for both men and women satisfaction with the following body characteristics was most often related to self-esteem: complexion, distribution of weight, waist, nose, body build and face.

What body characteristics were not important? For men, unimportant features included height, ankles and chin. For women, hair texture, teeth, arms

and mouth were among these.

In a questionnaire given to 62,000 people (see *Ch 19*), almost everyone was happy with their face. Almost 50 percent of the women and 35 percent of the men were unhappy with their weight, and twice as many women as men were very dissatisfied (21 percent versus 10 percent).

People worried about their weight were also unhappy about their abdomen, buttocks, hips and thighs. Some 36 percent of the men were concerned over their "spare tires." Women worried about the size of their hips – 49 percent were dissatisfied. **EH**

her menstrual cycle. The shift from the more voluptuous form of years past toward the lean look of the modern woman is, therefore, having long-term emotional and physical effects on women growing up in the 1990s.

Coloring the picture

Another factor that we take into account when we judge other people is their coloring and this too is susceptible to a range of stereotypes. We tend to associate certain characteristics with certain shades; for example, Caucasians who are too pale are considered anemic; those who are too rosy, excitable, and so on. These stereotypes seem to be based slightly more firmly in reality insofar as a pale skin may well indicate that a person is tired or ill, and a rosy flush may be the result of anger or embarrassment. But, on the other hand, a deep tan, commonly interpreted in the past as a healthy glow, really gives very little indication of someone's underlying state of health.

Every body is different

There is no single "best" way to look. All of us have both positive and negative features. To enhance our self-image and the image we project to others, we need to recognize which of our features are most positive and to emphasize them. By anticipating others' initial reactions, we can aim to modify them by dressing or behaving in ways that will improve the image we project. Persistence in projecting a positive and self-confident image of ourselves is probably the most effective way of breaking down the inaccurate stereotyped images other people may have formed of us and encouraging them to see beyond our most obvious physical characteristics. Other people's preconceptions should eventually begin to be replaced by the images we choose to present to them.

Bodyshape is one of the most important features in the overall presentation of ourselves. If we have the idea that our own bodyshape is usually seen in a negative way, we can compensate by adopting behavior that minimizes those perceptions. If you are overweight, for instance, the obvious solution seems to be simply to lose weight, but this is only part of the issue. Experiment with projecting yourself as

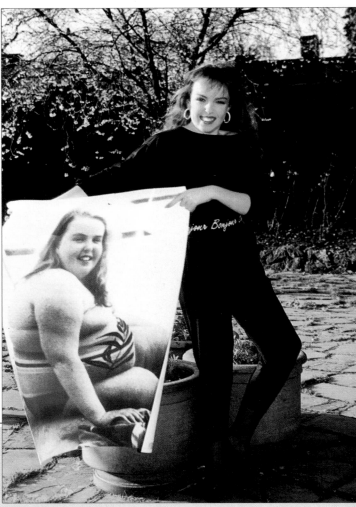

Changing your mirror image

■ If you are not satisfied with your body, stand in front of a full-length mirror with a hand mirror to help you check your appearance from all angles. Make a list of all the things you do not like about yourself and give each item a code:
I Impossible – something such as your height or bone structure that cannot be changed, though it could be disguised.
P Professional – something that would require professional help to fix, such as crooked teeth or bust size.
C Change – something you know can be changed such as your haircut or your weight.

First check the Cs on the list. Do you care enough about these things to take action to change them? If the answer is yes, underline them and make a firm decision to take action. If they are not important enough to you to do anything about them, there is no point in worrying about them any more and you should cross them off your list.

Next, look at the Ps. Are they really a possibility? Can you afford the cost of professional help? Is the problem really that important to you? Again, either decide to do something about it and make some inquiries, or choose to accept it.

Finally, count the number of impossible dislikes that are left. Then take another look at yourself in the mirror and, this time, make a second list of all the things you like about yourself. Go on writing until the list of your likes is at least as long as your list of impossible dislikes. Make a decision to begin to appreciate and accentuate your positive features and not to dwell on the others. The more you focus on your good points, the less you will notice or even care about the things you do not like.

▲ **A program of change** for improving your bodyshape can be realized with patience and self-discipline. When assessing aspects of your appearance that you would like to change, it is important to be realistic. Excess weight need not be a permanent condition, but even the strictest regimen will not alter bone structure.

more socially confident, self-reliant and energetic. You might try dressing in a way that does not necessarily hide the fact that you are heavy, but reduces its significance. If you are too thin, try to project yourself as relaxed and comfortable in social situations.

As with other stereotypes, prejudices about height can be overcome through behavior and presentation. We cannot do anything to change our height but we can change our attitude toward it. Rather than trying to compensate for it, we should attempt to diminish its importance by not being overly sensitive about it and by projecting confidence in ourselves in spite of it.

Coloring, like height, is something that usually does not change in the long term, although makeup and hair color can accomplish temporary changes. Overcoming the stereotypes associated with particular colorings may require us to avoid behavior which might reinforce the negative stereotypes ("dumb blonde," "temperamental redhead," "sultry brunette") and, instead, emphasize behavior more commonly seen as positive.

Before you can begin to project a positive image you need to develop it in your own mind, and that means spending time re-acquainting yourself with your body and tuning in to its needs. Your body's needs are your needs; it is not simply a machine that occasionally lets you down. When you feel ill and tired your body might be trying to tell you that you have eaten the wrong foods, perhaps drunk too much or been working too hard. Rather than spending all your time worrying about the things you do not like about your body and wondering why it is letting you down, put your energies into taking care of it and focusing on the good things. As your awareness increases, you will find yourself able to avoid many health and beauty problems. You will also find increased energy that can transform both your self-image and your lifestyle.

The first step is to accept your own body. Everyone has things they do not like about their own bodies but it is important to put your dislikes into perspective.

Be realistic about what you can change and what you cannot. You have no control over your basic skeletal and muscular frame but there is a great deal you can do to improve the way you look, walk and feel. You can do this by losing any excess weight, toning up your muscles and improving your posture. The reward for this exercise when it is done in a spirit of self-acceptance is that you can relax about your body and focus your energies elsewhere. **DC MK**

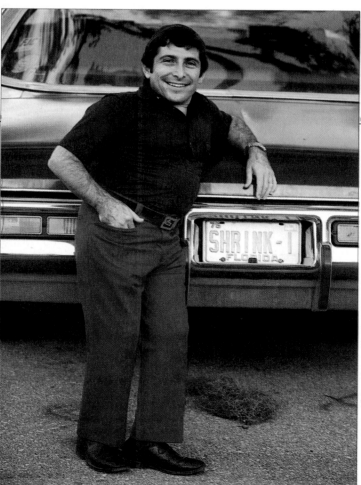

◄ A sense of humor has helped this psychiatrist to accept his short stature. The license plate on his car broadcasts a pun on his profession and his height.

The height dimension

■ Tallness, especially for men, is a social advantage. A survey at the University of Pittsburgh showed that shorter men might be shortchanged on job opportunities and salaries: Pittsburgh graduates between 188cm and 193cm (6ft 2in and 6ft 4 in) received average starting salaries 12.4 percent higher than those under six feet.

Tallness is often associated with power, but behavior labeled "competitive" in a tall man is seen as evidence of a "Napoleonic complex" in a shorter one. Unusually short people are often judged to be less attractive on a variety of levels, while taller people are deemed to be higher in status and more persuasive.

A woman who is much taller than average may be labeled "ungainly," and in relationships, it is commonly believed that women prefer tall men.

However, research has found that women prefer medium-tall men and generally like men to be about four to five inches taller than themselves. A man might, therefore, be ill-advised to overestimate his attractiveness to women simply because he is tall. Similarly a man of medium height should not underestimate his appeal.

21

What Clothes Say

Your clothes are a public advertisement of your attitude about yourself ● *We are all quick to categorize each other based on what we are wearing, but the message received may not be the one we intended to send.*

"WHAT AM I going to wear?" You probably ask yourself this question every day, consciously or unconsciously. The way we dress affects the way we feel, and we, in turn, make assumptions about others from the way they dress. Many of us would claim to be interested in clothes and fashion, yet we also tend to regard dress as a rather frivolous subject. People who show excessive concern about what they wear are commonly regarded as shallow and superficial. Even in the way we dress, we mask our interest in clothing: really stylish dressing is supposed to be casual, uncontrived and not obviously new. Paradoxically, achieving this effect requires considerable attention to detail and a knowledge of the social significance of clothes.

What are clothes for?

If asked, most of us would say that clothes keep us warm and dry, and cover up the more intimate parts of the body. Whether we really want or need them for protection is debatable: within living memory the natives of Tierra del Fuego, living at the southern tip of South America on the nearest continental land to Antarctica, clothed themselves only in paint and were perfectly adapted to life in rough weather without any clothing at all. Covering up for the sake of modesty is a cultural variable. The women of Bali used to expose their breasts as innocently as Western women bare their faces, and in the last century women's skirt lengths have risen from their ankles to their upper thighs. Our ideas about what is or is not "indecent" are highly adaptable and easily influenced.

Dress signaling

Perhaps the most important and universal purpose of clothing is to send messages about ourselves. When we choose one item in a store out of a thousand others, we are planning our appearance to be seen by others. We share this attempt at communication with Afghani tribesmen, wearers of Paris couture and police officers.

Research into decoding dress shows that much information we hope to convey in clothing gets lost along the way. In a recent experiment in Oxford, England, groups of women stated that they chose clothes that suited them, conveyed the right image and sent the right message. Much of their detailed impression-management was not successful, however. The women were asked to wear clothes that expressed their personalities and qualities, and to write down the message they were trying to convey. They were also asked to write down interpretations of what others were wearing. There was little correlation between most of the women's intended messages and the messages the other women said they received, although distinctions in social status and occupation were clearly understood.

In cultures where the clothing alternatives are few and the rules governing their wearing are strict, this sort of mixup is much less likely to occur. In Ethiopia, the way a toga is wrapped around the body expresses quite specific moods that would be hard to misinterpret. Part of our problem may be that in industrial countries the range of clothes is enormous, and the "rules" about the way we wear them – fashion – change very fast. Keeping up with the language of clothes in our society is like trying to follow a conversation

Power dressing for men

■ Men are lucky in having a widely acceptable style of dress – the suit – which works well for all business occasions. But the male wardrobe can be a bit dull, and that may not be an advantage in business. It can be spiced up in a number of ways which will make you look smart but not excessively trendy.

There are three basic cuts to the male suit: English, European and American. The European cut is highly tailored with sharp shoulders. The American style tends to be more generous, with little obvious shaping through the body of the jacket. The English cut is more tailored than the American, but is looser throughout than the European and has more rounded shoulders than either style.

If you have always worn one or other of these styles, experiment with one of the others – you may find you are better suited to another. You might also experiment with single-breasted and double-breasted styles, and single or double back vents. Try styles and shapes different from those you usually wear to see which might look best on your frame. You can also experiment with color. Gray, black and navy are standard colors for male suiting, but there are many variations within these shades. Use tailor's fabric swatches to judge whether you would look best in strong, clear shades, or whether more muted tones suit you. Do the same with shirt and tie colors.

Always buy the best quality you can afford. Men's suits are highly tailored, and the better they are made, the better they will hang on you. A cheap suit looks awful and does not mark you out as a high-flier. The same thing is true for accessories. Discreet but interesting colors for shirts are crucial. You do not need many ties – get rid of the unsuitable ones, even if they were presents, and buy three or four good-quality silk ties in colors that go with your skin, hair and eye color. A good waistcoat, matching your suit or in an interesting wool or suede, can extend your wardrobe and add a dash of interest. Buy only good leather shoes, handmade if possible, and keep them highly polished. Wear only well-designed, modest jewelry. You will look younger, healthier, sexier and more successful.

in when the speakers are continually switching into a different dialect.

So how do we use the language of clothing to express ourselves, if everyone has problems understanding us? Even if the things we are wearing are difficult for others to interpret, we can still "read" and enjoy our own clothing, and much of the psychological impact of wearing clothes comes from the feelings of self-confidence and attractiveness that we get from wearing things we like. If the other messages we are trying to send get scrambled, the projection of an assured personality will probably still get through. When we want to be quite clear about meanings in situations such as job interviews, important meetings and parties where first appearances are important, we need to try to make a statement with our clothes that is distinct and appropriate. Some styles of dressing continue to give out unambiguous messages, no matter how often fashion changes; "classic" clothes are among these.

Power dressing for women

■ The urge to succeed spawned a definitive dress style for business people in the late 1980s. "Power dressing" involves dressing not just for your current position but for the position above that – even for one that you hope to achieve in several years' time.

Women's working attire has changed in the last ten years as women develop a distinctive business look. At first women copied the powerful people whose jobs they hoped to step into by wearing rather masculine, loosely-cut suits in dull colors, relieved only by a bow at the neck. The look was unattractive and too unassuming to indicate power or status. Women soon began to choose suits that were more sympathetic to the female form, and abandoned the shirt for well-cut blouses, silk T-shirts and sweaters. These looked better under the tailored, rich-looking but sober suits with knee-length straight skirts that had become the female version of power dressing.

The secret of power dressing is to have a good look at what the people above you on the career ladder are wearing, and try to emulate that as closely as possible while remaining appropriate for your position. Always choose quality – it shows in the cut and fabric of a suit. Power dressing also requires immaculate grooming. The style is sharp and smart, and poor haircare or sloppily applied makeup will ruin the effect. You want to look both striking and discreet: a difficult thing to achieve, but it can be done by balancing sober tailored cuts with unusual colors or accessories.

151

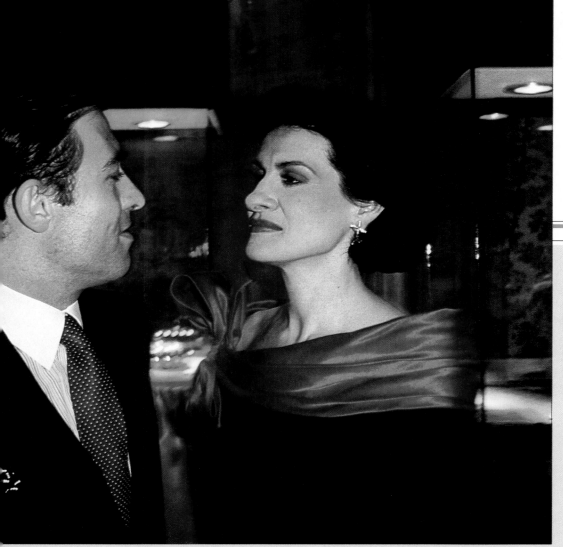

◄ **Successful attire** *for any occasion makes a point about the wearer, attracting attention and admiration. Your look will be more striking everywhere if you choose high-quality, well-cut clothes. The relative lack of variety in men's clothing means it is especially important for them to buy the best they can afford. Add personal details, such as Paloma Picasso's signature red and black, shown here. Correct posture lends authority to any outfit and makes you stand out from the crowd.*

Clear clothing messages

We associate traditional, slightly old-fashioned clothes – dark suits for men, dresses for women – with being conservative and conventional. Clothes cut in a similar style but with a slightly sharper, more fashionable look – tailored suits for both women and men – are associated with success in the business world. "Radical," politically liberal or socially unconventional people or those in creative fields of work signal their interests fairly clearly by breaking these rules of dress, wearing the same styles in unconventional colors or materials (corduroy suits for college professors is an obvious example) or by leaving aside items of clothing that signify formality. In a formal situation, not wearing a tie with a suit, or women wearing trousers, is usually a definite sign of a desire to express unconventionality.

Certain colors are also unambiguously associated with dress messages. Wearing bright red or yellow signifies forcefulness or cheerfulness, though this can range from the hint in a bright tie or socks to the aggressiveness of a woman's red suit. Navy, gray and black suits are associated with sobriety and reliability, though black may be unconventional in some situations. Women should pay particular attention to the meaning of black clothes, which will often depend on the style of the garment: a severe, modest black suit creates a very different impression than a short, closely fitting one, or one that is extremely trendy.

The secret of sending the messages you want through your clothes lies in understanding clothing messages and learning how to apply them to fit your physical type and the various situations you will encounter. Obvious power dressing may be right for some job interviews and wrong for

152

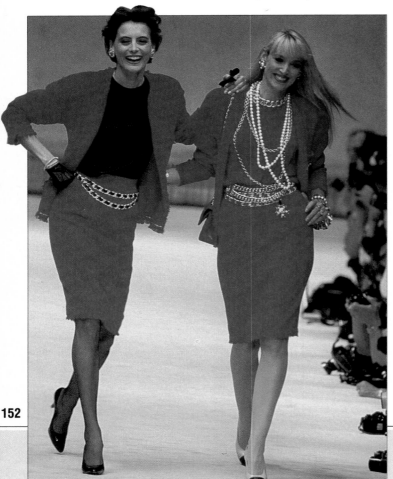

▲ **Even world-famous models** have good and bad colors. Olive-skinned, dark-eyed Ines de la Fressanges looks radiant in true red and other colors in the Water range. Blond Jerry Hall cannot be said to look unattractive, but she would probably look better in a Fire red such as red-orange or bright coral. Most blondes are either Fire or Air, but their range depends on their skin tone more than their hair or eye color. Olive-skinned, Asian and black people are usually Waters, the only people who can wear black and true white successfully. Earths should avoid gray, pink and most shades of blue. Fire people can wear almost any color except black and pure white, as long as it is clear, warm and not too strong. Air people look best in pastels – vivid shades overwhelm their delicate coloring.

Four elements of color

■ Wearing the colors that suit you best makes an enormous difference to your appearance and to your confidence as well. Everyone can wear most colors, but the correct shade should match your hair, eyes and skin tone.

The chart of colors below divides colors into four elemental ranges that apply to both men and women. Earth and Fi colors are warm; Water and Ai are cool. You may be able to wear colors from more than on range, but the ones that look best on you will depend on whether your underlying skin tone is blue (cool) or yellow (warm). An Earth man who is reluctant to part with his classi

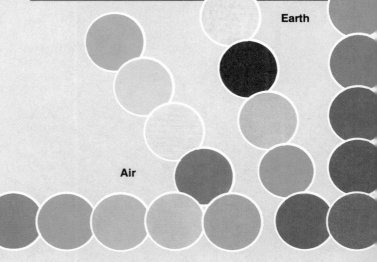

Earth

Air

others; you will not worry so much about impressing your close friends with your clothing as you will a new date. Most importantly, you need to learn to please yourself. If you are happy with your clothes and the way you look in them, your confidence will shine through even if your messages are misinterpreted.

Dressing for effect

When your outfit makes you feel better or more confident about yourself, then it is likely you will also make a more positive impression on others. That is most people's intention in dressing carefully. We are constantly putting on dramatic performances to manipulate impressions of ourselves in the minds of others. This is done by individuals and by groups, from families to social cults (hippies, for example), particularly when we are on show – on formal occasions, when we are motivated by the desire for immediate gains (getting a job at an interview) and to project an idealized version of our self-image. We hope others will accept this picture of us, which in turn will enable us to believe in it ourselves.

Clothing is a form of self-presentation that is difficult to achieve in words. You may choose clothes that announce, "I am glamorous and rich," but if you attempted to make the

same statement in conversation, your audience's reaction would probably be the opposite of admiration. Such messages can be conveyed more effectively with clothes than with words and there is plenty of evidence that people do try to present themselves in this way. When asked, the vast majority of people confirm that they choose their clothes carefully to convey an image. People who are ambitious will

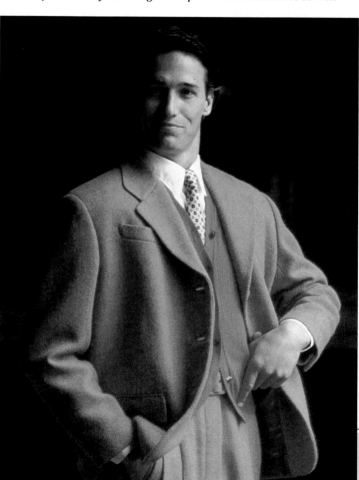

vy or gray suits (Water colors) ould keep in mind that a shirt tie chosen from his correct nge will look better than tching Water ones.

Earth colors are always ong, with rich gold under-es. Olive and kingfisher blue Earth colors.

Fire colors are not all yellow or red, but have warm yellow undertones. They are bright and clear, light to medium in intensity. Ivory, peach and camel are Fire colors.

Water colors are clear and sharp. Black, white, true blue and true red are Water colors.

Air colors are more delicate than Water colors, often pastel versions of the same shades.

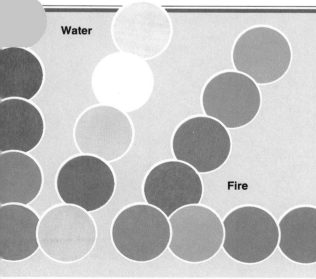

Water

Fire

▲ **Men's elemental colors** *are in the same four ranges as women's, but men should keep in mind that the brighter colors are for accessories and casual wear while the dark and neutral colors are for business or formal wear. This man's olive complexion would be more flattered by the classic men's colors of the Water range – black, navy and gray.*

153

If the messages we send with clothes are often lost, how can we use clothes to express ourselves? What you are wearing may not be as important as the way you wear it. If you are happy with your clothes and the way you look in them, your confidence will shine through, and others will respond positively to that.

adopt the clothes of their superiors or other people that they admire. A foreman at a factory, for example, might wear a suit instead of overalls to indicate that he sees himself as part of management.

The theory of self-presentation might imply to some people that the image we are trying to present is a false or shallow one suggesting, perhaps, an intention to deceive. But this does not appear to be the case. The researcher Efrat Tsëelon has found that most women feel their clothes truly express their real identity or their realistic aspirations and are in no way deceptive. Even if they wear quite different clothes on different occasions, they are still likely to feel that all of these clothes express their self-image reasonably accurately. **MA**

Do glasses make you look intelligent?

■ Wearing glasses gives the impression of intelligence, but only at first sight. The studies that have been conducted suggest that brief exposure to a photograph of a person wearing glasses will enhance intelligence ratings for that person, but a longer exposure seems to neutralize any initial advantage glasses may give. Interestingly, wearing glasses may make more of an impression on the wearer than on the observer. Researchers asked a group of people who normally did not wear glasses to perform a

number of tasks, in some cases wearing glasses and in other cases not. They discovered that wearing glasses did not make the volunteers perform any better, but they believed that they had done better. They also described themselves as more stable, scholarly and competent when asked to complete assessment forms while wearing glasses.

However, the old adage seems to remain true: most women are perceived as less attractive if they wear glasses. **M K D C**

What makes you choose the clothes you wear?

Work among college students suggests that there are connections between clothes selection and personality. One research project found that men who were highly clothes-conscious tended to be more deliberate and traditional when rated on standard personality tests. Men who professed to be unaware of clothes were more likely to be aggressive and independent. Women who were highly aware of what they wore tended to be inhibited and anxious, but also kind and sympathetic. Women with little clothes-consciousness were more likely to be forceful, independent and dominant. A fondness for wearing bright colors and daring styles correlated with sociableness, confidence and independence in both sexes.

Practically stylish

Finally, the people being assessed were asked whether they were more interested in practical or stylish clothing. Men who preferred practical clothing were also found to be more inhibited, cautious, rebellious and dissatisfied. Practically oriented women were clever, enthusiastic, confident and outgoing. Men who preferred beauty over practicality were more success-oriented, mature, forceful, serious and analytical. Women who opted for beautiful clothing tended to be more self-centered, independent and detached.

These results suggest that there may be a connection between our attitudes about clothing and our personality traits and it may be possible to gain insights about ourselves from what we wear. These results are not definitive and do

In a poll of company executives, 91 percent thought that applicants' clothes and grooming indicated their attitude to the company, and 95 percent perceived clothing as a definite aid to career advancement. Are your clothes having a direct impact on other people, or are they influencing the way you perceive and therefore project yourself to others?

▶ **Defiant dressing** *sends a clear message. It is not necessary to say or do anything further to create an impression of unconventionality. This may involve wearing unusual or even inappropriate attire for a certain occasion, or simply using a consistent personal style to set ourselves apart from others. A man might choose to wear an earring, never wear a tie or adopt an unshaven appearance. Groups who adopt deviant clothing are usually making a statement about their dissatisfaction with society, but more important is their identity as a group.*

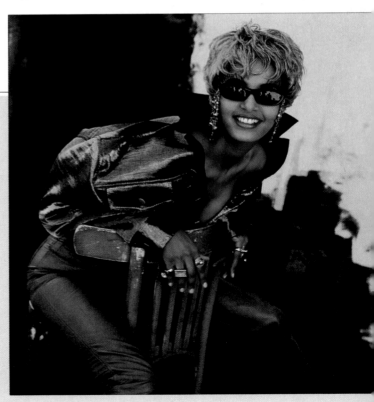

not make clear-cut relationships between personality type and clothing preference, but they do suggest an avenue for self-discovery through the wardrobe.

How clothes can affect your behavior

Personality affects how we choose our clothes, and it might also be true that our choice of clothes could alter our behavior. Wearing tight or uncomfortable clothes may put people into a bad humor and cause them to be more brusque and impatient than they might normally be. If we leave home in the morning wearing something that we do not like, we often feel self-conscious and will be uncomfortable until we can get home and change. We may continually focus on what we are wearing and what is wrong with it, and we begin to worry that others can see our discomfort, or that we are inappropriately or unflatteringly dressed.

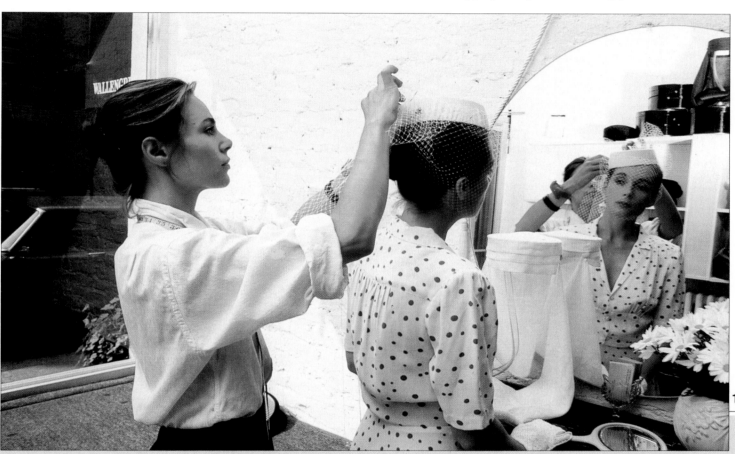

155

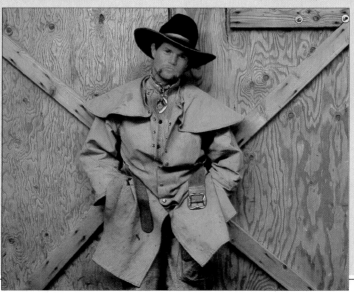

▲ **Women's hats** are no longer a staple of their wardrobes. In Europe they may still be seen at formal occasions, but they are worn much less in North America, where they have become an accessory worn for fun. It has become perfectly correct to attend a church service, wedding or funeral without one. Nevertheless, Europe dominates women's haute couture and hat shops such as this one in New York are enjoying renewed popularity.

◄ **The romance of the range** is kept alive by a modern cowboy. Cowboy clothes were originally designed for practical purposes; the ten-gallon hat kept out both the rain and the sun as the cowboy rode over hundreds of acres in all weather. This cowboy is a rancher by profession and belongs to an association of cowboys dedicated to preserving their heritage through costume and poetry. Other men adopt this style purely for fun and leisure – possibly because they like to be identified with an active lifestyle so glamorized in movies.

Being preoccupied, we may also become less productive, more insecure and increasingly uneasy, and we may even find ourselves going out of our way to avoid others so that we do not make a bad impression.

On the other hand, if we are particularly pleased or proud of what we are wearing, we might go out of our way to talk to others and show ourselves off. We feel confident and happy, and others respond to that. The aim of all fashion designers, "you should be able to put it on and forget about it," refers to this confidence about the way you are dressed. If you are constantly checking and adjusting your clothes it will make you worried and self-conscious. Really good clothes set up the first impression you make and then leave you free to get on with other matters. Choosing clothes that convey the image you want to present, fit your personality and make you feel good may take a little trial and error at first, but a few simple rules and guidelines will go a considerable way toward helping you put together a wardrobe that is in really good shape.

Dress for success

Most of us want to make a good impression at work, and the largest part of our clothing budget will be spent on that unless we wear a uniform. But while most of us feel confident about what to wear to a party or a sporting event, we may find it difficult to decide on the best thing to wear to work, particularly if we are changing jobs or entering the work force for the first time. Understanding the impact of clothes on others, and what they can do for you, will help you to develop a successful working wardrobe.

Clothing is the aspect of your appearance that is most likely to be noticed first. In a Roper Organization survey, 35 percent of those asked reported that they noticed dress first, ahead of eyes, figure, build or face, when meeting someone of the opposite sex. When meeting someone of the same sex, 41 percent noticed dress first. Dress is most effective in making a successful first impression – after that, studies show that attention to dress begins to fade on a conscious level, unless major changes are introduced. The best dress

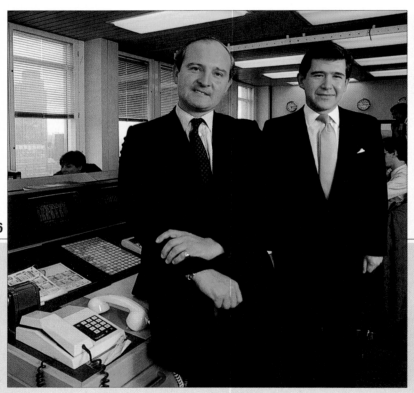

156

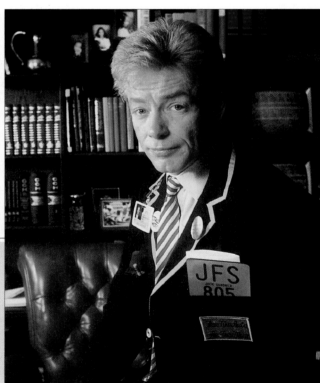

One research project discovered that salesmen who wore a suit with a shirt and tie had 43 percent more sales than when they had on just trousers with a shirt and tie, and 60 percent more than if they wore just trousers and a shirt.

▲ **Assumptions of trust** are often made on the basis of personal attire. People whose work depends on contact with the public should keep this well in mind when dressing for work. Appropriateness in choice of clothes is never more important than on the job. We expect a bank manager to look like a bank manager – conservative,

cautious, serious. Classic suits LEFT are most effective in relaying these qualities without words. The humor of the unexpected frivolous touch in a highpowered business setting RIGHT is something that may be appreciated in a senior executive but frowned on in a middle manager, and unthinkable for a junior member of

staff. Loud or very trendy clothing for men is associated with fast-moving, possibly unstable professions, and frequently with insincere or untrustworthy personalities.

Choosing the right suit for you

■ A good suit is an investment. It is worth spending time and money finding the right one.

● If you are long and lean, you can probably wear almost any style and look good by today's aesthetic standards. Broad-shouldered cuts will widen you all over; pinstripes will make you look like a beanpole. Double-breasted suits will probably look good on you.

● If you are inclined to be a bit top-heavy, choose a jacket that is fitted, without obvious broadening details like extended shoulders, gathered-in sleeves or wide lapels. Trousers and skirts will look better if there is some pleating around the hips, balancing your lower and upper half.

● If you are pear-shaped (a problem some men have, as well as women), ensure that your suit shoulders are as wide as your hips, to even out your proportions. Choose slim-fitted trousers and skirts to complete the effect.

● If you have a bulky waistline, do not draw attention to it. Avoid belted styles. Choose longer, fuller jackets that end well below the waist. Pin-stripes look slimmer.

■ **There are three golden rules to follow**:

● Buy the best suit that you can afford.

● Make sure it is roomy enough – tight suits are uncomfortable and look badly fitted. If necessary, buy a larger size than you would usually take.

● Choose a shade that matches your own coloring.

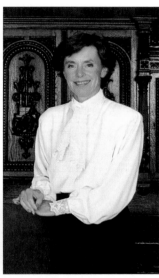

■ **Looking the part**. *Rules for women's business attire are not as strict as for men's, but women who expect to be taken seriously in a professional setting should dress accordingly. A ruffled blouse ABOVE may soften the effect of a severely tailored suit without compromising dignity. The sleek hair and conservative dress and accessories of this woman LEFT would fit in at most levels of an office environment – she would not look out of place as a legal counsel or a senior secretary.*

A uniform effect

■ Uniforms are designed to give absolutely clear information about the status, authority and purpose of the person wearing them. In the industrialized world these are the most unambiguous types of clothing available, and they have the greatest effect upon how others react to the wearer. In a study measuring compliance, a researcher had four men dress successively as ordinary middle-class men (sports jacket and tie), milkmen (uniform jacket, white pants and carrying milk bottles) and guards (uniform and cap but no official insignia or badge and no gun).

▼ **Hero worship** *often surrounds those who wear a prestigious uniform, such as the stunt pilot who is offering his autograph to a young fan. Any special costume worn in public draws attention to the person wearing it. The pride and authority of such glamorous uniforms may be used to attract young recruits into the profession.*

These men then stopped people walking along the streets of Brooklyn, New York and asked them either to pick up a bag, put a dime in a parking meter for someone else, or stand on the opposite side of a bus sign. The guard had by far the greatest compliance rate, even though his uniform clearly suggested a private guard, not a policeman or public official. People in official-looking uniforms that convey authority are able to influence others more than those in ordinary clothing or in uniforms that do not convey high status.

As a result of such studies, more and more businesses are putting their workers who have high contact levels with the public into official-looking uniforms rather than ordinary clothing. They claim it makes the workers more confident about their own authority, raises morale, gives the company a high profile and makes contact with the public easier, as people are more willing to accept the statements of a person in a uniform. **M K D C**

157

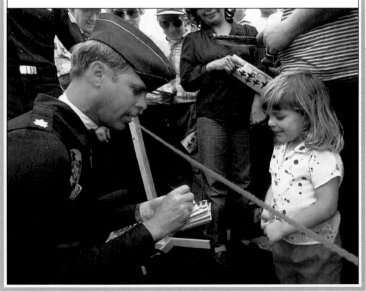

strategies take advantage of this fact, and aim to make a strong initial impact while, at the same time, taking into account what is appropriate for the situation.

Looking the part for the job you do

Dress also helps to persuade others of your effectiveness. An overwhelming majority of Chicago personnel executives believe that dress is influential in selecting job applicants.

Clothes can also affect your standing and authority at work, and dressing incorrectly may cost you a promotion. Despite her degree and obvious acumen, the heroine of the popular film "Working Girl" found it impossible to advance her career because her clothes and accessories clearly labeled her "working class secretary." With a change of image, she was able to make her mark in the business world.

In working situations, a willingness and ability to adapt to the standards of dress is very important – most of all we need to be aware of what is appropriate. We are more likely to project a positive image of ourselves and have a positive impact on others if we understand what is and is not proper for any given situation. A person wearing an expensively tailored suit might be treated with respectful admiration or envy at a meeting of professional people, but in a poolroom or garage that same outfit might provoke ridicule or mild amusement because the suit would be out of place. In the first situation the clothes communicate taste, style and wealth, while in the second they may communicate an attempt to put on airs or impress others.

Knowing what is appropriate

In a business setting, dress is not always spelled out in the form of a dress code, but rules and norms still exist. In a study which focused on masculinity and femininity in dress,

it was found that regardless of occupation, men and women who wore "masculine" clothing – usually strictly tailored outfits – were judged as being more successful in those occupations than people wearing "feminine" clothing (softer, frillier items, pastel colors and dresses rather than suits). Also, those who wore high-status, well cut and expensive clothing were perceived as more attractive, regardless of sex or physique.

This may seem to suggest that masculine high-status clothing is what we should wear if we want to be successful. However, a more likely interpretation may be that the judges were indicating a preference for more conservative businesslike appearances in both men and women. What the researchers probably received from the judges were their

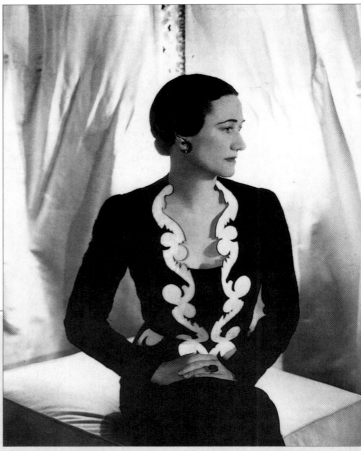

■ **Why do we follow fashion?** *If clothes are a way of sending messages, why do we keep changing the signals? It may be that features of our attire which might initially be distinctive become routine over time. Contrast the stiff formality of the Duchess of Windsor's day ABOVE with the exaggerated playfulness of the 1960s RIGHT and the relaxed style of the* early 1990s FAR RIGHT. *Clothing is also an indicator of social status. High fashion usually begins in elite circles and filters gradually down and across different groups. By the time it has become established, the fashion-makers are ready for a change. Fashion may confuse the language of clothes, but it also keeps it alive.*

Letting their hair down

■ Fashion editors, makeup artists, and others whose business is beauty often care very little about their own appearance.

Recently a fashion and beauty magazine organized a meeting with scientists to review the latest research on the importance of good looks. The audience consisted of presidents of perfume, cosmetics and clothing companies. The academics expected to be the only casually dressed people there.

The experts, they thought, would be "dressed for success." However, the professionals in

the beautycare field, who know more than anyone about projecting a good image, took the opportunity of a day off to relax in their old clothes.

Many commented in discussion that in their own lives, they cared more about the kindness, sense of humor and intelligence of their lovers, friends and colleagues than their looks. Surrounded by the world of beauty, they could often see more clearly than others what improvements to personal appearance can do and what they cannot substitute for.

perceptions of the normal style of dress for business rather than strictly masculine or feminine clothing. In other kinds of work, appropriate dress is also more important than masculinity or femininity. Successful construction workers will be expected to dress like construction workers, cooks like cooks – not like executives.

Sharpening up your working wardrobe

There are five basic steps to evaluating your working clothes, and they need not involve spending any money at all, depending on what you have hanging in the closet. First, take out all the clothes that you might wear to work and lay them out so you can have a good look at them. Find pictures of yourself in working clothes and lay those out as well. Next, think about how others dress at work, especially your immediate superiors whose jobs you might be in line for. What sort of "clothing language" functions at the place you work? This is particularly important if you are about to start a new sort of job or are hoping for promotion. Many people make the mistake of using a dress strategy that worked in one sort of job but is inappropriate for another.

Take a good look at your own clothes. Do they fit your job, or are you dressing wrongly for the part? Are there clothes that you should discard? Are there some good suits there that you should wear more often? Be ruthless – throw out any clothes that are wrong, set them aside for the thrift shop or relegate them to weekend wear. Finally, consider the makeup and hairstyle that you normally wear. Will they fit with a sharper image, or should they be adapted too? Try on the clothes you have decided to keep and use, and experiment with new makeup and hairstyles to see what suits best. As long as you are honest with yourself you will soon have a look that will boost your own confidence and may help you get along better at work. **M K D C**

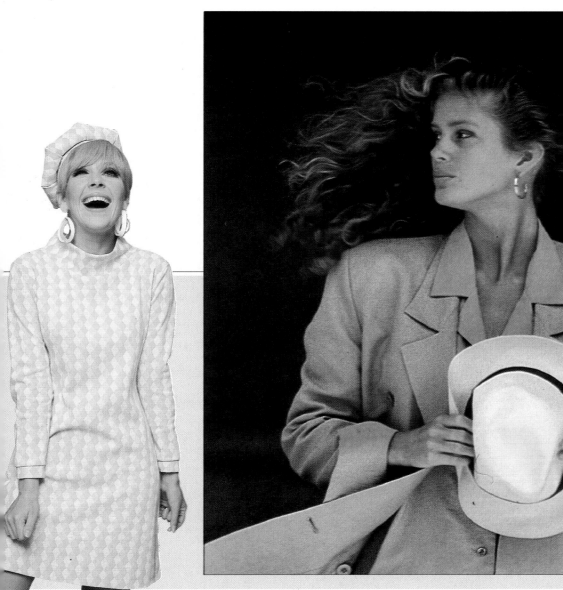

159

22

Bodytalk

The most fluidly changing features of your appearance tell people the most about you
● *Postures, facial expressions, movements of limbs, tones of voice and touches reveal our emotions and much more.*

WE CAN LEARN a lot about our own and other people's emotions and attitudes by observing signals from various parts of the body. Friendliness and warmth, sexual attraction, feelings of dominance, even mental disturbances can all be read in the cues given by the various channels of nonverbal communication – what we often call "body language."

Rarely do we have any difficulty in decoding these body signals accurately. We all implicitly understand the "display rules" that influence the signals: we know that there are some emotions that people will feel impelled to control or even hide, especially intense dislike or sexual interest. Sometimes, however, our true feelings slip out in the form of nonverbal messages. We are sensitive to these even when we cannot see them, and in extreme cases display rules may break down altogether. For example, researchers have found that if they put seven or eight students into a small room about 3m by 3.5 (10ft by 12), in pitch darkness for an hour, display rules about controlling emotions are broken. The students begin to allow a great deal of body contact to take place.

Facial types and facial expressions

Most people tend to link a person's face with their personality – an idea borne out by various types of psychological research. Men with shallow-set bright eyes and light brows we judge to be carefree, easy-going, cheerful, honest, warm-hearted and with a sense of humor. Young male faces, with a few wrinkles are considered energetic, conscientious, patient, honest, warm-hearted, friendly, intelligent and easy-going. Young women with narrowed eyes, a large red mouth, smooth skin and with a well-groomed appearance are considered highly sexual. People who have "baby faces" – small chins, large wide eyes, high brows, smooth skins and large foreheads – are considered to be dependent and immature, qualities traditionally thought to be more desirable in a woman than a man. Just as biologically we want healthy mates, so youthfulness is an

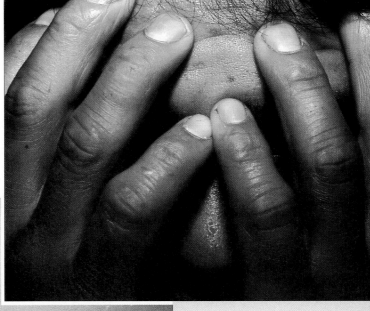

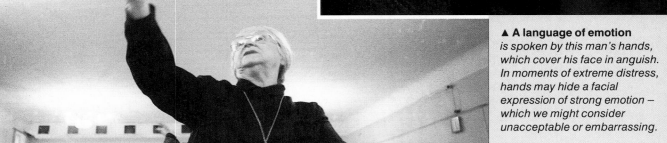

▲ **A language of emotion** *is spoken by this man's hands, which cover his face in anguish. In moments of extreme distress, hands may hide a facial expression of strong emotion – which we might consider unacceptable or embarrassing.*

◄ **A language of gesture,** *employed particularly expressively by a ballet expert. The position of her whole body gives her point far more emphasis than words could alone.*

advantage in females and maturity and physical strength in males. We cling to certain stereotypes when linking face and personality. High foreheads or glasses are taken to denote intelligence, and thick lips sensuality.

The expressions on our faces show emotions and attitudes to others. We show pleasure or anger, friendship or hostility by smiles or frowns. Our faces also reveal depression, anxiety, disgust, surprise. Smiling is the most effective positive facial signal and can act as a powerful reward. However, we do control these according to specific rules.

People normally find it easy to read eye signals correctly. We regard people who make direct eye contact more favorably, and are more inclined to rate them as competent, friendly, assertive and socially skilled. Those who avoid our eyes we think of as cold, neurotic or submissive. People in love stare into each other's eyes a lot. Dominant, powerful

people stare more while talking and less while listening. Staring can be threatening – animals in the wild use it to intimidate each other, and rival gangs of youths or other people in a hostile situation often use staring to the same effect.

The language of gesture and posture

Gestures punctuate and reinforce what we are saying. On the whole, women use finer and more expressive gestures. Mental patients use gestures for self-stimulation rather than communication. Dominant people use gestures to reinforce their power. Courtship involves many levels of touching, including self-grooming. There are also a host of rude and colorful gestures to indicate hostility and derision.

In the main, posture signals indicate levels of relaxation, tension, self-confidence and anxiety. Dominance and

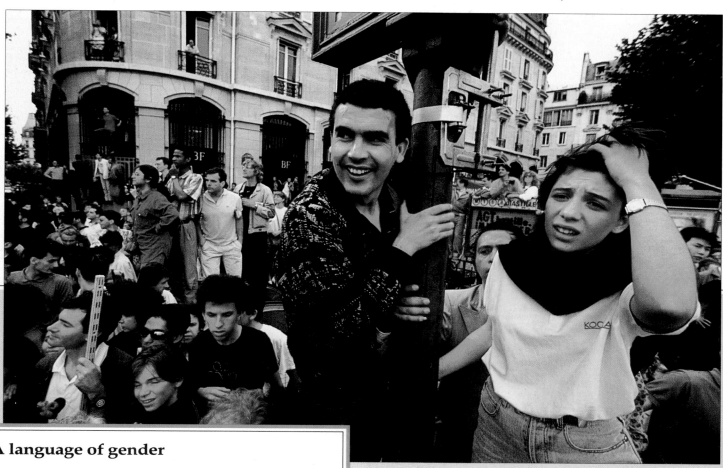

161

A language of gender

■ Men and women typically use various distinctive body cues, which often become signals for masculinity and femininity. The main differences are that women smile up to 50 percent more than men, and use a wider range of facial expressions. They have higher-pitched voices and use direct eye

contact much more. They require less personal space and approach others more closely . Men hesitate, stutter and use the wrong words much more than women. They also interrupt more and are much louder. They appear more restless and they take up more space, especially when sitting.

▲ **Reactions to the same situation** *can vary with personality, gender and personal experience. Much depends on what you think you are seeing – is it something funny or something distressing? An important influence is your own notion of the "display rules" that apply in* *your case. Do you feel permitted, because you are a woman, to show distress? Do you feel obliged, because you are a man, to look tough?*

friendliness, for example, have distinctive body positions. When two people like one another or have grown up together, they often adopt mirror-image postures. Sometimes we deliberately present an image through posture, posing as a soldier with a military bearing or an intellectual, with a slouched stance or slightly eccentric way of gesturing.

Speaking your mind

It is surprising how much personality is expressed through the voice. Extroverts tend to talk loudly and quickly, with raised voices and no breathiness. Depressives speak softly and slowly, in a low pitch. Aggressive personalities speak loudly, quickly and with explosive emphasis. Voices can smile, frown, be friendly, hostile, depressed or worried. Dominant voices are slow, loud and low. Persuasive voices are fast, loud and expressive. The voice is a very flexible channel of communication – much more flexible than the face. It is possible for our voices to be both dominant or persuasive and friendly at the same time, for example. If we tried to do this with our faces we would be trying to smile and frown at the same time.

Reactions to voice styles are also often based on stereotypes. For instance, we tend to think of nasal speech as undesirable, but a throaty voice is sophisticated and mature. Someone who has a resonant voice, we regard as energetic and interesting. Accent gives us an accurate clue to the social class of the speaker and only time or theatrical training can help us to acquire a new accent.

Personal space

We all need personal space and feel uncomfortable if anyone comes within about 50cm (18in) of us. Women tend to allow others to come closer, as do extroverts. Violent prisoners need up to three times more space than others. We allow people we like to invade our personal space. This cue means much the same as smiling or gazing and indeed these body signals can act as substitutes. Body contact is a very powerful signal and touch can be both exciting and disturbing. We show friendship by special kinds of touch,

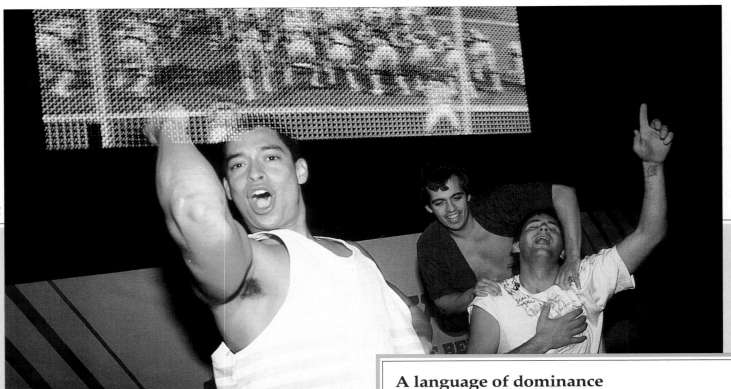

▲ **A language of triumph.**
As the video projector shows a replay, a football fan identifies himself with the success of the team he supports. The leap in the air and the shaking fist strongly suggest physical dominance while the finger in the air is a gesture of authority similar to those used by an orator. The prevailing sense of machismo permits a degree of physical contact between the two men in the background.

A language of dominance

■ Dominant people in a group typically announce their dominance with their bodies. They occupy high status spaces, such as the head of the table or a raised position – the pulpit in a church or the judge's chair in a court. They may stand at full height, chest out, hands on hips – but where their dominance is clearly accepted by the group, their whole body is relaxed. They present a serious face to colleagues. They use a lot of powerful direct eye contact, and enjoy staring the others down. They talk loudly taking every opportunity to interrupt, and punctuate their speech with emphatic gestures.

usually with our hands or arms. People who touch a lot are considered to be warm and affectionate and are usually widely liked. We do not, on the whole, like being touched by strangers and in particular women dislike being touched by male strangers. Touch also adds to social influence, if combined with a request or, for example, if used by nurses in therapy sessions. Encounter groups sometimes use touch in an attempt to overcome psychological isolation.

Broken body language

People within a wide range of mental disorders share certain body cues that are visible signs of their illnesses. They rarely smile and they hate people to get too close to them physically. They use very few gestures designed to communicate with others. Instead they touch themselves a lot, hand to face or hands clutched together. Their body movements are also directed toward themselves, with a lot of fidgeting or scratching. But people with different mental illnesses also display characteristic styles of body language.

Schizophrenics have a generally untidy appearance.

Some twist their faces into distorted expressions. They need two or three times more personal body space than other people. They dislike being touched or touching, and touch only themselves. Their gestures appear random and are often divorced from what they are saying at the time. They make very few body movements, sometimes becoming deliberately immobile in some kind of symbolic stance. Their voice has a monotonous quality, is often breathy, and their words are often indistinct.

Those suffering from depression have a generally drab appearance, tending to wear dark-colored clothes. They rarely smile and smile weakly when they do. They avoid eye contact, keeping their eyes downcast to the floor. Their general body posture has a downward direction, with dropping shoulders and bowed head. They may talk loudly, in a low-pitched voice that often sounds dead or listless.

Among neurotics, manic or hysterical patients tend to wear striking, colorful clothes. Neurotics also tend to withdraw, smiling little, and looking away from others. They usually talk quickly, indistinctly and little. **MA**

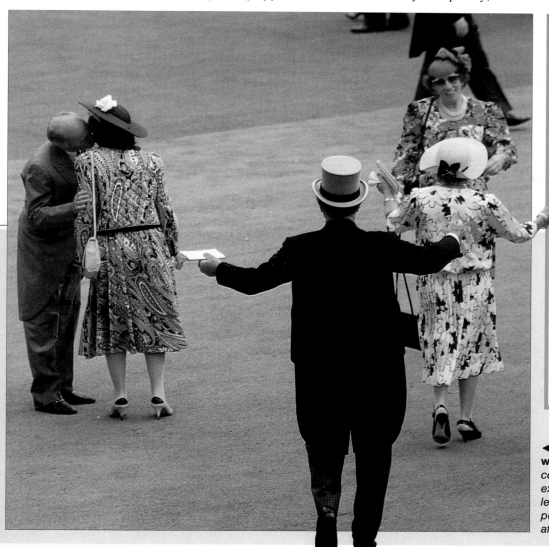

A language of liking

■ When people like each other they tend to exchange very distinctive body signals and facial expressions to indicate friendliness. They sit or stand close to each other and they are not afraid to make frequent eye contact. They touch, and make lively body movements. They converse in moderate tones.

If they are also sexually attracted to each other, these body cues are heightened. They gaze into each other's eyes, the pupils dilate, giving a wide-eyed look. They fiddle with their clothing or hair and a lot of self-grooming, (straightening clothes etc), takes place, especially by women. Touch can include hand-holding, stroking, embracing and kissing. They might perspire or blush, both signs of sexual arousal.

163

◄ **Open arms are a gesture of welcome,** *inviting someone to come nearer. The kiss being exchanged by the pair on the left suspends the boundaries of personal space, indicating affection and trust.*

23

Personal Style

Having a strong sense of personal style and wearing the latest fashion are not the same thing ● Feeling confident about the way you dress means expressing your own personality as well as looking right for the occasion.

RECOMMENDATIONS about enhancing your appearance can be useful, but if followed too slavishly they can result in a boring, predictable look that says nothing about you as a person. We are all individuals with our own quirks and unexpected qualities, and you may want to communicate these facets of yourself as well as a generalized image of competence or attractiveness.

We have all known people who have closely followed all the fashionable trends in appearance but never quite make an impression. Their look is boring and forgettable, because they are missing the spark that marks them out from the crowd. They have followed all the rules but they have no personal style.

What is style?

"This is a classic jacket style." "They have real style!" We use the term frequently, but it is hard to say exactly what we mean by it. In the first sentence, the term "style" refers to a set of features characterizing a type. The second refers to a much more elusive quality, valued in itself but not specifically marked by particular features – this sense of style can be applied to all sorts of people who look quite different.

Many books and magazines talk about clothing, cosmetics and hairstyles as falling into a number of distinct styles. These can range in number up to 20, but three basic categories appear to be universally recognized in western clothing:

Classic/professional. Plain, traditional styles and colors, simple lines and a somewhat formal air.
Romantic/artistic. Unusual details or colors, especially with an "ethnic" or bohemian flavor; slightly eccentric.
Country/sporty. Casual, informal style and muted colors; practical clothes suitable for working in.

These categories of style as a guideline can help to pull a whole look together, but following any one of them too slavishly will result in a uniform look, not personal style.

Understanding style means understanding why we dress up, put on cosmetics and experiment with hairstyles. The touchstone is appropriateness: fitting the look to the situation. On that basis we build up a look from two angles: communication and self-expression. Appearance is a way of sending messages to others about who we are and what our intentions and interests may be. But clothes are also a way of celebrating our own sense of self. The secret of personal style lies in achieving all three aspects of appearance at the same time: appropriateness, communication and self-expression.

What makes a style personal and individual is the aspect of self-expression. A personal look allows the wearer to feel the confidence of being properly dressed and the comfort of being "at home" in this look. If it is overemphasized your look may not be clearly readable by others and it may not adapt itself well to situations; you may appear eccentric instead of stylish. But without it you will look boring or simply remote. Unlike the rules of appropriateness and

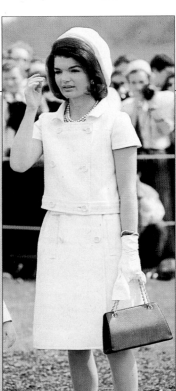
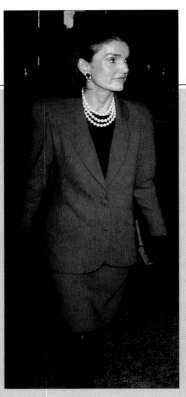

◄ **Defined and confined** by other people's taste, Jacqueline Kennedy as First Lady FAR LEFT was demurely dressed as the image of the president's wife. Even with her formidable poise, she did not always look at ease in her clothes, which did not express a personality but a concept about public life. Later LEFT, as Jackie Onassis, she was free to choose her own clothes, not only to look her best at public functions but also to suit her individual taste. She had never looked better than she does here – confident, elegant, vital, relaxed.

► **The three basic styles** leave you room to show who you are while fitting comfortably into your surroundings. The romantic-artistic look RIGHT uses color boldly and finds distinctive, sometimes eccentric, combinations. Country-sporty styles TOP RIGHT are for the outdoors and for activities where comfort and practicality are especially important. The classic-professional look FAR RIGHT is most common for business, especially for men, but may still permit personal flourishes, such as cufflinks or a brightly colored pocket handkerchief.

communication, there are no firm rules about self-expression in appearance. Developing personal style means experimenting and having fun with all the aspects of your appearance (clothing, cosmetics, jewelry, hairstyles), and not being afraid to make mistakes, until you find a look that makes you comfortable and confident.

Adapting to the occasion

Appropriateness is the basis of all good style. The clothes that we wear, the sort of makeup we put on and the hairstyles we choose vary a great deal between different social situations, and act partly as signals about how we relate to the particular situation we are in. Any good personal style allows for a variety of looks to fit all the aspects of our lives.

If people are asked to group situations into clusters, rather broad groupings emerge like work, leisure, formal and domestic. Each of us needs a look for all these different parts of our lives. Proper appearances for work vary

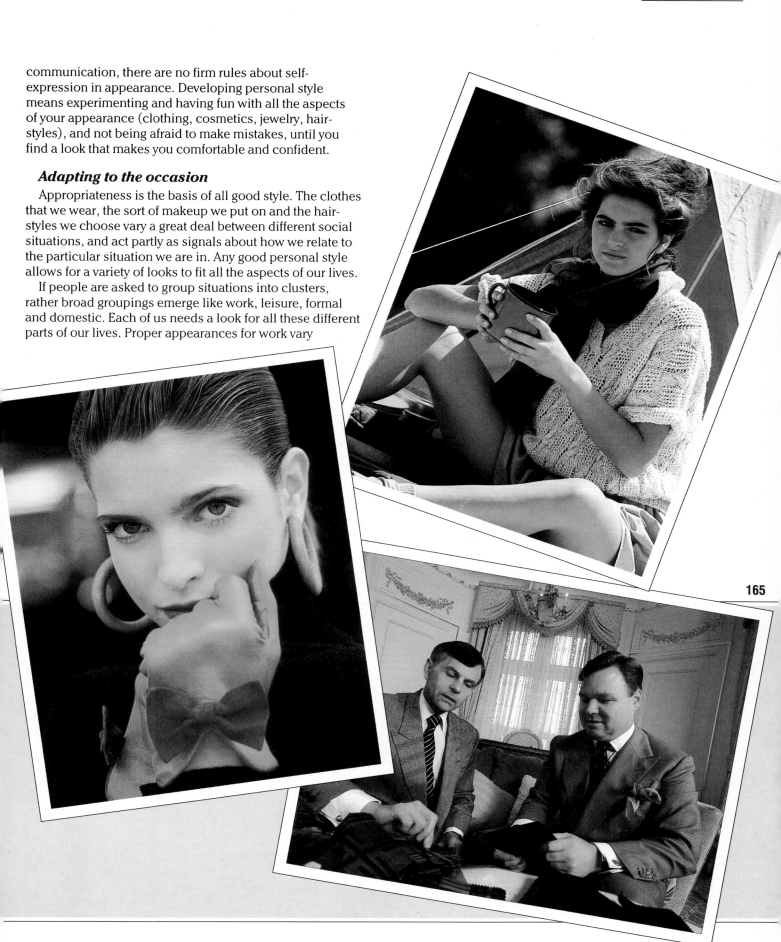

165

depending on the job; construction workers have quite different requirements from business people. Leisure style is usually associated with loose, informal clothes, minimal makeup, and simple hairstyles. A number of special situations have strict rules about appearance – funerals, weddings and graduation ceremonies, for instance.

Adapting appearance to situations may seem to be a restriction of personal style, but it is in fact an important aspect of self-expression. After all, the situation you are in is a result of your being who you are. Doctors have to look like doctors, bank managers like bank managers, or their clients will not trust them. People who feel unhappy in "professional" clothes, even after a year of wearing them regularly, may also be unhappy with the job that goes with them.

In any case, appropriateness need not mean conformity. A man can express his individuality in a work situation by choosing a somewhat unusual cut of suit, and a woman might choose unexpected colors in hers. While still being appropriate, their look will also be individual and distinctive. In fact, real dressing for success requires this individual touch; it is the difference between looking like a cog in a wheel and looking like a high flier.

Especially in managerial and professional roles, adopting a clothing style to suit your career helps others to identify and place you. In one research study, when newscasters wore sober, professional-looking suits, viewers were more likely to remember the news and were more inclined to believe it.

Social-skills training may involve suggesting that a client change clothing styles to improve how he or she is judged and treated by others. In one case, a psychologist employed in a mental hospital was constantly being mistaken for a patient. He had long hair, wore medallions, and an oriental shirt open to the waist. People found it difficult to accept him professionally. In another case, a young female student looked and sounded rather dull and eccentric and was understandably having problems with her social life. In the second case a change of style was attempted and it immediately improved the student's popularity and well-being.

Dressing appropriately helps you to have successful social interactions and to feel comfortable in role. However, if professionals in the caring professions, such as social workers, are working with people in very different circumstances from their own they may do better if they dress like their clients. People tend to like and be more influenced by a person who is dressed similarly to themselves as they feel that such persons will be better able to "understand" them.

Class and style

We sometimes say that a stylish dresser has "class." Really stylish appearance used to be restricted to the upper levels of society who had the time and the money to spend on clothes, cosmetics and haircare. Up until about 200

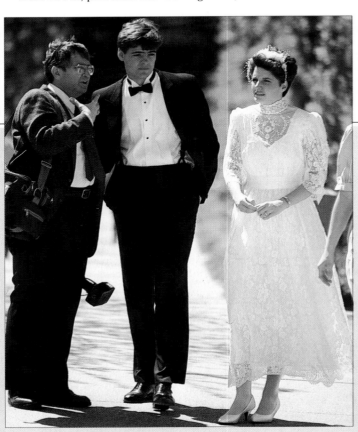

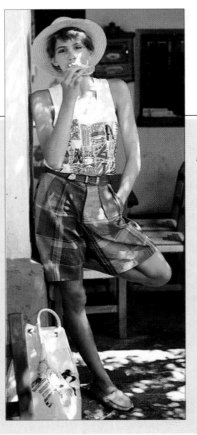

◄ **The style of the occasion** *may restrict you or leave you totally free to express individuality. A church wedding, such as this one at the Mormon Temple in Salt Lake City* FAR LEFT, *may demand a strict observation of tradition and etiquette. They are usually once-only experiences and so offer the principal participants little opportunity to learn how to bring a personal style to their role. Vacations allow the most leeway in dressing for the occasion* LEFT; *riotous color combinations, fabrics and accessories may appear, offering the maximum opportunity for creativity and release from social convention.*

years ago many societies had laws prescribing the clothes and cosmetics which could be worn by people of different social ranks. Even after the old clothing laws had fallen into disuse, styles trickled down the social classes. The very rich wore the latest styles, the middle classes copied last season's style, and the poor wore hand-me-downs several years old.

The historian Veblen formulated a well-known "theory of the leisure class," suggesting that wealthy people engaged in conspicuous consumption of goods, adopting an appearance of obvious richness and impracticality for serious work, which marked them out as members of the

élite. Only people with considerable money and time were able to put effort into appearance, and personal style was a monopoly of the wealthy – hence the relationship in our language between "style" and "class."

Fashion, style and money

Class differences in appearance are now much less obvious. Rising standards of living, more leisure time, and the increased cheapness and availability of good-quality clothing and cosmetics have made it possible for anyone to be stylish. Since the late 1960s top designers have been inspired by the dress, makeup and hairstyles they see on

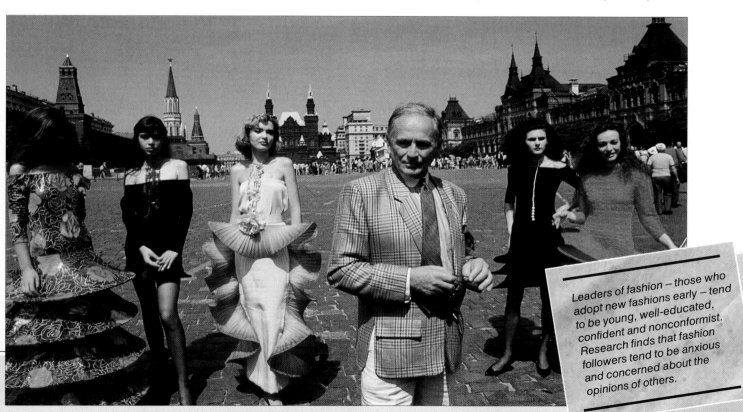

Leaders of fashion – those who adopt new fashions early – tend to be young, well-educated, confident and nonconformist. Research finds that fashion followers tend to be anxious and concerned about the opinions of others.

▲ **Very classic yet individual,** Pierre Cardin's menswear bears little relation to his fanciful creations for women's haute couture, seen here in Moscow's Red Square on Soviet models. The jacket, trousers and tie he is wearing are distinctive but could be worn in a variety of situations. The dresses, designed for once-only wear on very fashionable occasions, would be out of place in the wardrobe of most women, as well as far beyond the reach of their budgets.

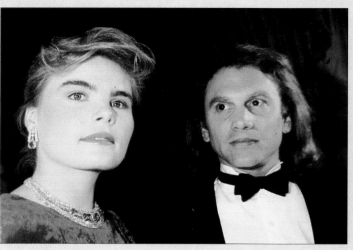

◄ **Eyebrows – a personal trademark.** The model Marie! Hemingway was urged to pluck her thick eyebrows, but she resisted and they became a feature marking her as an individual. They made her instantly recognizable and projected a strong, forthright, unaffected character. This may have helped to open the door for the more natural, individual-looking models enjoying successful careers today.

ordinary people in the street, and some of the most stylish clothes now are old-fashioned working costumes – overalls, Levi 501s, and cowboy boots, for example. No one now needs much money or the right social background to have style.

Fashion, like class, is sometimes confused with style, but it is certainly not the same thing. It is perfectly possible to be stylish without being fashionable, or to be fashionable without being stylish. The messages that clothes communicate change, just as a language changes, over the years. Fashion is the articulation of these changes. There are many explanations for the phenomenon of fashion. In part it is always connected to a country's economy; the more money that is available, the faster fashions tend to change, as people can take up and abandon different appearances more easily. Today, however, all sorts of people from pop stars to street people initiate fashion; it is no longer related solely to class or wealth.

We may change appearance because we want to attract attention. Appearance makes the most impact in the first few minutes of meeting; after that, although it still matters, it ceases to have the same effect, and changing styles may be a way of refreshing the eye and renewing the focus of attention. However, slavish following of the latest styles can create "fashion victims" – people who wear what is new regardless of whether it is appropriate to them or their personality and situation.

When creating a personal style you cannot ignore fashion, because appearances do change meaning. In the late 1950s, for instance, thick white ankle socks were a sign of being daring and carefree. Now they indicate a relaxed, sporty look. Many aspects of look for men and women have, however, remained stable since the 1920s with only minor differences in detail, and continue to present a coherent,

In vogue

■ The late Diana Vreeland, shown here with Yves St Laurent, editor of Vogue and later curator of the New York Metropolitan Museum of Art's clothing collection, is probably one of the best examples of personal style this century. She was never a beautiful woman, and attempts in her young days to be conventionally attractive merely made her appear plain. Later she threw aside attempts to soften her harsh bone structure and began to exaggerate it. She pulled her hair severely off her face and wore only red and black, in cosmetics as well as clothes. To many she looked like an exotic bird, but she was always memorable and always herself. Her extreme appearance fitted her enthusiastic, adventurous personality, and grew out of her immense confidence in her own taste and judgment. While few will want to imitate her actual look, her strong sense of personal style is still a source of inspiration.

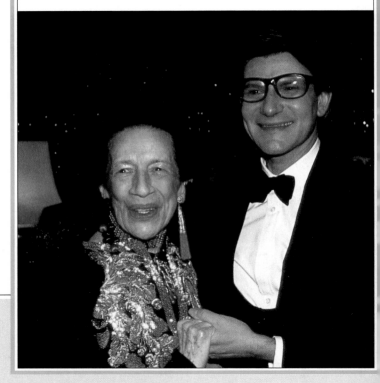

Painting a public face

■ Different cosmetic styles are closely associated with particular situations, researchers have found. But women are just as likely to choose cosmetic colors to fit their different moods and express their personality as they are to adapt them to a situation. Most people have quite clear ideas about what colors and styles fit with each mood. Nearly everyone agrees that intense, flamboyant colors look wrong in the office or the supermarket, but are perfect for a party or dinner out.

Correlations between particular makeup styles and situations are so clear-cut in our minds that just putting on bright fuchsia lipstick can put us into a partying mood. In a test run by the psychologist Judith Waters, photographs of a woman before and after a cosmetic make-over were assessed by recruiting agencies. To make the test fair, one of the sets of photographs had to be discarded because it was impossible to match the woman's depressed expression in the "before" photographs with the radiant look of her "after" photographs. The cosmetic change had completely lifted her spirits.

The immense range of cosmetics available, however, indicates that matching colors to mood and situation is not entirely straightforward, otherwise, we would all use identical colors and makeup styles. Some people simply cannot wear certain shades. Bright red lipstick is universally acknowledged to be intensely seductive, but on some faces it looks silly, not sexy. Restrained browns are recommended for work and professional situations, but they can make a dark-skinned woman look dull and uninteresting. For a color to affect your mood and fit a situation, it has to fit you first.

Self-expression also plays a part in makeup choice. Many women have found a cosmetic strategy that is distinctive and makes the most of their looks, and they wear it in all situations, because it is adaptable and always makes them feel their best. They may have found a particular lipstick shade which suits them very well, or they might concentrate on distinctive eye makeup balanced by sober cosmetics on the rest of the face. **JAG**

readable style. Constantly changing your look to fit the latest fashion craze may prevent you from expressing your individuality and may prevent you from communicating clear images to others and adapting to different situations.

Developing a personal style

So how do you develop a personal style? Have a good look through your wardrobe and other personal possessions. Look at old pictures of yourself. How many "looks" have you managed to collect?

Most people have a whole range of appearances from romantic to sporty to professional, and they use these very different looks to try to express different aspects of themselves. Wearing jeans and cowboy boots one day and a severe suit the next only leads to confusion, both in how others perceive you and in how you view yourself. While we need different outfits for different pursuits, it helps if they add up to a coherent statement.

Which styles make you really feel most comfortable? Make a list of what you like to wear for work, leisure and formal occasions. You will soon find that certain elements keep cropping up – a preference for sober, severe types of clothing, makeup and hairstyle, or a tendency to choose bright accessories.

You may like to wear a hat, or have a fondness for paisley ties. Once you have a clear idea of what makes you feel happy and confident about your appearance, you can get rid of all the alternative styles cluttering up your image and your closet. You will be left with a simple, flexible and above all clearly recognizable style.

Accepting yourself

The final and most important point about developing a personal style is to accept yourself. Most of us have features that we would prefer to minimize or mask because they do not fit in with conventional ideas of beauty. But as we reproportion our bodies and recontour our faces we may all begin to resemble each other. After all, the really delightful thing about people is their infinite variety. Whatever sort of features you have, there is nothing wrong or right about them; there is no recognized council that sets standards for human beauty. Style is about freeing your personality.

Of course, many people have a physical feature that makes them uncomfortable, and some conditions, such as acne, will always be a problem. There are times when camouflage is beneficial (see *Ch 26*). One course is to play up a defect – make a feature of broad shoulders or a big nose. Think about the people you know with a distinctive personal style. What they all have in common is confidence in themselves and in their own judgment. They like and accept themselves. Style can grow out of confidence, but trying to develop personal style can, in turn, help you to be more confident and value yourself more, because it assumes a belief in your self-worth and attractiveness. **JAG**

169

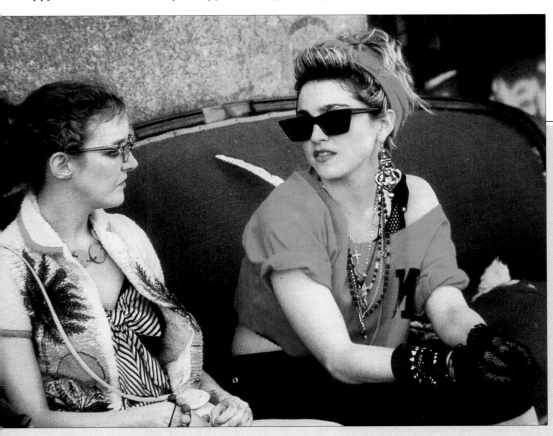

◄ **Vintage Madonna**. *The rock star's name is synonymous with bold and highly individual personal style. Changing several times a year – from short platinum-blond waves to long dark curls; a torn sweatshirt and leggings, to Marilyn Monroe look-alike – she might hide behind dark glasses, but the look – however unexpected or contradictory – is always unmistakable. Having a personal style is a matter of developing a distinctive look and making it work across the whole range of situations that you appear in.*

24

Looking Better With Age

Looking good is not necessarily a preoccupation of the young ● We feel dismayed when the years begin to take a toll on our appearance ● But looking better with age is achieved in the same way as looking good in youth.

OUR BODIES change as we grow older. Find an old photograph album and look at some pictures of yourself as a child, a teenager, a young adult and an older person. How have your face and body changed? Are your facial bones more prominent, or is your nose longer? Have you developed the classic pear-shaped body? Do you have any wrinkles? These changes are part of the pattern of growing older. Some of them can be delayed or eliminated; others

are unstoppable. Some are desirable – no one regrets the disappearance of adolescent skin problems – and others make us less happy.

Aging and self-esteem

All these changes affect the way we think about ourselves. We tend to assume that the heyday of attractiveness is the twenties, and after that it is "all downhill," especially for women. People often say of an older woman, "you can tell she was a great beauty once." We do tend to judge the attractiveness of *others* partly in terms of how well they age; but "old" does not have to mean "unattractive." In terms of our image of *ourselves*, young, middle-aged and elderly people are equally satisfied with or critical of their bodies throughout the lifespan.

In a survey of 62,000 Americans, scientists asked men and

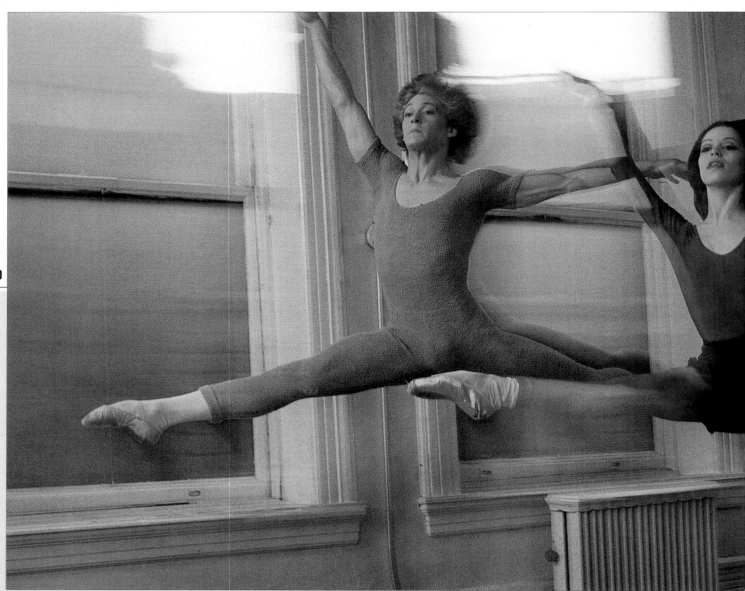

women from three major age-groups – 24 and younger, 24 to 44, and over 45 – how they felt about their looks. The results were astonishing. Young adults, despite the generally held view that this age-group is the most physically appealing, seemed to be no more satisfied with their own looks than the elderly.

How do good-looking people age?

Good-looking men and women are probably more affected by age than average-looking or unattractive people. Two popular but conflicting theories about age and handsomeness jostle for our attention. Some people maintain that "a thing of beauty is a joy forever," and that men and women who are good-looking in their teens start with an advantage that they maintain throughout their lives. A second theory holds that beauty is short-lived, and good

looks are soon ravaged by time. People who are stunning in youth are tempted to rely on their good looks, and when these external attributes fade, they are left with empty lives and poor self-esteem.

The truth presents a somewhat different picture from both these theories. Social psychologists asked women and men ranging in age from 10 to 90 how attractive they were in childhood, adolescence, young adulthood, middle age and old age. They also asked them how happy they were at various ages and how happy they were at present. People indicated their general satisfaction with life on a ten-point scale ranging from "living an ideal, happy life"(10) to "living the worst possible life" (1).

This study showed a clear link between good looks and happiness. Childhood and adolescent attractiveness went hand in hand with early happiness. The child or teenager who felt unattractive was also miserable. Childhood beauty or homeliness had little connection with a person's later happiness or unhappiness, however. By the time people

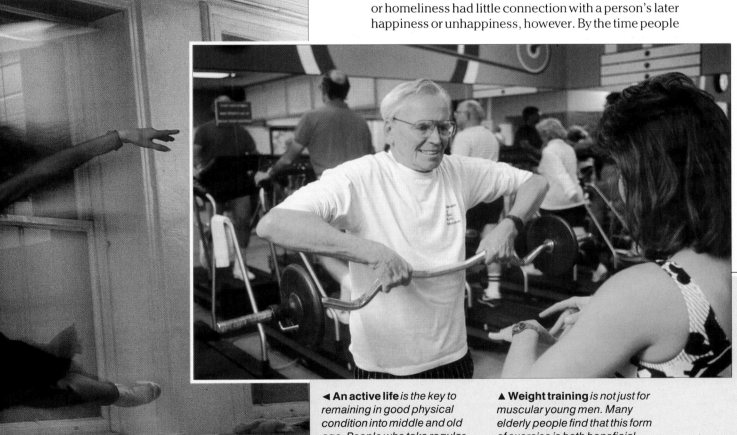

171

◄ **An active life** is the key to remaining in good physical condition into middle and old age. People who take regular exercise, as well as athletes and dancers who continue their activity past their prime, will feel younger than those with sedentary lifestyles. Good physical health contributes to good mental health. Both of these promote an active and rewarding life.

▲ **Weight training** is not just for muscular young men. Many elderly people find that this form of exercise is both beneficial and enjoyable. It is especially helpful in building and maintaining bone density in women, who are more likely to suffer from brittle bone disease (osteoporosis) in later life (see Ch 2).

reach college age it seems to make little difference whether they were attractive as children or not. On the other hand, adolescent attractiveness or unattractiveness seems to leave its mark forever. People who were unattractive as teenagers were affected by low self-esteem related to their looks, and had low happiness ratings, regardless of how they rated their looks at a later age. People who were attractive as adolescents maintained good self-esteem and happiness over a significantly longer period.

Body image and life satisfaction

Nevertheless, people who were handsome as teenagers do tend to experience a drop in general feelings of happiness from middle age. The decline is not great and levels out by old age, but it does seem that people who were attractive adolescents find it more difficult to cope with the effects of aging in their middle years. Homely teenagers, on the other hand, tend to get happier as they get older, with their self-esteem ratings increasing dramatically in the middle years (though they never quite draw equal with those who were attractive adolescents).

Keeping up appearances is just as important to mental and physical health in older people as it is for the young. The elderly who feel their looks no longer matter and "let themselves go" are usually depressed and unhappy. With effort, personal appearance can be changed for the better when we are older as well as in early life. **EH**

Growing old gracefully

Body image is just as important in old age as it is in youth. It is a good idea to keep working on your appearance even when you are past the age when, formerly, these things were thought to stop being important. Attitudes are changing – you do not have to be young to be beautiful anymore.

Though the body is getting older, it is still the same body, and most of the care it requires is contained in the good health habits we established or tried to establish in youth. A healthy, moderate diet, regular exercise and avoidance of smoking and drinking are more important, not less so, as we get older. The older body is less resilient and supple, so it reacts less favorably to abuse and takes longer to heal; older people also have a slower metabolism and gain weight more easily than their younger selves.

Even if a person has been careless, a great deal of the damage caused by an unhealthy lifestyle can be reversed or

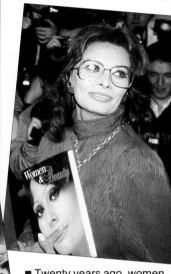

Well-preserved women

■ Twenty years ago, women over 40 were thought to be old. Today women well into their forties and beyond are fighting for the title of "Most Glamorous Woman in the World."

All these famous women are past 50, and while we might think that their attractiveness stems, at least in part, from the fact that they look younger than they really are, theirs is not the beauty of young women but has a quality of its own.

While improved makeup and skin care regimes have allowed women to keep more youthful looks, one of the main reasons for this social change may be the demographic changes of the last 20 years. The bulk of the population is no longer under 30, as it once was. The "baby

Does smiling give you wrinkles?

■ How does facial movement affect the development of wrinkles? Certainly we call the wrinkles that run from nose to mouth and the crinkly marks at the corners of the eye "laughter lines," because they do parallel the wrinkles that appear on our faces when we laugh or talk animatedly.

One school of thought proposes that to prevent wrinkles we should try not to screw up our eyes, squint, frown or laugh too much, and should avoid touching our faces, leaning a cheek on the hand, etc.

But laughter is healthy and good for the spirit, and a person afraid to respond to emotion for fear of creating a few wrinkles would be very uninteresting. After all, wrinkles are not unhealthy, just a sign of expression through the years.

■ **Another school of thought** holds that wrinkles develop along laughter and expression lines because of the way skin drapes over our facial features, not because of excessive facial expressiveness, and that exaggerated facial movements exercise facial muscles and actually prevent the skin from sagging and wrinkling.

A number of facial exercise regimes include the repetition of exaggerated frowning, smiling, and grimacing to exercise the face, claiming that this tones and invigorates the skin and muscle. It probably does stimulate circulation in the skin, but our facial muscles probably get enough exercise in the course of daily interactions. Keeping the skin moist and supple probably does more for it, allowing the skin to stretch and contract freely when we laugh, cry, and talk. **JAG**

halted by adopting good habits later in life. Older people do need to be careful about exercise, taking things a little more slowly and allowing themselves more time to warm up and cool down. But otherwise the rules of a healthy lifestyle are the same: take regular exercise, eat a balanced diet, avoid smoking and drink only in moderation.

Adapting your skin care habits as you grow older is another main strategy for maintaining a satisfying appearance. For details, see Chapter 25.

Age and stress

We think of our later years as a time to sit back and rest, but older people are prone to stress and suffer more seriously from it when it occurs. Ensuring time to relax is just as important for the older retired person as for the busy working person in mid-life. Although surveys show that retired people overall are happier than those still at work, retirement itself can be frustrating, especially for those who have been very active and worked all their lives. Even women who do not work outside the home may find their husbands' retirement stressful if they have been used to having the

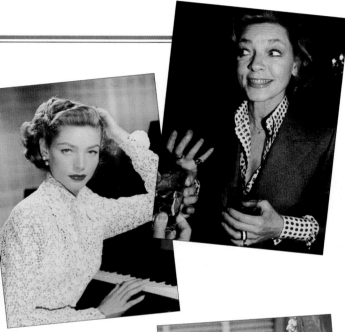

■ **Touched by the hand of time**, *these famous actresses have still retained their looks past middle age. Sophia Loren FAR LEFT, elegant and sophisticated at 32, had not changed much at 50. At 29, Lauren Bacall LEFT was cool and imposing; at 55 LEFT she favored a classic style but was more relaxed and outgoing. Jane Russell at 32 LOWER LEFT was a well-known sex symbol. At 67 BELOW she had the same inviting smile. While some older women may feel the need for surgical procedures such as face-lifts, proper diet and exercise and a happy lifestyle are the best weapons against the ravages of time.*

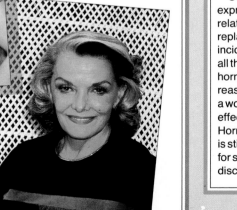

boomers," people born in the postwar birth explosion of the 1940s and early 1950s, are no longer children. This group is large enough to dominate social outlook, and their favorite icons are, naturally enough, no longer young people.

The teenage era is said to have been created in the late 1950s, when baby boomers ceased to want to look like their parents and developed a youth look and a mass market of their own. With advertising, sales and social developments all directed toward this aging group, we may again see a time, in the not too distant future, when teenagers try to look like their mothers and fathers, rather than parents attempting to appear as young as possible.

Hormone replacement

■ Hormone replacement therapy was originally developed to help women cope with the more distressing symptoms of the menopause, many of which are caused by an excessive drop in estrogen production. The treatment is sometimes regarded as a way to combat the aging process in women (there is no male equivalent).

Hormone replacement can improve skin condition and stop the development of excess facial hair and loss or thinning of scalp hair. It is more useful medically in preventing severe loss of bone mass, (osteoporosis), a condition that can lead to fragile and easily breakable bones, especially in elderly women.

Some doctors have expressed concern at a possible relationship between hormone replacement therapy and the incidence of breast cancer. Until all the results are in, taking hormones for purely cosmetic reasons may be unwise, unless a woman has experienced the effects of aging very rapidly. Hormone replacement therapy is still a very valuable treatment for serious menopausal discomfort and osteoporosis.

173

house to themselves most of the day. The inevitable aches and pains, the fears about bad health and a growing awareness of being unable to manage alone can also induce stress in the elderly. Using relaxation techniques to reduce stress and anxiety can be extremely beneficial for the health of the elderly person.

Correcting vision and hearing

Good health and a relaxed attitude are the groundwork of attractiveness, but there is much more the elderly person can do to improve body image and self-esteem. Many elderly people feel cut off from life around them, and may appear dull and uninteresting. Decaying vision and hearing may be among the causes of this. Older people should have frequent vision and hearing tests – as often as once every six months, if they suspect problems are developing – to keep prescription lenses adjusted and fit a hearing aid if necessary. Taking an interest in the world and in other people, a prerequisite of attractiveness, is much easier if we can see and hear what is going on properly.

Youthful posture

■ Posture can make or break your appearance, at any age. People who slouch or are round-shouldered tend to look sloppy and unself-confident most of the time.

In old age, the inevitable loss of bone mass and the shrinking of cartilage in the backbone and joints can also lead to poor posture. Stiff muscles and joints due to lack of exercise, or diseases like arthritis and rheumatism, which tend to be common in the elderly, can have the same effect.

Exercise, and treatment for diseases of the joints, will help you retain your suppleness and improve your posture to some extent, but a good look in the mirror can be very beneficial too. Are you standing and sitting up straight, or do you tend to slump and hump your shoulders?

Make a conscious effort to pull yourself upright. You may find that you still have a waist and that your "widow's hump" is due partly to the way you are standing. Good posture is better for your internal organs, your muscles and bones, and it can make a difference to your appearance.

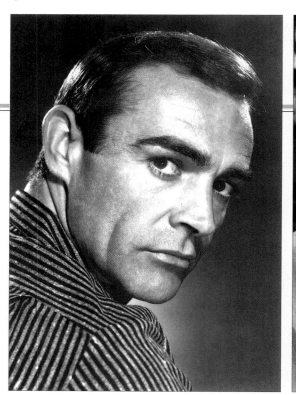

Well-preserved men

■ Men have always been thought to age more gracefully than women, and male film stars in particular did not face the same decline in roles and popularity as they got older.

In fact, male skin appears to be more resistant to the effects of weather and sun than the thinner, more delicate and drier skin of women. Especially before the advent of readily available moisturizers and skin creams, men's skin did seem to take longer to show signs of aging than women's.

Perhaps more importantly, however, male attractiveness in a purely physical sense has never been thought to be as important as female beauty. Older men are more likely to have money and power, and it is likely to be these things that will attract other people to them rather than their looks. Although this attraction equation between males and power and females and physical beauty has been changing as the social relationships of men and women alter, it still remains a powerful influence over how we evaluate people in relation to their appearance.

■ **Longevity favors leading men,** *who continue to have career opportunities as they progress to distinguished middle and old age. Their careers may expand, allowing them to take on a wider scope of roles than when they were typecast as handsome heroes. At 33, Sean Connery* LEFT *was well established as a screen idol. In middle age* CENTER *his roles reflected not only his good looks but also strong character. The trend continued as he approached 60* RIGHT.

Dress, makeup and hair

Older people need to pay as much attention to dress, makeup and hair as their younger counterparts do, but what suited a person when they were young may look washed-out or garish in old age. Skin tone and hair color change and we have to adjust the way we dress to suit these changes. Colors like beige and gray may have looked good on you at 20 but skin loses its glow and hair gets lighter in color. Brighter colors may suit you more as you get older, or deeper richer shades of the same colors you used to wear.

Careless dressing can look charming on the very young, but it does not suit elderly people. Good, simple tailoring for men and women is the answer. Frilly and baggy clothes are aging, but an older woman can look elegant in a simple dress and an elderly man can still look good in a beautifully cut plain suit.

Makeup has to be adjusted as well. Dramatic eye shadow and rich lip colors can look silly on an older woman, because the skin has become too delicate to carry them. Lips shrink and eyes grow hollow; vibrant shades can merely emphasize this. Older women usually look better with less makeup and should wear more subtle shades than they used to as young women.

Many people find the loss of hair color difficult to cope with, and have it dyed to match their original shade. After the age of 60 this has to be handled carefully. The change in skin tone may mean that your original color now looks too dark and harsh. You can still dye your gray or white hair, but it is better to choose a lighter shade to give a softening, rather than a harsh, contrasting, effect on the skin.

Growing older is not the end of looking your best. There are some aspects of aging that no one can escape, but many so-called "inevitable" characteristics of aging are actually the preventable results of poor self-care. However, there is no need to be mutton dressed as lamb – balance is the key.

As the average age in the industrialized world mounts, we are beginning to appreciate that age has its own tranquil and delicate beauty. Just like youthful attractiveness, hand-some old age can be cultivated and encouraged for our own benefit and the delight of others. **JAG**

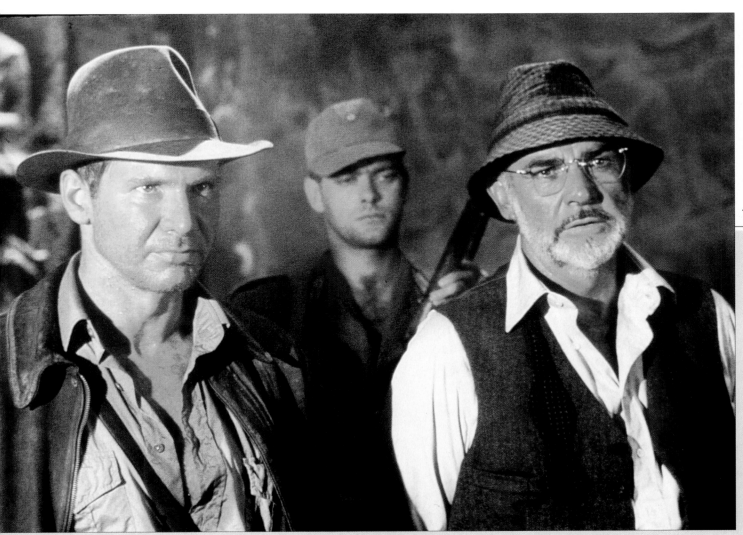

25

Skincare

We spend more on skincare products than on any other cosmetic ● The best skincare is overall health and well-being ● Good, clear skin has a positive effect on others and makes you feel good about yourself.

THE APPEARANCE of your skin is a crucial element in whether people perceive you as attractive. We worry much more about the way our skin looks than we do about its health, even though its health and appearance are in fact closely related. For many years an even tan was supremely desirable, despite warnings from skincare specialists and dermatologists that too much sun was related to skin cancer. Only when sun exposure was related to the effects of aging did people begin to pay serious attention to what dermatologists had been saying for years.

Our bodies are covered in skin; the average adult has about 6sq m (20sq ft) of it. It is our most obvious feature and its condition can enhance, detract from or disguise any other element of our appearance. Skin also bears the brunt of our physical environment and reflects the state of our health and emotions. So it is not surprising that we pay a good deal of attention to it, and spend more money on skin preparations than on any other cosmetic aid. Skin that looks clean, healthy and cared for makes an immense difference to our overall appearance, while spotted, damaged or dull skin can ruin the looks of an otherwise very attractive person.

Your general health is reflected in your skin. Any illness you have is likely to make your skin dull and tired looking.

Both smoking and alcohol inhibit the supply of oxygen to the skin and will damage its appearance in the short term as well as over a period of time. A poor diet prevents your skin getting the nutrients it needs, and too much refined food will overload it with waste products. Lack of exercise may mean that skin circulation is sluggish. Really healthy skin requires good general bodycare.

Because the skin is so responsive to your mental and physical state, it is extremely vulnerable to the effects of stress. Anxiety has a direct influence over hormonal secretions, circulation and nervous reactions, and all these functions are closely connected with the health and functioning of the skin. Many skin conditions such as shingles, scleroderma (hardening and calcification of the skin surface), psoriasis, acne and even some allergic responses have been shown in clinical trials to be greatly relieved or exacerbated by stress levels. Just as a blush may betray a shy or nervous nature, a tendency to break out in a rash or spots may be a signal of an anxious temperament.

Toward a healthy skin

If your skin looks well-groomed and cared for it improves the reactions of others toward you and makes you feel better about yourself. Taking care of skin can itself be an enjoyable activity that encourages feelings of well-being. Unfortunately, some common practices that appear to improve the look of the skin may damage it in the long term. We need to understand how the skin works in order to help it stay healthy and glowing. The condition of the skin reflects the health of the body, because many physical and medical factors can contribute to premature aging.

In China, Korea and other Asian countries health is frequently diagnosed by looking carefully at the skin. Texture, color and even odor are analyzed to give clues about internal problems, and the results are often extremely accurate.

Psychological repercussions from a skin problem can occur at any age, and the intensity of emotional disturbance is not necessarily proportional to the severity of the skin problem. One small wrinkle or spot can have a big emotional effect.

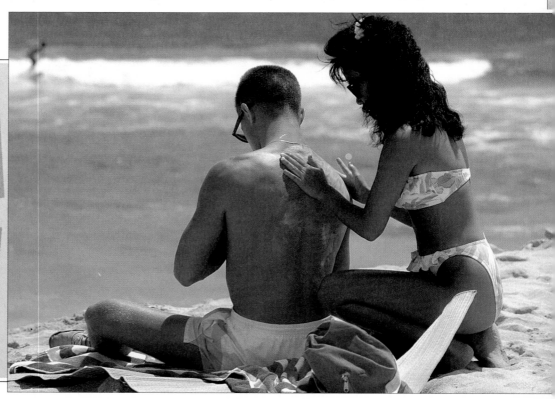

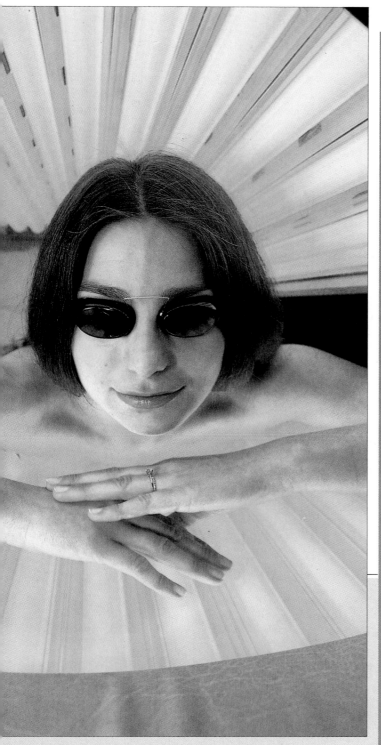

How to assess your skin type

■ Identifying your skin type is very important in treating it correctly and selecting the right products for it.

● **Dry** – central heating, air conditioning, strong sun and harsh winds can all contribute to robbing the skin of its natural moisture. Dry skin feels taut, flaky and can have a crepe-like appearance. It is usually more prone to lines, wrinkles and

▼ **Clay and cucumber** *are two popular natural skin care substances. Face masks consist of a double layer of clay which is spread on the face. As the outer layer hardens the rise in temperature brings out the healing properties of the minerals contained in the inner layer. Cucumber contains substances that moisturize sensitive skin and soothe the eyes.*

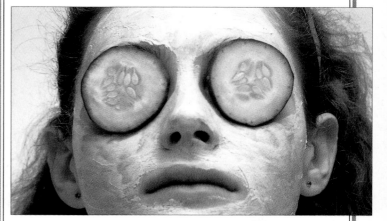

broken veins. Use a cleansing cream, a mild skin freshener, a moisturizer under makeup and a nourishing cream at night.

● **Oily** – oily skin is usually a problem in adolescence when the change in hormone levels causes the sebaceous glands to produce too much sebum, but it can be a problem for people of any age. Skin feels greasy and is prone to spots, pimples, blackheads and even acne. It has a shiny appearance and may also be sensitive or allergic to certain products. Use a milk or clarifying lotion to cleanse, followed by a slightly astringent toner. You might choose to replace these two stages with a wash-off cleanser. Even oily skin needs a moisturizer, so use one that has been specially formulated for this skin type.

● **Sensitive** – sensitive skin can be dry or oily. It may be allergic to many skincare products and usually reacts badly to harsh

weather and sometimes even to washing. As well as exhibiting signs of dryness or oiliness, it will also show signs of irritation which may appear in patches or in an overall redness. It may have flaky areas that are dry and very red and can also be prone to broken veins. Use products that suit the basic skin type but select those that have been specially formulated for sensitive skin and contain no perfumes, colorants or anything that might irritate the skin.

● **Combination** – this is the most common skin type. Many people have dry areas at the sides of the face and an oily panel down the center. The skin will appear to have patches of dryness and oiliness. The oily areas may have spots and pimples and the dry areas may look flaky. Treat the two areas of the skin quite separately, using dry-skin products on the dry areas and products designed for oily skin on the center panel.

■ **Ultraviolet radiation,** *always present in ordinary sunlight, is a mixed blessing to our skin. Both men and women spend hours in the sun every summer to bake their skin to a fashionably dark shade LEFT caused by ultraviolet (UV) radiation. In less sunny weather a UV-producing sunlamp ABOVE has the same*

effect. Artificial UV is also prescribed as a remedy for some skin disorders. But the problems caused by UV outweigh its benefits. Overexposure to UV light is a cause of skin cancer, and frequently tanned skin will age more quickly than skin that has been protected from the sun.

Research conducted on elderly men has shown that those with prematurely aged skin tended to be older by biological measures of health and resilience. Men who looked old for their age judging by their skin were in fact physiologically older as well in terms of the state of their heart, lungs, etc. Longer-term follow-up studies indicated that men with younger-looking skin actually lived longer too. Caring for your skin may not reverse the internal problems that are reflected there, but it can give an enormous psychological lift, and regular attention to your skin may also alert you to symptoms of illness which are reflected in it. **JAG**

Taking good care of your skin

The most important care you can take of your skin is promoting good general health: eating properly, exercising, avoiding alcohol and tobacco, and keeping stress to a minimum. A healthy lifestyle provides your skin with the benefits of a strong body and mind. Since skin is so sensitive to the internal condition of the body the best skincare is overall well-being. People who live in warm climates and wear little clothing seldom even need to wash their skin to keep it in good condition, so long as their nutrition is well-balanced. In industrialized countries, standards of hygiene,

What is skin?

The skin is more than just an envelope that keeps our bodies together. It is actually a specially adapted bodypart that regulates a number of important bodily functions. It is an organ of the body just like the kidneys or liver. Because it also has intimate connections with all the other parts of the body, it tends to reflect many specific internal conditions as well as our general health status. The skin protects our other body parts, registers and transmits sensations, absorbs, formulates and secretes various vital substances, and regulates body temperature.

The skin consists of two chief layers, lying over a deeper layer of subcutaneous (under-the-skin) fat. First comes the dermis, containing blood vessels, nerve endings, hair follicles, a lymphatic drainage system to remove waste products, sweat glands and sebaceous glands. Next comes the epidermis. It begins with a basal layer that produces cells at an enormous rate to replace those shed by the epidermis. The epidermis is a thick, dense layer of cells which contain most of the skin's pigmentation, moisture and oil. The very top layer of the epidermis is a harder layer of dead skin cells which flatten as they reach the skin surface.

The skin is fed by the blood vessels which transfer nutrients to its living cells. Good circulation is of enormous importance to healthy skin, as blood will be diverted away from extremities to vital organs if circulation is impaired. The outermost layer of dead skin is kept supple by the oil (sebum) produced by the sebaceous glands, which also keeps hair in good condition. In addition, skin needs moisture to stay smooth and supple, and will absorb water from the air as well as fluid from the deeper layers.

The skin is a major sense organ, and it relates to the sense of touch as the nose relates to smell. It is full of nerve endings and blood vessels that register the most delicate sensations of touch, transmitting information to the brain and central nervous system. This is why skin massage makes us feel so relaxed and calm, and why skin irritation is so distressing – there is a very high concentration of nerve endings being soothed or aroused. Such nerve endings are so plentiful that we rub or agitate an injured area of skin to excite other nerve endings and to interfere with any pain messages being sent.

These nerve endings also receive and transmit sensations of heat and cold that help the skin perform its most important function, that of controlling body temperature. Mammals (including humans) keep their body at

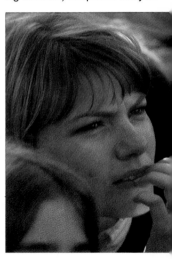

178

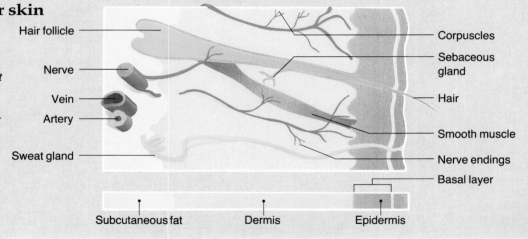

The structure of our skin

■ *Skin is essentially an impervious barrier. The outer layers of skin will absorb a certain amount of oil and water, but the deeper layers can only be penetrated by extremely small molecules, and very few chemical or bacterial substances can reach the blood vessels of the skin. Whether a substance is helpful or harmful, it is unlikely to do much good or evil deeper down unless the skin has been damaged in some way.*

Hair follicle

Nerve

Vein

Artery

Sweat gland

Corpuscles

Sebaceous gland

Hair

Smooth muscle

Nerve endings

Basal layer

Subcutaneous fat   Dermis   Epidermis

cold weather and heavy clothing make our skin drier and dirtier, and it needs good surface care as well as internal nourishing.

Our bodies are usually encased in clothing, and air seldom has a chance to circulate around them freely. Dirt, sweat and bacteria remain in close contact with the skin, so even if we do not actually see marks on our skin it still needs regular cleansing. The body should be washed once a day, and the face, which is often exposed to the sooty air of urban environments, should be washed in the morning and evening.

Most people like the clean feeling that they get from soap and water, but if your skin is dry, soap will make it feel tight and sore, and you may be happier with a creamy nonsoap cleanser. Bath foams and bubbles are pleasant but they can be very drying on sensitive skin. If you are wearing water-proof cosmetics, you may need to use special removers. Whatever you use, massage it well into the skin and rinse thoroughly. Alternate splashes of warm and cool water help the circulation and give the skin a fresher appearance.

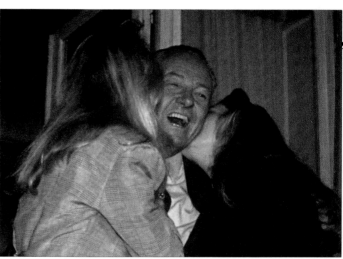

round the same internal temperature. By regulating bodily systems our bodies maintain an optimum temperature at which all our physical structures function best (around 37°C, 98°F). The body can do

Touching our own skin *is something we do all the time – rubbing our hands, stroking our noses, resting the chin on the hand, scratching our ears – specially when we feel nervous. The touching both hides and diverts our agitation, and reassures us by reminding ourselves of our own presence. It can induce spots or irritation by pressure or the transmission of bacteria, however, and if you often get pimples where you rest your face on your hand, you might want to try to break this habit.*

"Skin like a baby's" *is a phrase often used to describe a perfectly healthy and beautiful skin. A very young child has extremely elastic and supple skin with a visible sheen. These are qualities central to any healthy, attractive skin. Smooth, supple skin with a good moisture content is best able to protect the body by responding quickly to the environment, and this is also the condition in which the skin feels most comfortable.*

this easily in all but the most extreme climates. Most mammals control body temperature by breathing, eliminating heat through the lungs, but human beings regulate temperature mainly through the skin.

The body produces heat constantly, generated by the activity of our organs. This heat is conducted to the skin by the blood, where it is lost by exposure to the cooler air. In very hot conditions, the sweat glands will become activated and exude moisture through the skin; the moisture evaporates and cools the body quickly. If it is very cold, the skin responds by contracting its blood vessels to slow down heat loss, and will even set off involuntary muscular tremors which we experience as shivering, in an attempt to create heat by means of muscular activity.

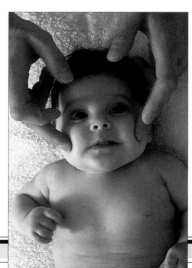

Changing color with emotion

■ The skin responds to and reflects the emotions we feel. We go pale with fear or fatigue, blue with cold, red with embarrassment or effort, gray or green with nausea or shock, and flushed when pleased or sexually aroused. Skin produces sweat when we are nervous or overheated, and goes cold when we are afraid or surprised. The tiny strands of muscle it contains can make skin go rigid or goose-pimply, and cause the hairs to stand on end, when we are afraid. These effects show most strongly in light-skinned people because their skin shows the flow of blood which regulates these changes most clearly, but we all exhibit the same range of skin reactions to emotions.

We frequently "read" other people by the state of their skin; it is often a better guide to their real feelings than their words. Novelists sometimes explain a

▲ **The flush of emotion** *shows up clearly on the face of this politician. The surprise of having heard good news and the feeling of having achieved a personal victory contribute to a state of emotional arousal. His reddened face contrasts with those of his daughters who are less affected by the excitement.*

situation by simple descriptions of a character's color change, and artists can tell a whole story in the skin tones of their subjects. Acting out violent emotion on stage can be inhibited by the actors' difficulty in changing their own skin tone to fit the feelings of the characters they play. The audience subconsciously expects to see this change, and a whole range of lighting and make-up techniques may be used to give the right appearance to a scene of extreme grief or joy. **R R**

179

Rubbing the skin with a loofah or towel has the same effect.

Rubbing the skin will also remove the topmost layer of dead skin cells. As we get older we tend to lose this layer more slowly, and the skin can look dull and lifeless. Exfoliating creams are commercially available which will gently buff away this skin while simultaneously aiding the circulation. Some people find exfoliating creams easier to use than a loofah or brush on its own, which can feel uncomfortable. You can make your own cream from a mixture of coarse sea salt and almond or baby oil. Remember that dry skin will lose moisture if it is exfoliated too frequently; once

a week is enough. Oily skin benefits greatly from exfoliation several times a week, as sebum too can build up in the dead skin layer, attracting bacteria. Do not stimulate the skin too vigorously though, or it will produce excess sebum.

"Cleanse, tone, moisturize" is the litany followed by almost all male and female skincare regimes, but some dermatologists are doubtful about the benefits of toning. Toners are astringent lotions that may vary in strength, and often include substances like alcohol which make the skin feel tighter and fresher, and remove surface oiliness. If you have rinsed your skin properly you should not need a toner after you have washed but they are useful in removing traces of cleansing cream and lotions. Some people, particularly those who have combination skin, with an oily panel around the nose and mouth but dry cheeks, find toners useful as a way of freshening the skin during the day.

Even the driest skin usually produces adequate sebum, but every type of skin can be lacking in moisture. The point of a moisturizer is to restore water to clean skin and help it retain and attract water. Moisturizers are produced in different ways to help different skin types. Rich emulsions known as water-in-oil creams are good at preventing moisture loss. Oil-in-water emulsions are lighter in texture and contain less oil but they contain agents called humectants that attract atmospheric water. They are best for use on combination or oily skins or under foundation which will have some moisturizer in it.

What are free radical scavengers?

■ Many new cosmetic skin products term themselves "free radical scavengers." Free radicals are atoms or groups of atoms that are highly likely to have chemical reactions with other atoms in order to pair an unpaired electron. Ultraviolet light from the sun has the effect of turning oxygen atoms in and on the skin into oxygen free radicals which will then seek to combine with other atoms in a chemical reaction known as oxidation. Over time, thousands upon thousands of oxidizations will eventually lead to degeneration of the skin characterized by dryness, leatheriness and wrinkles. Free radical scavengers are mostly vitamin compounds such as A and E which bind oxygen free radicals.

Dermatologists outside the cosmetics industry do not seem to be completely convinced of the value of free radical scavengers, although the theory is sound as far as it goes. A healthy diet should contain enough vitamins without the need for supplements, and surface application may not be able to prevent free radical damage at the deepest skin levels where serious damage takes place. Research into the effectiveness of free radical scavengers in the top skin layers is still continuing.

Skincare for men

■ Male skin is thicker and oilier than female skin. It often suffers from irritation due to shaving followed by overharsh aftershave products, and may be prone to spots even in later life. Male skin needs thorough cleansing, gentle, careful shaving techniques (see *Ch 28*), and a good light moisturizer to remain in good condition. Like female skin, it benefits from exfoliation with a cream or loofah.

Because male skin is thicker it tends to accumulate more dead skin layers, and can often look dull and rough. Shaving will remove some of these dead layers, and skin here may look brighter than on the rest of the face, but it can also be sensitive to irritation. Aftershaves usually contain alcohol and can damage the newly-shaven skin. Shaving balms designed to soothe skin are much better.

Male skincare used to be something of a joke, but it has become acceptable in recent years. Now more and more men are trying to improve the condition of their skin, especially as they find it helps them feel much more comfortable.

A number of skincare lines formulated for male skin are now available. It is better to invest in these than to borrow your partners's skin prepara-

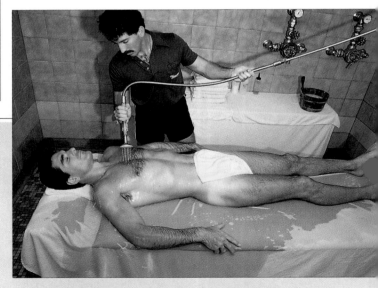

tions; women's cosmetics are not intended to treat male skin and may be either too rich or too gentle. As male grooming becomes more important, good skincare is becoming a crucial aspect of any man's self-presentation. Take the time to take care of your skin, and it will take care of you.

▲ **Cosmetic treatments for men** *were once derided but are becoming more popular now that improving your looks is regarded as part of the same process as health care. This spa offers salt water treatment which invigorates the skin making it look and feel healthier.*

Massage is one of the most beneficial treatment techniques known. It is good for the skin and relieves stress and tension. Touch is the most important way we communicate caring; stroking a baby or animal can immediately soothe it. Stroking brings the same sense of calm and pleasure to adult humans. Massage also stimulates circulation, relaxes muscles, rubs moisturizer deep into the skin, and may help to keep wrinkles and sagging at bay.

Massage techniques are easy to learn. Use a good-quality cream or oil to moisturize the skin and prevent friction. Press the thumbs gently into the area to be massaged to guide the movements of your hands, and work along the skin in firm but gentle circular movements, moving from the extremities toward the heart. Use a stroking massage movement to finish, passing the hands along the skin in long smooth strokes. These techniques can be used on any part of the body, from a shoulder rub to a full massage.

Problems under the skin

The exact causes of many skin conditions are unknown. In some illnesses the poor state of the skin may be a symptom of disease, and other skin problems may have multiple

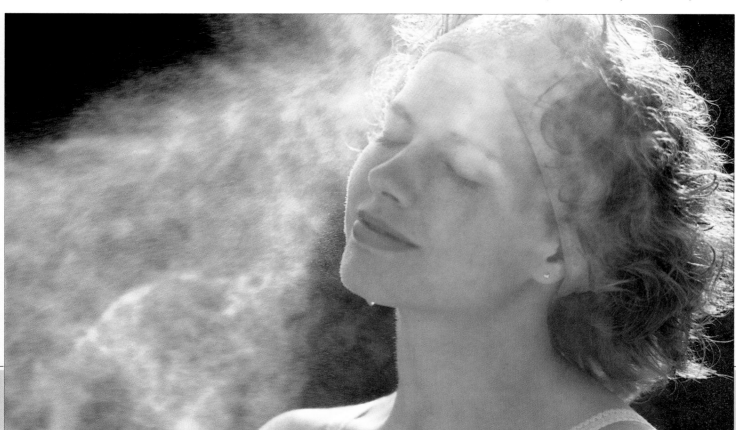

181

Giving yourself a facial at home

■ Giving yourself a facial every four to six weeks will deep cleanse your skin and keep it in good condition. Prepare a large bowl of hot water and sprinkle into it a few herbs such as rosemary or peppermint. These will scent the water and help to open the pores.

● Cleanse your skin thoroughly with your usual cleanser.

● Expose your face to the hot water vapor for three to four minutes if it is oily, seven to eight if it is dry.

● Now that the skin is warm and soft, you can examine the pores for impurities. Inspect your face closely in the magnifying mirror. If there are any blackheads, dab them with antiseptic, cover your fingertips with a tissue and squeeze gently. Dab with antiseptic again.

● Massage your face with a treatment cream suitable to your skin type. Dot the cream all over the face and neck and, working from the base of the neck, massage in small upward circular movements from the collarbone to the chin and face right up to the hairline.

● Remove all traces of cream with damp cotton wool.

● If you normally pluck your eyebrows do so now.

● Apply a face mask and relax with slices of cucumber over your eyes or cotton wool pads soaked in witch hazel.

● Rinse off the mask and finish with your usual moisturizer.

▲ **Water vapor treatment** *is a reliable way of ensuring that your skin gets thoroughly cleansed. The warm vapor opens the pores of your skin, releasing particles of dirt trapped inside. In its simplest form the treatment requires no more than a basin and a kettle, though for a more thorough job you can buy specialized equipment that directs the vapor at your face and includes a heating element to maintain the temperature of the water.*

sources. Boils, for instance, are caused by an infection but also become more likely with poor nutrition. The skin is also sensitive to mental tension, perhaps because it has so many nerve endings. A number of neurological diseases are often accompanied by eczema.

All skin conditions can be helped by sensible eating, gentle but thorough skin cleaning, and stress reduction but there are also many specific aids to cope with individual skin problems. If a skin condition arises it is important to have it properly diagnosed so that the real cause can be understood and treated. Dermatologists are constantly pushing back the frontiers of skin treatment, and many serious conditions can be cured or managed successfully.

Spots and acne

Most teenagers develop some form of skin eruption after puberty, when the surge of hormones into the young body overstimulates the sebaceous glands. Excess sebum builds up in the skin and attracts bacteria; the bacteria cause the inflammations we call spots or pimples. In some teenagers this condition is quite mild and lasts only a short time, but 50 percent develop chronic inflammation, or acne. There are many forms of acne, ranging from extremely serious infection of underlying skin layers to an excess of simple surface pimples.

Acne usually begins to recede in the later teenage years and disappears during the 20s, but acne is persistent in

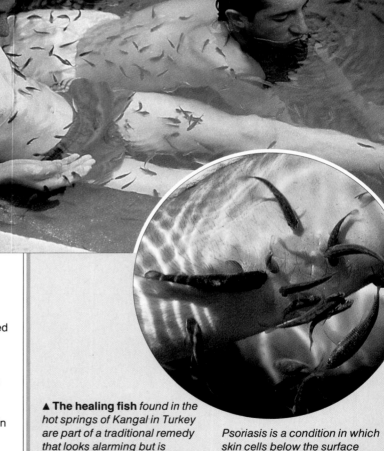

▲ **The healing fish** *found in the hot springs of Kangal in Turkey are part of a traditional remedy that looks alarming but is apparently effective. Patients suffering from the chronic skin complaint psoriasis relax in the pools ABOVE while the fish indulge in their taste for dead or diseased human tissue INSET.*

Psoriasis is a condition in which skin cells below the surface reproduce themselves faster than the natural rate of skin loss from the surface. The removal of skin by the fish restores the balance.

Coping with skin conditions

■ Beautiful skin is essential to an attractive overall appearance, and most people find skin problems particularly disturbing. Anyone with a serious or chronic skin condition, even quite a common one, often suffers mentally as well as physically. They may report feelings of being dirty or unclean and they frequently suffer from low self-esteem and depression. Promoting good general health and skincare is particularly important in these circumstances. If sufferers understand that good self-care is crucial to the management of their skin problem they will be motivated to carry out a new regime, and this will aid both their skin and their health. Looking after yourself promotes self-esteem. It also gives ill people a sense of control over their problems, relieving the frustration which often stems from chronic skin conditions.

■ **Your skin may respond to mental suggestion**. In one test, patients were given a series of pills which they were told would at first cause mild skin irritation

and then relief. In fact the pill was a simple sugar pill or placebo which could have no physical effect. Nevertheless many of the subjects developed mild skin irritations.

A classic case of skin treatment through psychological suggestion used hypnosis. An adolescent boy with a severe skin condition was instructed under hypnosis to "tell" his skin to return to normal gradually, and over a series of sessions his skin did recover permanently. Teenagers with severe acne have also responded to relaxation techniques.

some people, and women will often continue to experience brief flare-ups of the condition around the time of menstruation, probably in reaction to the release of hormones into the bloodstream at this time. Acne can lead to facial scars and seriously affect the appearance, so it needs to be treated seriously. Keeping the skin very clean, and avoiding surface stimulation of the sebaceous glands will help. Many people are helped by sunlight and sunlamp treatment; most drugs prescribed for acne (including Retin-A, recently publicized as a possible wrinkle-reducer as well as an acne treatment) use Vitamin A and also zinc, which seem to dry up the sebaceous glands.

Eczema or dermatitis

Eczema, or dermatitis, is a chronic condition in which the skin is itchy, prone to inflammation, and often very dry. Its exact cause is unknown, but it is not infectious, tends to run in families, can sometimes be related to poor diet or other

skin irritants, and is almost always made worse by stress. Thyroid problems or sensitivity to light can also lead to eczema. About one in twenty people are affected by eczema, so the search for an effective treatment goes on, but unless allergy is the cause it is seldom entirely cured.

Anti-inflammatory steroid creams are frequently used to control bad outbreaks of eczema, but they can have unpleasant side effects and are seldom recommended on a regular basis. One of the best strategies is to find out what triggers eczema in any one person, and avoid it as much as possible. In addition, a good diet is essential. Increasing your intake of essential fatty acids (found in cold-water fish like mackerel and sardines, and in oil of evening primrose) helps many people. Specially formulated zinc oxide creams can be used to protect and soothe itching skin directly.

Psoriasis and seborrhea

Psoriasis is another chronic skin condition characterized by scaly red patches on the skin of the body. Seborrhea occurs only on the scalp, but is similar in appearance to psoriasis and shares with it a basic phenomenon. In both conditions the skin cells reproduce as much as 1,000 times faster than normal. Cells are pushed to the surface before they have died and hardened, and as a result the surface of the skin becomes flaky, sensitive, itchy, and prone to infection. In severe cases the entire body is affected and the skin may be unable to control body temperature successfully.

Fortunately such severe episodes in the condition are rare. Nevertheless psoriasis and also seborrhea are disfiguring and distressing illnesses. Their cause is not known, though they seem to be in part genetic and may be triggered by stress. Treatment with ultraviolet light, steroids, and tar applications may help, and a diet rich in vitamin B6, zinc, sulfur, and essential fatty acids is often recommended.

183

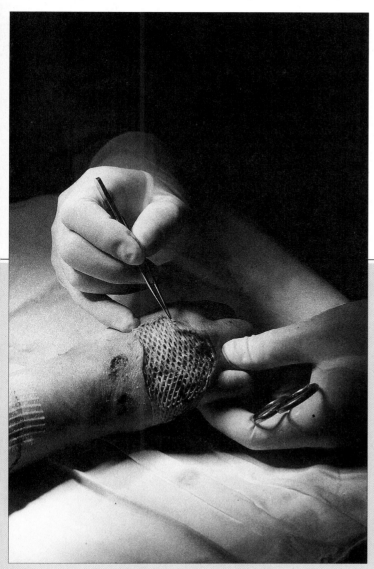

◄ **Skin grafts** are necessary if a large area of skin has been damaged at a deep level and is unlikely to replicate itself afresh. Because grafting is a painful and dangerous process with a high risk of infection it has only been used in serious cases such as burns and major skin cancers. New developments, however, have made it possible to perform grafts more safely and successfully, thanks to cultured skin. Now a small fragment of skin can be "grown" in the laboratory in a solution of essential nutrients and used to cover extensive areas of the body without having to remove skin from an equally large area elsewhere. It is made to grow in a lattice pattern in the laboratory. When applied to the human body LEFT the lattice grows into a continuous sheet of skin to cover the affected area. The culture can be made from the patient's own skin, or, if a graft is needed immediately, it can be taken from a bank of donor skin. The operation is carried out in thoroughly sterile conditions to cut down on the risk of infection. Victims of psoriasis and skin cancer, as well as burns patients, may benefit enormously from new grafting techniques, and the greater understanding of skin structure which grafting has led to may have some interesting cosmetic applications in the future.

Skin condition and age

We tend to associate beautiful skin with both youth and attractiveness. This is partly a result of the youth craze of the sixties and seventies, when the majority of the population was young, and as the "baby boomers" are now reaching middle age manufacturers of skin preparations are using older, more mature models. More and more mature women appear to challenge the association of youth and beauty, but in fact perpetuate it because they look so young for their age. Their skin is soft and unlined.

Research indicates that in the elderly, skin condition remains an important factor in attractiveness. A panel of women ranging in age from 60 to 90 were photographed and rated for attractiveness by a panel of judges (also elderly). The judges tended to rate the women as attractive or unattractive depending on how well or badly the subject's skin had aged. Those with poor skin condition, especially with age-related defects such as undereye bags or hollows, brown spots, wrinkles and sagging were quickly relegated to the unattractive category, but those with a better color and fewer wrinkles tended to be much more highly rated.

Stop your skin from aging

While some aspects of physical aging cannot be avoided, taking care of your skin now will help it to age better. Adapting your skincare regime as you get older, allowing in particular for your skin becoming drier, will keep it in good condition. The most important thing you can do for your skin at any age is to avoid excess exposure to the sun. Wear a sunscreen or cover the skin with clothing, scarves and hats if you are going to be outside for any length of time. This is just as important in the winter as in the summer. Sun damage is cumulative but it is not irreversible; skin can repair itself once it is no longer exposed to the sun.

184

Retin-A

■ Retin-A has been hailed as the new wonder drug for combating the effects of aging in the skin. Originally developed to help reduce acne, Retin-A also proved to have some effect on wrinkling and leatheriness, and is now being tested for use as an anti-aging serum. It is also known as Retinoic Acid (hence Retin-A) or tretinoin. It seems to provide the most impressive results on middle-aged skin that is just beginning to show the signs of wrinkling and fine lines. It cannot correct sagging or take the place of a facelift, but it can improve the color and the texture of skin if used regularly.

Retin-A can cause surface skin irritation – dryness, scaling and sensitivity – and it should be accompanied at all times by a sunscreen, as the skin becomes particularly sensitive to ultra-violet light. It is also known to lighten skin pigmentations such as freckles and small moles or melasma as well, and seems to inhibit the development of precancerous growths.

Retin-A is a powerful drug, and research into its effects is still continuing. Use it for purely cosmetic reasons only under medical supervision. **JAG**

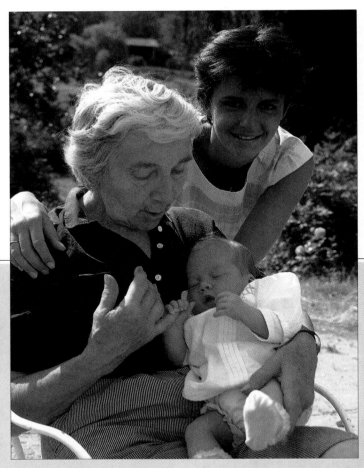

The problem of aging skin

■ From the smooth skin of infancy through an adulthood of suntanning and cosmetics, to old age, RIGHT it is perfectly natural for the skin to wrinkle and sag as we get older. These conditions are not caused by disease nor do they affect the health of the skin. Aging can lead to excessive dryness, delicacy, and loss of suppleness, but this can be countered by proper cleansing and thorough moisturizing. Even badly-wrinkled skin can preserve something of the glow and elasticity of its youth. Nevertheless, people often regard wrinkles as a problem, and aging skin is judged as unattractive.

When wrinkles and sagging are severe plastic surgery is sometimes used. Face lifts continue to become more and more sophisticated and successful, but they still involve temporary bruising and swelling, possible disappointment with the results, and the risk of infection. A face lift is, after all, major surgery with all the risks that involves. The best way to prevent wrinkles and sagging is effective skincare.

Good skincare really starts in babyhood, but it is around the age of 30 that wrinkles and lines begin to form in the skin's deep structures, and care should begin. There are many very

expensive cosmetic preparations available to treat wrinkles and prevent their formation, but the two most important guides to good skin in old age need not be costly. Avoid the sun and always use a good moisturizer

morning and evening, especially if the skin is dry. Sun damage and loss of moisture are the main cause of the skin losing elasticity. Gentle massage may also help by toning the muscles that support the skin.

Older skin and sun-damaged skin are both likely to be dry. Applying a good moisturizer morning and evening keeps the skin strong and supple and can prevent some wrinkling. Wearing a moisturizer throughout life is probably one of the best skin treatments you can have, but you can still aid your skin by starting to use one regularly at any age.

Cold, dry air and biting winds can rob your skin of moisture causing the outer layer to thicken and leading to the formation of thread veins on the cheeks and around the nose in old age. Using a moisturizer just before you go out will coat the skin with a thin film which will help protect it from the elements. For women, makeup also provides protection against cold and wind. Wrapping a scarf round the face or wearing a broad-brimmed hat will also help in very cold and windy weather.

Lifestyle is another major factor that affects how well we age. People who spend most of their lives out of doors are more likely to have wrinkled, leathery skin than those who have been office workers. The amount of smoking and drinking you do will also affect the way you look as you grow older. Both smoking and drinking affect the circulation, introduce toxic substances to the body, and rob the extremities (including the skin surface) of oxygen. Even in the elderly, cutting down on smoking and drinking can lead to a rapid improvement in skin texture.

Caring for aging skin

Aging skin tends to be dry and leathery. You may need to use more moisturizer than usual. Take care not to drag the skin when you are washing and moisturizing it; handle it gently. Older skin is also more likely to be sensitive because it is thinner. Protect your hands from harsh cleaning fluids by wearing gloves to do the housework, and switch to hypo-allergenic skin products.

Older skin is prone to certain problems, some of which respond well to treatment. Most elderly people, especially the fair-skinned, develop thread veins. These can be removed by laser or by electrocoagulation if you wish. Small red vascular growths, known as cherry angiomas, also may appear; these can be treated quite easily with liquid nitrogen or electrosurgery. Many older people also develop "skin tags" – small, soft, wart-like growths, often on the neck or around the eyes. When they are darkly pigmented they are known as seborrheic keratoses. These can be successfully treated by a doctor – either cut off or frozen off with liquid nitrogen.

Skin cancer is now appearing in younger people due to excessive sun exposure, but it is mainly a disease of older skin. Watch out for abnormal patches of skin or changes in moles, and report them to your doctor immediately. Pink or tan patches with a rough, scaly texture – solar keratoses – may develop into malignancies. Moles appearing suddenly or turning jagged at the edges, often very dark in color and asymmetrical in shape, may be cancerous. A growth with a somewhat translucent appearance with a small ulceration at the center may be a cancer of basal skin cells. When you shower or bath keep a check on any skin markings, and remember to look at your back in a mirror. If caught early, skin cancer can be easily treated and cured, so report anything unusual to your doctor. **RR**

185

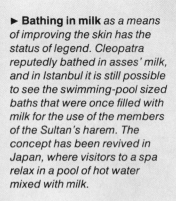

▶ **Bathing in milk** *as a means of improving the skin has the status of legend. Cleopatra reputedly bathed in asses' milk, and in Istanbul it is still possible to see the swimming-pool sized baths that were once filled with milk for the use of the members of the Sultan's harem. The concept has been revived in Japan, where visitors to a spa relax in a pool of hot water mixed with milk.*

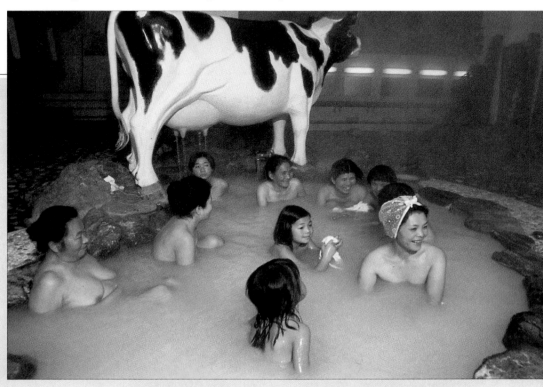

The sun and your skin

■ Some exposure to the sun is healthy, even vital, for everyone. It provides us with most of our essential vitamin D, and ultraviolet light from the sun can act as an antibiotic, killing off much harmful bacteria that thrives on shaded skin. Sunlight undoubtedly induces a feeling of well-being, and some people, deprived of sun, develop severe mental depression. Only small amounts of exposure are necessary to benefit us, however.

A total of 30 to 60 minutes daily (depending on how direct the sun's rays are) will allow you to reap all the benefits of exposure to the sun. Being near a window for much of the day or outside on a cloudy day can be just as good as 30 minutes in full sunlight.

Too much sun, on the other hand, can damage the skin. Ninety percent of the damage your skin suffers throughout your life is a result of the environment: wind, rain, cold and especially exposure to sunlight. The damage can be cumulative, building up over the years. We often underestimate just how much sun exposure we get in a day. Sitting within 10 feet of a window touched by sunlight counts as sun exposure; so does that quick dash to mail a letter or walk the dog. If your home has large windows, then even on an overcast day spent indoors you may be getting your full quota of sunlight.

What is a tan?

After a certain amount of exposure, the ultraviolet rays of sunlight begin to irritate and overheat the skin. The skin responds by producing more melanin, the pigment contained in skin cells that gives skin its color. The outer layer of skin also tends to thicken and toughen with regular exposure, to prevent the rays from reaching the skin's deeper layers.

If you spend too much time in strong sun the skin will burn. If your skin is fair and lacking in natural protective pigments, it will burn that much sooner.

If the sun is weak or your skin has sufficient melanin, the skin will gradually grow darker and thicker, without burning. Children are particularly vulnerable to sun damage and should always be protected from overexposure.

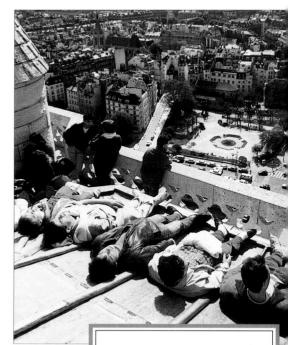

► **Soaking up the winter sun.**
Our urge to make the most of whatever sun we can get during the colder months stems in part from a need for vitamin D. The skin is amazingly efficient at manufacturing vitamin D, and very little sun exposure is needed to produce enough. However, before the days of vitamin D supplements in milk, children growing up in dark, narrow streets in northern Europe, and black children growing up in cities in the northern United States and Canada, often developed rickets (a bending of calcium-deficient bones).

Cumulative sun damage

Successive exposures to too much sun will build up an accumulation of damage, known as photo-aging. As the skin thickens, it sheds dead cells from the surface more slowly, making the skin look dull. This thicker layer of surface skin is slow to absorb moisture because of its toughness, and is less elastic because of the changing nature of its protein strands. Just like a piece of meat that is left in the oven for too long, the skin becomes leathery, wrinkled, dry and hard.

The changes that exposure to sun can bring about in cell DNA are more alarming. A cell's DNA carries the chemical instructions for how the cell is to work. Ultraviolet energy from the sun is readily absorbed by DNA. The impact of this energy transfer can cause a rearrangement in the chemical bonds holding DNA molecules together. This may result in changes in the chemical properties of the DNA, which means that normal control over a cell's functioning can be disrupted.

Disruption may simply mean that the cell dies and the body loses one skin cell, or that the cell lives out its life at less than normal efficiency. The body can easily cope with such losses.

Sun and vitamin D

■ About three-quarters of the vitamin D needed by the body is manufactured in the skin, the product of a chemical reaction promoted by sunlight. Vitamin D is toxic in large amounts and cannot be stored by the body, so a daily supply is necessary.

Vital in the body's maintenance of calcium levels, which support strong bones, teeth and nails, vitamin D can be obtained from some foods, such as liver and fish oils, but the surest dietary source is the supplement now added to almost all milk commercially available in industrial countries.

It is likely that the need, especially in children, to manufacture adequate vitamin D during short winter days was the chief evolutionary pressure that made primitive northern European crop-growing populations fairer than southern Europeans. Many northern hunter-gatherers, such as the Innuit, seem to have obtained enough vitamin D from meat and fish.

However, the affected segments of DNA are sometimes those that prevent excessive cell division or those that prevent the cell from adhering if it comes in contact with a tumor. When combinations of defects like these occur in a skin cell, it can become the parent of a skin cancer.

Skin cancer is increasing rapidly among the fair-skinned people of the industrial world, as more and more seek a golden tan. Skin cancer may not manifest itself as a tumor until years after the damage has been done, but generally the fairer the skin and the greater the exposure, the more rapidly skin cancer develops. In Australia and the United States, people in their twenties may develop skin cancer. In Europe most sufferers are in their forties.

Preventative measures

Although photo-aged skin that is later protected from the sun can sometimes repair itself, and skin cancer is easier to detect and treat than many other cancers, it is better to take steps to prevent the damage in the first place. You can protect against photo-aging by using a moisturizer, wearing a sun screen, and avoiding intensive exposure to the sun. Wind, rain and cold also rob the skin of moisture. Replacing moisture makes the skin stronger and more resilient. Sun screens and sun avoidance protect against cancer.

Sun screens are available in various Sun Protection Factor (SPF) ratings, which are unfortunately not standardized. Follow the maker's instructions. **JAG**

▼ **Total sun blocks** – *usually zinc oxide creams – physically prevent any sunlight from reaching the skin. These are useful on areas that burn easily, such as the bridge of your nose or on the lips. Wearing a hat with a brim and keeping the shoulders covered will also prevent the sun reaching vulnerable areas. Remember that sun exposure can be just as damaging in the winter as in the summer – protect your face and other exposed areas of the body.*

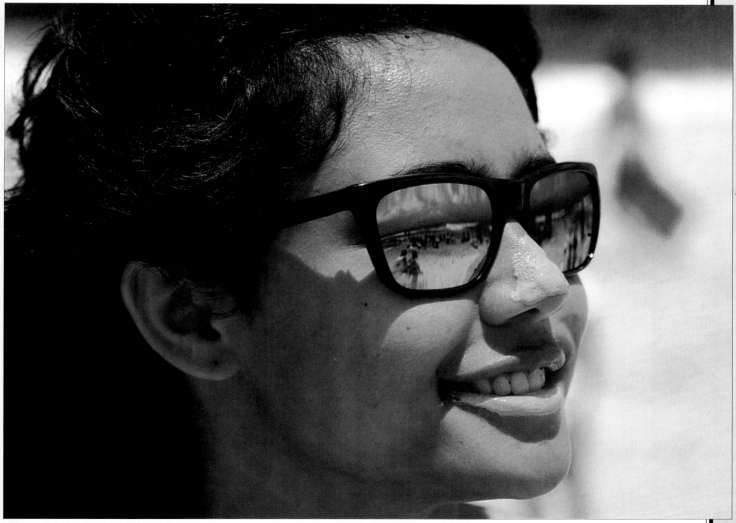

26

Putting Cosmetics to Work

Cosmetics make us feel better about ourselves
● *They can bring out the best in your physical appearance and enhance your self-esteem*
● *Cosmetic therapy builds confidence by masking deformities and accident scars.*

"COSMETIC" solutions to problems are often mere cover-ups – superficial strategies that change the appearance of things without tackling the underlying reality. Painting over the rust on your car is a typical example, or pretending to balance your household accounts merely to cheer yourself up. But not all cosmetic solutions are unworthy of us – for example, filling and papering over the cracks on the living-room wall (so long as they are not signs of a structural flaw that needs more serious attention). This does no harm and makes the livingroom a more pleasant place to live in. Putting on makeup to improve the way you look is a similar example: it can make you more effective in your job or make an evening out a greater success.

Cosmetics can even do a lot to overcome injustice. Being attractive brings with it social advantages – we all tend to react more favorably toward attractive people, and only when we think about it do we remember how unfair this is to those who are less well endowed by nature. With skilled use of makeup, most of us who are only average-looking can improve our appearance enough to gain some of the advantages that attractiveness brings. People with physical defects or blemishes, especially on the face or hands, have even more to gain. Defects bring negative reactions – by disguising them these reactions can be minimized.

The value of making up

Experts have found that many people would welcome more information on how to choose and use cosmetics to greatest advantage, as there are clearly tremendous benefits to be gained on the psychological as well as the physical level.

A great deal can be accomplished with simple makeup tools: foundation can be used to diminish the effect of wrinkles and other signs of aging; blusher can shade and contour a face that is too full; lip-color adds youth and vitality; skillful eye makeup wakes up tired-looking eyes and enhances attractive features. Color can make rapid and dramatic changes. Research has shown that we have powerful psychological responses to color cosmetics, both on ourselves and on other people.

In one study, a questionnaire was used to explore women's personal experiences of using makeup to color their faces. The women, who ranged in age from 18 to 60, were asked to talk about the changes they commonly experienced when using color – how they felt, their image of themselves, expectations, attitudes to other people and the impressions they hoped to make.

The study showed that certain responses were universal, regardless of age – for example, "I feel more confident with makeup on," "I feel better about myself," and "I feel prettier." Other responses were associated with health. Women thought they looked pale or ill when little or no color was used; according to their answers, they often used color to disguise pallor. Looking better helped to lift a depressed mood, or to deflect attention from a physical health problem.

Makeup can also have a remarkable effect on how others

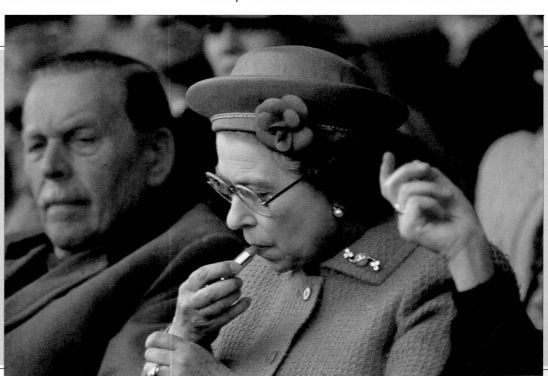

▶ **Putting on your face in public** *is a fairly uninhibited thing to do. This photograph has caught Queen Elizabeth in an uncharacteristically intimate pose, retouching her lipstick during a formal engagement. Although most women feel uncomfortable if their makeup begins to smear or wear off while they are "on show" they will normally wait for a private moment to attend to it. Many will only feel comfortable taking off or putting on makeup in front of their partner or a very close friend.*

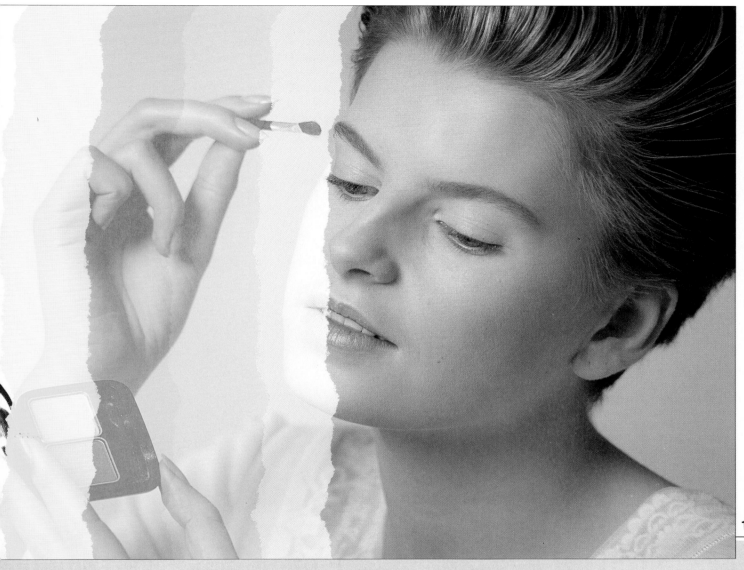

Putting on your colors

■ Essentially, using makeup is painting color on your face. Flattering shades and skillful technique can make a dramatic improvement in the way you look, while poorly applied makeup or colors that do not suit you can make your face look drawn or haggard. For most women, the overall effect of using makeup to best advantage is much more than a cosmetic one. Being happy with the way you look helps you to project a relaxed and confident image, and usually prompts others to respond more warmly. The reverse is also true, for men

as well as women. You wake up feeling below par and do not take any trouble over the way you look; you spend the rest of the day feeling miserable and every glance in the mirror confirms your worst fears about yourself. If, on the other hand, you take the trouble to dress smartly and spend some time on your hair and makeup, you can "put on a brave face" making yourself feel better and more self-confident, even if you are not at full capacity.

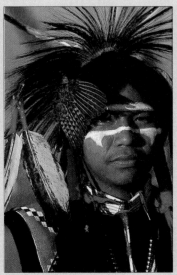

◄ **Men wear more facial makeup** *on special occasions than women do in many societies. Tribal ceremonies often give rise to elaborate painting. This American Indian of the Yakamah tribe, for example, is dressed for a Pow Wow. Celebration makeup often uses red and white paint and incorporates feathers, shiny leaves or shells. Painting has its dark side too. War paint is an effective psychological weapon among tribes in New Guinea where deep black markings and threatening designs convey power and aggression.*

perceive us. When women in their twenties and thirties of average attractiveness (assessed in a preliminary study) were photographed with and without a complete makeup, they were rated more positively with makeup rather than without it. Male and female judges in the same age group rated the women in the photographs as significantly more physically attractive, neat, clean, pleasant, feminine and mature when seen with makeup on. From the point of view of personality, they were rated significantly more secure, sociable, interesting, poised, confident, organized and popular. In another study, photographs of job applicants with and without makeup were shown to career consultants who were then asked to estimate the applicants' potential salary levels. Women who used hair coloring and makeup were judged on average to expect salaries 12 percent higher than those who did not.

Color transformations

Good facial makeup depends on a smooth, even base. Foundation will help to even out the skin tone, making your complexion appear firm and clear. Blusher "livens up" the face, adding color, dimension and a glow of health. A daytime look might include a light dusting of blusher over the eyelid and browbone, as well as the cheekbones. Gel or cream blusher is normally applied over foundation and under face powder; but powder blusher would be applied on top of face powder, together with any other powder cosmetic such as eyeshadow. For most face shapes blusher will look good applied in a "teardrop" shape along the cheekbone, starting below the pupil of the eye and tapering to a point toward the temples, then blended thoroughly until you cannot see where the color begins and ends.

A facial scar or blemish, however small, can affect your

Matching your skin tone

■ Sometimes you will be lucky enough to find a covering cream that already matches your skin tone and covers your blemishes well, but most people need to blend colors to get a really good match. The best way to do this is to use a palette rather like an artist's with a magnifying section allowing the user to view the skin closely. This allows you to blend the right shade using powders and creams mixed directly against the natural skin tone. If you cannot find a commercially made cosmetic palette, you can create one yourself at home using a plastic magnifying glass and a makeup tray or plastic artist's palette.

Place small amounts of cream or powder in the indentations around the palette. Using them from the palette instead of directly from the bottle is more hygienic as it prevents contamination of the container. Take one of the colors, place it on your magnifying section and hold this against your skin. You will be able to tell immediately if it is a good match. Blend with other colors until you obtain the shade you want and apply it direct from the palette.

■ **Surprising colors** can be used to neutralize skin tones. Red cream can be used to change a blue tone such as the

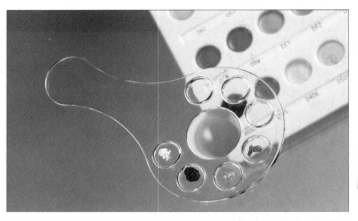

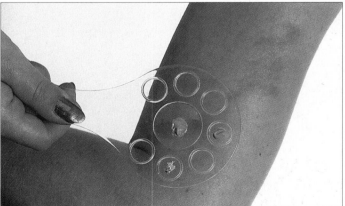

It is always better to use your middle or third finger to apply covering cream rather than your index finger or thumb. The pressure the middle fingers apply will be lighter, and the cover you achieve will look more natural. To achieve this, use two thin layers of covering cream rather than one thick layer.

pigment in a tattoo. Red can also be used with dark foundation to prevent a "gray" look. Green foundation will cool a ruddy complexion or the red discoloring of a port wine stain, broken veins or rosacea. Pink powder adds warmth and color

to scar tissue, and lavender neutralizes brown birthmarks, age spots and freckles. Yellow is used with brown and dark shades to enliven yellow-based or dark complexions. Alabaster, palest ivory or porcelain can neutralize and cover most

defects on young or fair skin, and will generally enliven the complexion.

■ **Any camouflaging cosmetic** needs to be fixed in place fairly firmly. There are a number of products, including lip and eye fixer creams and a spray intended for theatrical use, which are commercially available. Ordinary foundation can also be used as a fixer. Apply it to your face as normal and let it set before contouring. Camouflaging makeup like blushers or shaders will stick to it and set better than on bare skin. Apply foundation to the lips and eyelids, too – shadow and lipstick will last longer, and the foundation will prevent the color "bleeding" into wrinkles on the top lip or around the eyes. **RR**

confidence about your appearance. A concealer applied with foundation may help to cover up blemishes, broken veins and dark circles under the eyes (but not undereye puffiness). In addition, overall routine cosmetic care, including hair care, makeup and fragrance can provide a substantial psychological boost. Serious defects, however, may need heavier coverage using specially formulated products.

A cosmetic therapist can help you find the best products to disguise a defect, show the best ways to use them, and suggest ways to maximize good points as well as minimizing problems. Camouflage cosmetics will reduce the visibility of skin diseases such as acne, psoriasis or rosacea, as well as more permanent heavy discolorations such as "port-wine stains" and other types of birthmark. Pigmentary conditions such as vitiligo (*see Ch25*) can also be masked by a clever use of cosmetics. Camouflage is particularly helpful in disguising diseases such as lupus, affecting the appearance of your skin, which can require lengthy treatment and may result in some skin marking.

Covering up defects

Experts have put a good deal of effort into trying to measure the positive effects of successful cosmetic treatment. If clients are given a standard self-assessment test before and after a half-hour session with a professional cosmetician, they score remarkably higher in the second test for positive outlook and self-image, and say that they feel more like

meeting others and happier about being seen by them. The degree of change is quite significant both for people of average appearance and for those with facial deformity. All the evidence suggests that people benefit physically and psychologically from cosmetic camouflage.

Cosmetic camouflage uses specially formulated makeup, applied with techniques similar to normal daily procedures. However, it takes considerably more practice in the blending of color and more skillful application to get a really good result.

Large-scale camouflage involves covering an area of skin which is discolored as a result of disease, broken veins, a birthmark, burns or a scar. In some cases, normal foundation and concealer will serve to cover the area, but if heavier camouflage is needed there are many commercial products specifically intended to camouflage skin discoloration, some of which are available on prescription.

You will get the best information, materials and techniques by visiting a cosmetic camouflage consultant. Hospitals, doctors, beauty salons and support groups can refer you to someone in your area. Consultants may work in association with dermatologists and plastic surgeons, and thoroughly understand the nature of a cosmetic problem and how best to camouflage it. **JAG**

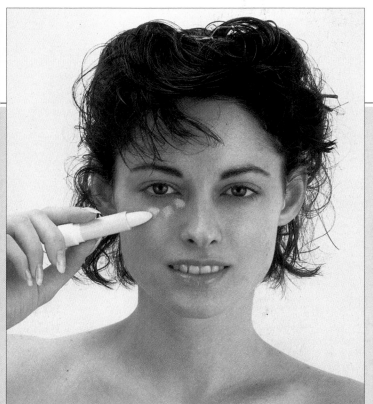

191

Covering scars

■ Raised or indented scars can be camouflaged using the basic principles of contouring. If the scar is discolored, use a covering cream, apply your regular makeup and then use the following techniques over your normal foundation or cover cream. A recessed scar can be made to look much less deep and noticeable by placing a light color along the center of the scar and a dark shade on each side of it. The opposite shading will flatten out a raised scar — place a dark shade on the surface and a lighter color on both sides. Use a brush to apply the shades precisely, and then feather across the scar to blend in the edges well. Almost any scar can be disguised or minimized in this way. Once the covering cream has been set with powder and a damp cotton pad, use your normal foundation over it or a second layer of covering cream.

◄ **Perfect translucent skin** *comes naturally to very few, but clever use of makeup can vastly improve the appearance of your complexion. Though relatively few of us need to learn heavy cosmetic camouflage, most will want to hide dark shadows under the eyes or minor blemishes. After applying moisturizer or foundation, dot very small amounts of concealor onto under-eye shadows and blend in well, using your ring (third) finger for a light touch.*

Always try to make up your face in the kind of light that you will be seen in, otherwise it will look unnatural. For the daytime, your bathroom light may be too strong. Make up near a window with the room light on, and it will look natural both outside and under artificial light. In the evening you can try stronger effects which look better in subdued or strong lighting.

Making cosmetic camouflage work

Makeup should always be applied onto a completely clean skin. If your skin is dry you may need to apply a moisturizer first. Give it a few minutes to soak in before you begin applying any makeup.

The purpose of camouflage cream is to cover a blemish with a fine "skin" of color that matches your normal skin tone and allows the blemished area to blend into the background. Use the pads of your fingers to press and pat the cream into your skin, beginning in the center of the discolored area and working outward. Some people prefer to use a damp sponge, also used to cover large areas. To cover small areas or finish a coverup, a brush can be used to feather lightly over a defect. Remember that all skins have irregularities, and if your cover is too matt or perfect it will look unnatural. A brush is particularly useful for blending the edges of a camouflaged area into the natural skin tone. If the skin you are covering is very much lighter or darker than the rest of your face, you need to "shade out" the area. Apply a darker color than your normal skin tone to a white patch or a lighter tone than your normal color to a dark mark. Take care not to go over the edges of the patch to be concealed. Then apply a second coat of cover cream that matches your skin tone over the area, this time blending the edges into your skin.

Using a powder will keep the covering cream in place and set a matt finish to your face. Allow a few minutes for the foundation to dry and then apply powder. Using loose powder and a brush, sweep or press the powder lightly over the covering cream in an upward movement, allow a few minutes to set and then remove any excess by brushing it downward, so that the downy hair on the face will lie flat.

Finally, set the powder by patting a damp cotton ball or pad all over the area. This removes any powdery effect and helps make the coverup waterproof. Once you have set your camouflage, the area can be treated just like the rest of your face and makeup may be applied with a light touch.

All cosmetic covering creams should be removed at night. You will need to use a cleansing cream, as soap and water will not be enough. Apply the cleanser in gentle circular movements in an upward direction. You may need several applications to remove it completely. Always be gentle with the camouflaged area. Use dampened cotton balls to remove the cleansing cream and follow with a soap and water wash if you wish.

Changing the shape of your face

If you have a full, round face and would really like sharper cheekbones, an application of darker foundation or powder along the sides of the face and in the "hollow" area below

Men with facial discolorations

■ Men suffer just as much as women from facial scars and markings, but cosmetics are still much less acceptable on men. In addition, they do not have the chance to develop the makeup skills that women do, so cosmetic camouflage problems are usually worse for them.

If the mark is not directly on your face, you may prefer just to leave it alone. The Soviet leader Mikhail Gorbachev has a large port-wine stain on his forehead. In early formal portraits, RIGHT, it was largely disguised with powder and foundation, and it was often airbrushed out of press photographs. One of the side effects of greater freedom of information in Soviet politics is that Gorbachev's birthmark is no longer concealed, FAR RIGHT, and it has long ceased to be a source of interest or comment.

The negative side of concealing a mark or flaw is that it puts

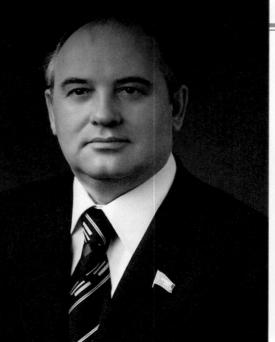

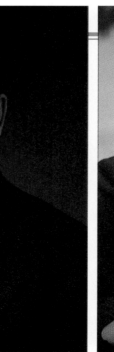

limitations on your lifestyle. Heavy rain, swimming, going to the beach or being seen early in the morning all present psychological threats and opportunities for painful embarrassment. However, you may feel that the

advantages of camouflage outweigh these factors, and if your defect is an obvious one near the center of your face a sympathetic cosmetician will help you learn the right techniques to correct it.

If the mark is in your beard area and has hair follicles, you might consider growing a beard or mustache – this will cover the defect and prevent irritation of skin that may be sensitive. **RR**

the cheekbones will help. The darker color will make these areas appear to recede, and your face will look thinner and bonier. A very long face can be shortened by using darker powder or foundation under the chin (the same technique can minimize a double chin), and lighter shades at the side of the face will make it look fuller. Never use a color more than one or two shades away from your base tone, and remember to blend the edges well. A cosmetic expert can teach you the tricks of facial contouring. These techniques were developed for use on the stage or in television and screen makeup, but they can also play down raised or indented scars, problems with bone structure or the kind of eye and lip defects which cannot be concealed effectively by covering creams.

Theatrical makeup was developed in the Victorian era to exaggerate facial features in the glare of gas footlights, which tended to "blank out" the actors' faces. Makeup mimicked the natural play of light and shadow over the face so that the expressions of the actors could be seen in the topmost balcony. Modern cameras and lights are more advanced, but most actors working in television, films or on stage wear some makeup to accentuate their features or to create the illusion of age, youth or some other effect.

Using makeup to alter appearance radically is a highly skilled art, and it takes time and talent to learn all the

193

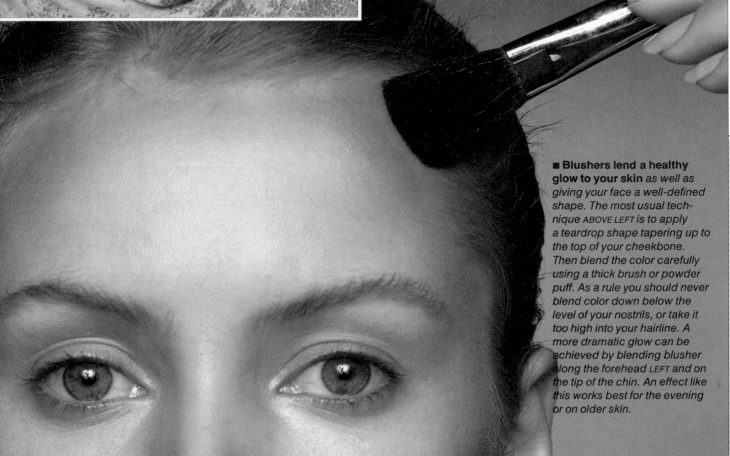

■ **Blushers lend a healthy glow to your skin** *as well as giving your face a well-defined shape. The most usual technique ABOVE LEFT is to apply a teardrop shape tapering up to the top of your cheekbone. Then blend the color carefully using a thick brush or powder puff. As a rule you should never blend color down below the level of your nostrils, or take it too high into your hairline. A more dramatic glow can be achieved by blending blusher along the forehead LEFT and on the tip of the chin. An effect like this works best for the evening or on older skin.*

techniques properly. Moreover, it is important to remember that these makeup tricks were developed for use in strong artificial light, and they can look extremely false and over-done in normal artificial or natural light. Many theatrical makeup techniques can be learned and adapted for daily use, and a good cosmetician can show you how to use the tricks of the trade to minimize a specific defect and completely mask small irregularities. There are also a number of makeup manuals, for both theatrical and general use, which will show you the basic techniques. Practice in front of the mirror to find the ones that work best for you.

Redesigning your nose

Light and shade are used in the same way on the face as in painting a picture. The play of light and shade can disguise or accentuate contours, so light tones are used to highlight a good feature, and darker shades can help to minimize a defect. Clever use of this principle in makeup can alter the entire shape of your face. People who have irregular bone structure can make the two sides of their face "match" by careful shading – filling out a sunken cheek with a lighter shade or regularizing a crooked jaw by using a darker tone on the more prominent side. The same techniques can be used to improve more regular bone structure.

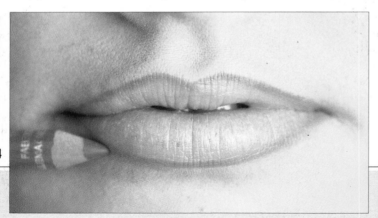

A long nose can be made to look shorter by brushing a little dark powder under the tip. If you have a thick nose you can make it look thinner by highlighting the bridge and applying a darker shade to the sides. Highlighting the bridge of the nose can also make your nose look longer. If your nose is crooked, applying dark shades to the one side of the nose and light shades to the other can straighten it out – experiment to see what looks best on your nose, remembering that dark shades recede, light shades come forward. A bump on the bridge of the nose will recede a little if a dark tone is applied over it and the rest of the bridge is highlighted. Make sure, however, that you blend the colors well.

Making up your eyes and lips

Eye makeup will vary considerably depending on the size and shape of your eyes, whether they are prominent or deep-set, close together or wide apart. Most women have preferences about how much eye makeup they want to wear. Looks might vary from a subtle makeup during the day to more dramatic looks for evening. Before applying eye makeup, check your eyebrows and remove any stray hairs from underneath. You might add a few light pencil strokes to add definition, or brush eyebrows upward for a "wide-awake" look.

Eye pencil defines the eyes. A line traced around the eye close to the eyelashes and then smudged with a brush or sponge-tip applicator will give a natural wide-eyed look. Eyeshadow may be applied all over the eyelid or in the inner or outer corners depending on the shape of the eye. Neutral colors look good for day or evening but brighter colors are likely to be chosen to go with what you are wearing rather than to match the color of your eyes. A touch of highlighter will add sparkle to an evening makeup and the effect can be completed with several coats of mascara.

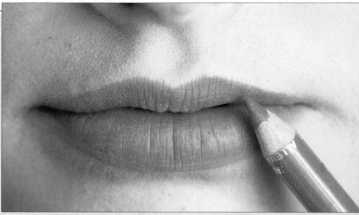

Reshaping your mouth

■ Very full lips became fashionable in the late 1980s, and in response many women have had collagen injections both to reduce the lines on their upper lip and to make their lips look fuller. Although effective in the short term, collagen injections need to be continued to maintain the improvement. Women considering this option have to measure the benefits against the trouble and expense.

There is no safe way of reducing lip size, but a great deal can be done to imitate the fashion of the moment or to camouflage a crooked pair of lips using lip color and clever makeup techniques.

A pale lipstick will make the lips look bigger and fuller; a dark color will minimize size. Using a lip pencil to draw an outline is a good idea on any mouth as it gives definition to the lips, and it can also be used to reshape them. A dark pencil applied to the inner edge of the lip will make them look smaller; a lighter but definite color applied to the outer edge will tend to make your lips look fuller.

If the mouth is crooked, penciling in the shape by using the pencil on the inner edge of the lip on one side and the outer edge on the other can help balance it. Make sure not to go too far over the edge of the natural lip line or the effect will be unnatural. Lip contouring cannot make thin lips into a Brigitte Bardot pout, but it can make significant changes to the appearance of a mouth.

Lip-color will add the finishing touch to your makeup. If you want to change the shape of your mouth, you might smooth a little foundation over your lips to disguise their natural outline and recontour them with a lip pencil. This can make thin lips look fuller and a full mouth appear less so. Color may be filled in with a lipbrush, blotted with a tissue and highlighted with a slick of clear lipgloss.

Accentuating your best features is just as important as covering your defects. Lovely eyes draw attention away from a crooked mouth and will make your face look positively attractive instead of just acceptable. Practice making up until you feel really confident about getting a good effect. If you are happy with your face, you will communicate self-assurance to others. The best makeup in the world will not cover up an anxious personality. People do react negatively to what is unattractive, but they can be influenced by your own sense of self-worth as well as by your makeup. Good cosmetic technique will certainly camouflage any physical defects, but the real benefit is that it can give you enough confidence to let your personality shine through. **RR**

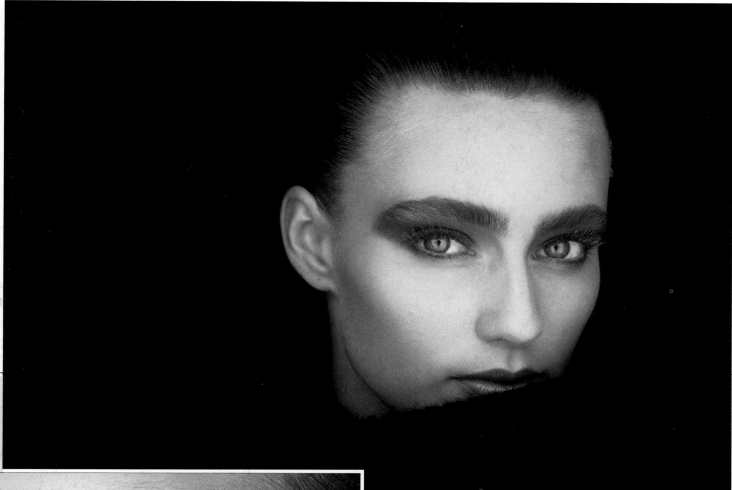

195

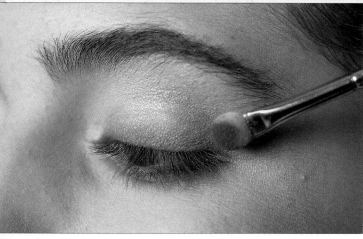

■ **Making eyes look dramatic,** or simply accentuating them in the face, probably causes women more uncertainty than any other aspect of putting on makeup. Colors that work best pick out the flecks of color in your eyes as well as complementing the shades that you are wearing. In recent years there has been a trend for more natural tones in eye makeup, warm browns and rust shades LEFT rather than the industry standard of the 60s and 70s – blue eyeshadow. A vast range of products is available if you want to experiment – colored mascara, kohl pencils, liquid eyeliner, and eyeshadow in powder, liquid or pencil form. For a result like the three-tone look using purple mascara ABOVE you will probably need a professional touch.

Living with disfigurement

■ Most people are appalled at the notion of discriminating against a person because of a physical deformity, but we very clearly admire the beautiful and recoil from the unattractive. While such feelings may not be openly stated or even consciously felt, research studies show that practically everyone reacts negatively to disfigurement, particularly if it is facial. We may tell each other that it is the inner self that counts, but disfigured people do suffer for their physical defects. Any cosmetic technique that makes them happier about themselves and favorably affects the reactions of others will be of real benefit, and will allow their personalities more expression.

People often cope better with physical impairments like the loss of a leg, blindness or deafness than they do with disfigurement. Strangers react less negatively to disability, but because disfigurement is a cosmetic, rather than a functional problem, doctors tend not to take it as seriously. People who suffer from blemishes or disfigurement also suffer the effects of discrimination, lowered self-esteem and depression.

Victims of serious injuries leading to disfigurement often experience tremendous adjustment problems due to their change in appearance and may find the stress engendered by this more prolonged and harder to deal with than any functional problems they have.

Disfigured people themselves report that they are handicapped in most "normal" life goals, and studies carried out by psychologists confirm that this is true. They have more problems than the average person encounters getting a job, are more likely to have troublesome family relationships, have difficulties making friends and organizing a social life, and have even more difficulty developing romantic attachments. Once disfigured people do get to know others, however, their friends will report that they hardly notice what was once an obvious cosmetic defect.

Not surprisingly, disfigured people may have low self-esteem, a poor self-image and generally few positive feelings about any aspect of their lives. Complete social withdrawal and even clinical depression

may result. Because they feel such despair about their appearance, disfigured people may neglect to take care of themselves properly, which makes their appearance deteriorate further. Lack of care leads to poor self-worth and the negative reactions of others in a vicious circle.

Research into the problems of disfigurement has helped doctors and psychologists to evolve a whole range of treatments, including surgery, prosthetics and cosmetic camouflage, to cope with them. In addition, a system of cosmetic therapy has been developed by experts as a way of raising the self-esteem and morale of disfigured patients.

Healing through cosmetic care

Cosmetic camouflage was developed largely during World War II, when large numbers of burns and injuries, especially among the flying corps, left the patients with varying degrees of disfigurement. Several organizations have since developed cosmetic camouflage services and referral agencies.

▼ **Accepting a disfigurement** *and learning to live with it is one psychologically healthy way of dealing with the problem. However, it takes considerable willpower and confidence, which few victims are able to muster – many unscarred people, even those who claim not to be prejudiced, treat the disfigured with revulsion. Simon Weston, badly burnt while fighting in the 1982 Falkland Islands war, has since devoted himself to campaigning for the rights of those permanently scarred in wartime or in accidents. He has become a well known public figure in the UK, which itself has done much to promote a positive image of disfigured people.*

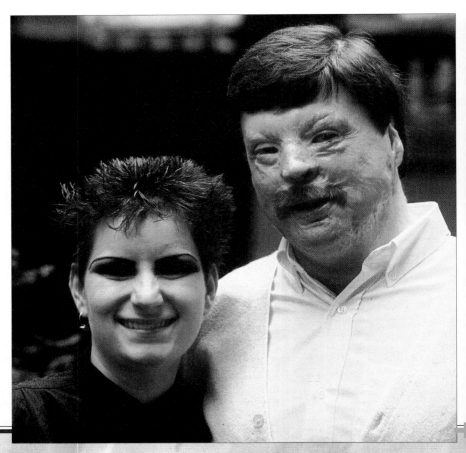

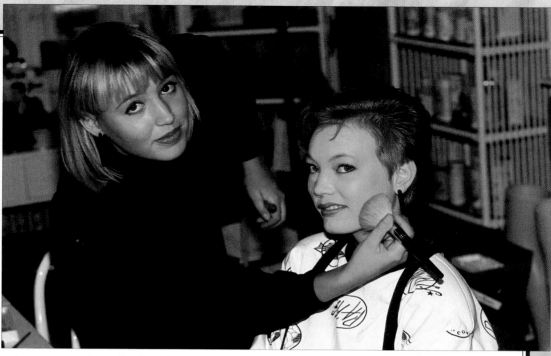

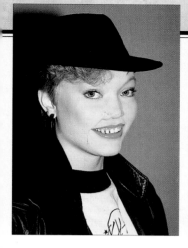

Cosmetic therapy

■ Therapeutic cosmetic treatments focus on removing or camouflaging blemishes or flaws in appearance and enhancing positive aspects. They can greatly reduce anxiety over appearance and revitalize the person concerned, presenting new possibilities for their lives. Here a woman receives cosmetic treatment to disguise a facial malformation which she has had from birth ABOVE RIGHT. The effect ABOVE is both to make the malformation itself barely noticeable, and to draw attention away from it by emphasizing her strikingly attractive eyes.

Cosmetic therapy in its most advanced form is not just a medical or mechanical procedure to correct defects, but an attempt to treat the whole person. Allowing disfigured people to discuss their fears, experiment with a new technique and ask questions about what concerns them provides them with some sense of control over the situation, which tends to raise confidence and self-esteem. Cosmetic treatment tells people that they are valuable and worth caring for – attitudes that have often become alien to disfigured people.

Even if a person's disfigurement is temporary, cosmetic treatment can be beneficial. Cosmetic help to cover temporary scars, bruises or wounds provides important psychological support through the recovery stage.

In many countries, the Red Cross performs cosmetic therapy in hospitals, training volunteers to use cosmetic treatment to boost morale for a wide range of patients. They have been running a camouflage service since 1975 to treat obvious disfigurement.

The Phoenix Society was set up in the United States and Europe to help burn survivors and their families, but is helpful in recommending possible surgical, cosmetic and prosthetic treatment for all sorts of deformities. The Society is particularly interested in the psychology of disfigurement and its conferences regularly report on new developments. Your local hospital may also provide instruction in cosmetic camouflage or may be able to refer you to an organization or therapist. University hospitals and special units for burns and plastic surgery can also help.

Facial scars and tattoos can be a definite social disadvantage. In one study, volunteers presented with a picture of a person covered with simulated facial scars judged the person not only to be less attractive, but significantly more dishonest, compared to their rating of photographs of the same person without scars.

Even one or two small scars have a negative effect. One young man opted for plastic surgery and cosmetic coverage of a scar he received after being attacked with a knife. He himself was not upset by his appearance, but people reacted to him as they might have reacted to his attackers.

Facial scars also seem to change the behavior of the person affected. A study of criminals with disfigurements showed that if these scars were removed their behavior in prison was improved and once released they were less likely to get into trouble with the law again.

The greatest distress is not necessarily caused by the largest disfigurement. Quite minor scars and irregularities can cause enormous problems for some people. Frances MacGregor, who specializes in facial deformity, studied several hundred plastic surgery patients whose problems ranged from the hardly noticeable to the extremely severe.

She found that most of the patients suffered from some sort of psychological disturbance, ranging from feelings of inferiority to psychotic illness, but that there was no direct relationship between the severity of their disfigurement and the severity of their psychological problem.

People who were born with a cosmetic defect often manage better than those who have acquired it later in life. Although children suffer from the same disadvantages as adults as a result of their appearance, those who have never known a different life have time to develop coping strategies before they face the rigors of the adult world. Teenagers may be extremely distressed by even mild facial problems because their concern with their appearance and with gaining the approval of their peers is so intense in adolescence. **JAG**

197

27

Being Made Over

A professional make-over is not just for the rich and vain ● *Expert techniques make the best of the features that are uniquely yours* ● *Others will respond positively to your good looks and increased self-confidence.*

A PROFESSIONAL make-over is one of the most effective ways for people to experience the full benefits of cosmetics. Skillful use of color can have a striking effect on the observer and make more lasting changes in the mind of the person using it.

Dramatic transformations of appearance can take place, but just as important are the increased confidence and improved self-image that result. Several recent studies have demonstrated how a professional make-over can transform the way we see ourselves.

In one of these, a 30-minute professional make-over was given to a group of elderly women, ranging in age from their sixties to their nineties. The women were asked to rate how they felt immediately before and after the make-over session. The results showed that they felt significantly more attractive, more socially confident and more positive, and that their self-image had improved.

The feelings of those who had a low attractiveness rating before the session improved more than those who had a high attractiveness rating, suggesting that the act of lavish-ing attention on your appearance plays as important a role in feelings of self-esteem as the actual improvement in appearance.

Assessment and examination

A professional make-over combines the twin benefits of improved appearance and a psychological boost with the sense of relaxation and well-being that comes from being attended by experts.

When you go for a make-over, you may have the services of a beauty therapist, a makeup artist and a hairdresser all working together to achieve the total look.

The beauty therapist will first assess your skin type and identify any specific problems that might need treatment. This stage is important because the condition of your skin reflects your general health, any medication that you have been taking, your diet, your lifestyle and the skin care routine that you have been following. From this, the thera-pist will be able to draw up a diet sheet which will include a vitamin program and will recommend a daily skin care and makeup routine for you to follow at home, together with any treatments for specific problems and products for improving the general condition of your skin.

Then the makeup artist will chart the shape of your face to see whether it is heart-shaped, oval, round, square or long. This will influence how your eyebrows should be shaped and determine whether or not corrective makeup is necessary. The hairdresser should also take the shape of

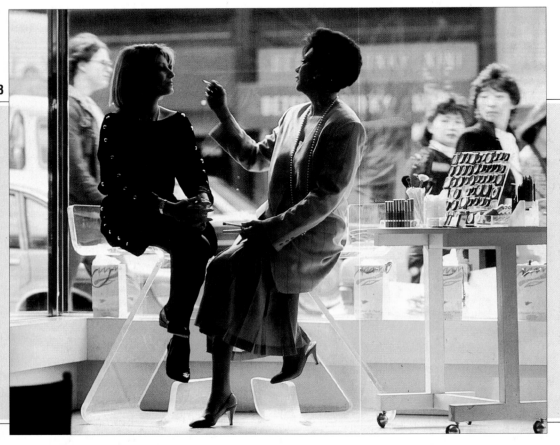

◄ **An individual consultation** *is the first step in a professional make-over. The total service may include beauty therapy (skin treatment), makeup and hairstyling all combined to create a complete, new and exciting look. Before trying any new style it is a good idea to discuss with the makeover artist what you are trying to achieve. The end result should utilize your best features and make you feel better about yourself.*

your face into account in deciding whether or not to cut, perm, color or tint your hair. But first they will make a full examination of your hair to assess its condition and texture and to identify any problems or special characteristics. Your skin tone will also be an important factor in the decision to use color on your hair.

Having a facial

When your needs have been assessed and a program of treatment decided on, the session will usually begin with a facial. The therapist might start by exfoliating your skin – that is, removing the top layer (epidermis) with an abrasive cream, sponge or face mask.

This will usually be followed by a deep-cleansing treatment – using a cleansing cream or lotion, the beautician will massage your face using light, feathery strokes and then repeat the process. When your skin is thoroughly clean, she will examine it carefully to assess whether it is dry, oily, sensitive or "combination" skin, and at this point she may also use a facial shampoo and a steaming process to unblock clogged pores and remove any impurities. She will then go ahead with the treatment that is appropriate for your skin type.

Electrotherapy is a new technique that is often used to improve the quality of the skin. Very dry skin may benefit from this treatment in which particles of the active ingredients of specially formulated cosmetic ampoules containing, for example, royal jelly or collagen, are

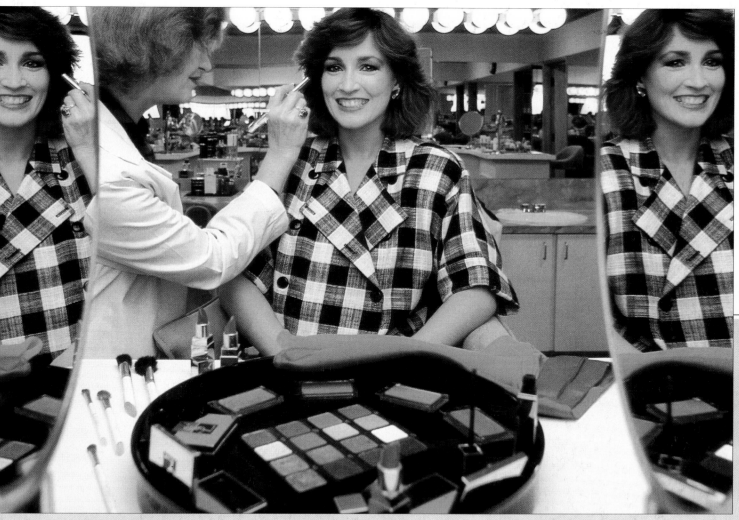

▲ **See yourself in a more favorable light**. *A professional makeup artist can make anyone look more attractive. They are experts at enhancing the good features and minimizing flaws. A good makeup artist will take into consideration skin tone and conditioning, total coloring (including hair color), the shape of your face and body, and your personal preferences. Working with all of these the makeover should achieve an improved version of the original – it is still unmistakably you, although you will probably never have looked so good. The increased self-confidence produced by a make-over is one of its most important benefits.*

diffused into the skin using electric currents. Another technique, disincrustation, uses the alkaline effects of a chemically produced electric current to remove excess sebum (oil) and impurities from very oily skin or skin that needs deep-cleansing.

In some clinics, vacuum suction and neon laser therapy treatments might be recommended to help regenerate the skin. Skilled massage techniques will improve the texture of the skin and soothe away tension and stress, giving the face a more youthful appearance. A face mask can also have a very soothing and beneficial effect. Face peeling with a chemical or vegetable face mask is often recommended to remove dead cells from the surface of the skin. Small areas of discoloration and surface lines can be improved in this way. Exfoliation has the added benefit of promoting new cell regeneration.

Some skin problems and blemishes can be dealt with during a make-over session. Others, like the treatment of broken veins and the removal of superfluous hair, can only be accomplished over a series of visits. Facial hair, however, can be bleached during a make-over, if you would like, to minimize a dark shadow on the upper lip or the sides of the face.

Choosing a new look

When it comes to deciding on the finished effect, the power of computer visualization is being used more and more to help people see how they will look with a different hairstyle or makeup.

An image of your face can be put onto a screen and a new hair color or style superimposed. In this way you can experiment with change without having to live with the results, you can decide which ones you like and really want to try, and, if necessary, the program can be saved and used again (see box).

With or without a computer, a makeup artist will bring a

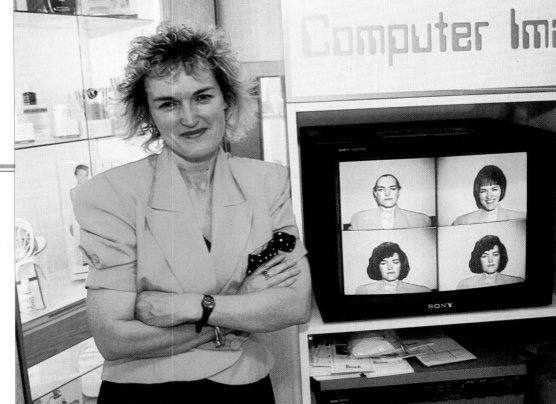

Computer visualization

■ Computers are bringing an increasingly professional, scientific approach to skin care, hair care and makeup.

Having a computer beauty analysis is becoming as easy as going for a medical checkup or having a birth chart drawn up.

One system on the market takes information from a skin imprint, rather like a dental impression. It is then magnified and projected onto a video screen.

From this the customer receives a diagnosis – a picture of her skin compared with the ideal condition judged against national or ethnic norms for her age, together with recommendations for treatment.

Another system prints out a personal "credit card" with the client's skin type in magnetic code. This means that the consultants of this beauty house can have the information to hand wherever they are in the world. Used once, skin analyzers provide skin typing and personalized beauty prescriptions. Used regularly, they can be a yardstick to measure how well products are working. Computer makeup allows you to try new colors without touching your face or removing your makeup.

▲ **Hairstyle options** are available for immediate inspection through the sophisticated imaging facilities of this computer system. Systems that allow you to visualize makeup options are also available.

fresh eye to the possibilities of your face and can lead you, step by step, to a new look. More than any other beauty treatment, the skilled application of makeup can transform your looks, the way you feel about yourself and, consequently, the way others see you.

But the process is not about completely changing your face or about making you look like someone else. A good beautician will work with your natural face shape, contours and coloring to help you bring the best out of your own natural good looks.

When having a professional makeup, it is a good idea to tell the beautician as much as possible beforehand about your favorite colors, the way you usually apply your makeup and any particular likes or dislikes you may have.

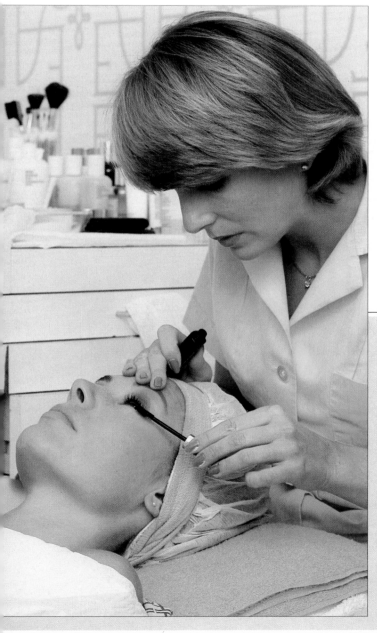

The makeup artist may use a palette to match your skin tone and apply a foundation. Blushers and face-shapers are used to correct any facial defects and bring out your best features.

The shape of the eyebrows and the color of the eyes can also be dramatized by a skilled makeup artist. Light and shade are used to give your features shape and contour. A lighter color can be used to highlight and bring out a good feature, a darker shade to minimize or disguise any area you might want to play down.

In a professional make-over all the colors chosen throughout are selected carefully in consultation with the client, taking into account hair and skin tone, eye color and personal preferences.

In the final analysis, a good make-over should achieve the aims jointly arrived at by the client and the professional consultants, exploit their client's best features to the full and correct or minimize any features that the client feels less than happy about.

It can take time for some people to accept a new image of themselves and to feel comfortable with a different makeup or hair color. For these people, a more gradual approach might help them to accept a new self-image as self-confidence and self-esteem become an established part of their personality.

Given the opportunity, most people would like to change something about their appearance. If you look good, you feel good and people respond to you in a more positive way. Improving your outward appearance can lift your mood, generate feelings of well-being, and attract positive responses from others, giving you confidence in yourself and making you more positive in your dealings with other people. You develop an upward spiral of confidence and enhanced self-esteem. **RR**

Showing your true colors

■ The expert use of color is a sign of knowledgeable application of cosmetics. Color counselors work on the principle that color gives you confidence. They will guide you toward shades that enhance rather than fight with your natural coloring. Contrasting shades can look dramatic but may well make you look washed out or overdone.

In a color-counseling session, analysis of your complexion undertone, hair and eye color will tell you which color group you belong to (see *Ch 21*), but good color analysts will not limit you to certain colors; you are encouraged to select shades you are attracted to or feel comfortable with.

Bringing out your true colors does not have to mean changing your whole wardrobe. Simply wearing something in your color range next to your skin will have the desired effect.

Color can have a profound impact on both the wearer and observer. In surveys, women frequently report that they feel more attractive and confident wearing makeup.

In job interviews cosmetics have been shown to influence interviewers' judgment to such an extent that women may actually earn higher salaries based on their makeup.

28

Hairstyle and Haircare

Your hair has an esthetic as well as practical function ● Healthy, shining, well-kept hair is a sign that you take care of yourself ● The right hairstyle can improve your confidence and the way others respond to you.

YOUR HAIR is the most flexible part of your body. It can be long or short, curly or straight; you can braid it, pin it up, gel it into fantastic shapes, or let it hang loose. Today with the help of modern products you can safely and reliably change its color and texture. Because hair can be changed so dramatically, it has long been a focus for shifting social statements and self-presentation. How you wear your hair reflects the mood of your own time, and it can be used to relay messages to others about who you are or who you want to be.

The significance of hair through the ages

Hairstyles have always been in the forefront of fashion, and the latest style always has a short lifespan. Roman and Greek artifacts can be dated accurately if they contain details of a woman's hairstyle. Ancient coins, which are dated, also show fashionably-coiffed women whose styles change every few years, and if a jug or statue has an identifiable hairstyle it can be dated almost as accurately as if the time and place of its making were stamped on it. In the same way, we can often put a fairly accurate date on a photograph by looking at both male and female hairstyles.

Because hair is so malleable, it can easily be manipulated to reflect what is happening in a particular culture. We have all seen pictures of the hairstyles worn by 18th century male and female French aristocrats, enormous constructions of natural and artificial hair, feathers, flowers, and stuffed birds. Such elaborate headdresses were used sometimes to reflect current events. One famous lady wore an entire model frigate on top of her head celebrating a famous naval battle. But the real meaning of these styles lay in their very elaborateness. They could only be worn by the aristocracy – those people with the time, money and leisure to spend on them. After the French Revolution much simpler "natural" styles of hair (worn down or loosely pinned and certainly not powdered and curled) became fashionable, reflecting the enormous change in social values.

Modern hairstyles for women and men reflect our ideas about what is good or admirable. Naturalness, functionability and ease have been notions crucial to Western life since the turn of the century. The emergence of the "bob" style for women occurred in tandem with the granting of women's suffrage, and it was certainly associated with freedom, ease and practicality. Some office firms advertising jobs for secretaries insisted that "no bobbed heads need apply." They feared such girls would be too liberated and even sexually adventurous if they had deliberately let down their hair. The bob has remained a popular hairstyle because it is easy to care for, suits many types of hair and looks neat and tidy – it fits the lives we lead and the messages we want to convey. The man's traditional "short back and sides" was developed in the Victorian era as a practical, sensible style and it remains associated with those qualities, just as periodic resurgences of fashionable long hair for men, whether in 1890 or 1960, are related to alternative or unconventional lifestyles.

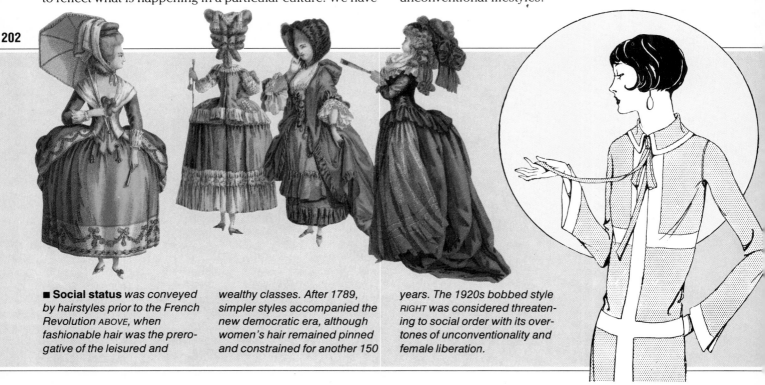

■ **Social status** *was conveyed by hairstyles prior to the French Revolution* ABOVE, *when fashionable hair was the prerogative of the leisured and* wealthy classes. After 1789, simpler styles accompanied the new democratic era, although women's hair remained pinned and constrained for another 150 years. The 1920s bobbed style RIGHT was considered threatening to social order with its overtones of unconventionality and female liberation.

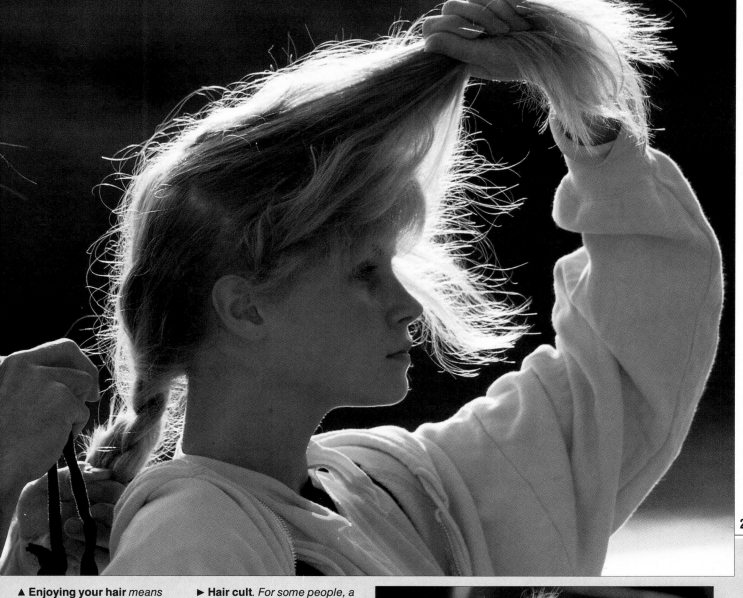

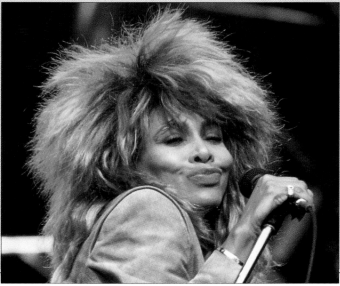

▲ **Enjoying your hair** *means wearing it with confidence. Attractive hair draws attention – it is a means not only of self-expression but also of sensual signaling. A head of glossy hair proclaims, "I take care of myself and I feel good." Begin with good care. Healthy, shining locks are a must no matter what length, color or texture. To find the right style may take some experimenting. The most fashionable style may not suit your hair type or your personality, and can make you look and feel uncomfortable and awkward.*

▶ **Hair cult.** *For some people, a hairstyle is not merely a style; it is an integral part of their personality, and in the case of Tina Turner, a trademark. Her mane accentuates her powerful presence and uninhibited style, a unique blend of soul and sophistication echoed by the combination of denim and suede she wears. "This is me – take it or leave it." When faced with confident self-assertion, the public is usually willing to accept the person or image offered, even if it is completely eccentric and might otherwise be laughed at.*

What does your hair say?

Most of us probably cling to certain stereotypes about hair length, style and color. Curly hair has connotations of frivolity and liveliness; blondes are supposed to be empty-headed, and redheads are widely believed to have fiery tempers. Because we can change our hair length, color, style and even texture, we often use these stereotypes to project a particular image of ourselves. Rock musicians cultivate long and tousled locks to appear rebellious and outside the establishment. Women who aim to do well in business may opt for a darker, more conservative hair color and a medium-length or short style to convey a picture of reliability and control.

Stereotypes, whether or not they have much practical relation to your way of life, tend to be reinforced by how others react. Princesses in fairy tales usually have long, flowing hair. This is one way that we have come to associate long hair with femininity, beauty, sexual appeal, romance and freedom. If you are a woman with long free-flowing hair, people may behave towards you as if you are romantic, feminine and sexually appealing, and you will tend to respond to such treatment by acting to type. On the other hand, you might resent their assumptions — and even change your hairstyle.

Haircare, psychology and personality

Using shampoo, conditioner, colorants and other hair treatments can have a significant impact on others, and also on ourselves. Successful haircare can substantially affect us psychologically and socially, and promote feelings of well-being. A number of interesting studies have shown how this works. In one of the first formal examinations of the significance of haircare, the researchers reasoned that by using standard hair maintenance procedures it should be possible to make an average-looking person look more attractive in the eyes of others. The results of the study bore out this theory, and highlighted the specific benefits of haircare.

The study used photographs of four professional working women in their late twenties and early thirties, all of average attractiveness. In the first photograph they were wearing no makeup and had given no obvious attention to their hair. In the second they appeared with just facial makeup. In the third hairstyling only was used to improve appearance. In the fourth, both hairstyling and facial cosmetics were used.

A panel of male and female judges of the same general age-group and background (to avoid class divisions in evaluations) were asked to rate the attractiveness and personality of the women in the photographs. In each set of photographs provided for rating, the women being judged appeared in just one of the conditions only, to prevent the panel members being aware of what exactly was being tested. Both the haircare and makeup used were fairly standard, hair treatment including shampooing, conditioning, cutting and styling.

The psychology of hair color

■ Fair-haired women are traditionally thought of as pretty but brainless, while fair men are sometimes associated with being shifty and untrustworthy. Theorists in the 19th century believed fair men to be "degenerate" and criminal. On the other hand, in women, dark hair has traditionally been associated with being more intelligent, complex and emotional. Though many of us would reject these stereotypes out of hand when we are asked about them directly, they still affect the way we evaluate others. Studies in the 1970s have shown that men asked to rate pictures of women for attractiveness consistently preferred women with lighter colored hair, and females tended to be attracted to men with darker hair and eyes.

However, in a similar study, a group of men were asked to look at pictures of a blonde and a brunette (actually the same woman in different wigs). The vast majority indicated that the blonde would be more fun to take out, but the brunette looked like someone they might marry. Red hair RIGHT, generally associated with a fiery temperament in both sexes, tends to be admired much more in women than it is in men.

With haircare, as compared to without, the same woman was consistently rated as more neat, clean, pleasant, mature-looking and more interesting. Ratings for femininity, warmth and kindness varied depending on whether or not makeup had been applied. But the study also showed that qualitatively different aspects of personality are affected by haircare compared with makeup. The softer, gentler aspects of personality are favorably affected by good hair grooming, whereas with makeup it is the outgoing, sociable, confident aspects of personality that are judged to be improved. Interestingly, though standard haircare produces a more subtle change than makeup, more rated characteristics were affected by haircare than by makeup.

Improving your image

One of the things that this study highlighted was the approval granted to looking cared for – neatness, tidiness, cleanliness and obvious signs of personal care all seemed to be related by the judges to aspects of attractiveness and personality. If you make yourself look well-groomed, people tend to assume that you have a number of other positive attributes too. This usually makes others more interested in you, and you may receive better treatment in various social situations, particularly when you have to make a good first impression.

Since research suggests that others believe that "what is cared for is good," then the chances are that you believe it too – about yourself. How does haircare affect your self-image? We should expect positive feedback from others if appearance and personality are judged more favorably when we look well-groomed, and that always improves self-esteem. More directly, you will feel increased confidence just by seeing yourself looking better. Knowing that you have taken the time to wash and style your hair for an occasion can make the difference between feeling passable or extremely attractive in any situation, and your feelings about yourself will be reflected by others' responses.

Most people, particularly women, often feel a lift of spirits after having their hair styled. If, on the other hand, their hair is "not right" they may feel cross and unhappy all day. For

Perming and dyeing

■ Treatments to change the color and texture of your hair do cause a certain amount of damage, but techniques and products are improving all the time. A permanent wave (perm) will curl straight hair or even straighten curly hair. Soft perms give a gentle wave and add body and bounce to the hair. They can also make fine hair look thicker. Curly perms can be used for "wash and wear" styles that do not require setting or elaborate styling. Root perming gives a lift at the base of the hair. Weave perming curls alternate sections of hair and creates a casual look that is easy to care for.

Color treatments range from temporary wash in, wash out products that give you the chance to experiment with color, to semi-permanent and permanent colors. The latter can cause an allergic reaction, and reliable hairstylists and good coloring kits will advise a skin test before use. Temporary and semi-permanent colors wash out over successive shampoos, and avoid a harsh line between the treated hair and the outgrowth, but they fade quickly and need to be refreshed more often. Highlights and lowlights are now the most common form of coloring. These pick out very fine sections of hair that are treated with lighter and darker shades to blend with your own hair color. The effect is more natural than a solid color, and grows out without being too noticeable. **RR**

■ **Apprehension** *is a common experience when people are having a change of hairstyle BELOW. Many women still harbor memories of home perms that went horribly wrong. Even a slight change of color can be a shock, and a drastic one RIGHT is only for the brave.*

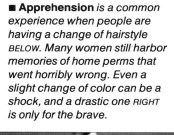

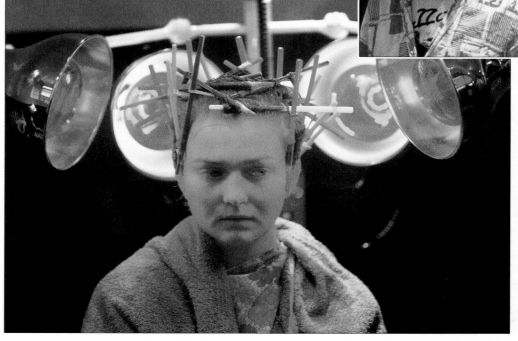

Hair under the magnifying glass

■ Trichologists are experts in the condition and treatment of hair. They are interested in the health and strength of your hair, rather than how to change it cosmetically. This is an area that has developed rapidly in the last 25 years, and trichologists now advise all major hair product suppliers about the best formulations for dry, oily and delicate hair.

Using magnification, a trichologist will examine the shaft of the hair to see if it is damaged in any way, pull gently on the hair to see if it is resilient or brittle and check the condition of the roots and scalp for oiliness or dryness. They can tell if your hair has recently been permed or colored, if you swim a great deal or wash it often, by looking at how the scales that coat the

outside of the hair are lying along the shaft.

You may wish to consult a trichologist if your hair feels chronically dry or brittle. They can advise for or against certain hairstyling procedures – they may suggest that you are using a blowdryer incorrectly, for instance, and will show you how to keep it far away from your scalp while still getting a good styling result. They will also suggest useful hair products.

Washing and conditioning your hair

■ Hair needs to be washed regularly. Oily hair should be washed often with a mild shampoo. If your hair is dry, wash it less frequently and use a more nourishing formula. Ask the person who cuts your hair for advice.

Before shampooing, massage the scalp with the fingertips or brush the hair to loosen dead cells. Wet your hair before applying the shampoo. Measure it out in your hand and mix it with a little warm water. Massage

shampoo into the scalp. Rinse your hair thoroughly. The rinse water will carry diluted shampoo through the ends. Rinse with cold water to make the surface of the hair appear smoother and shinier.

If your hair is dry you probably need to condition it every day. People with oily hair need less. If your hair looks dull use a deep conditioner that is left on for 15

minutes to half an hour, especially in winter when the air is cold and dry.

Mousse, setting lotion, gel and wax can help in styling your hair. Drying and heat styling can damage hair if used too much. Let your hair dry naturally whenever possible.

The best way to style your hair is to have a cut that you can manage easily at home. **RR**

Cooking ingredients can be used to condition your hair. A rinse of equal parts of lemon juice and water is good for oily hair and to enhance fair hair. Use 1 part vinegar to 8 parts water for dark hair. Egg yolk or olive oil is good for dry hair.

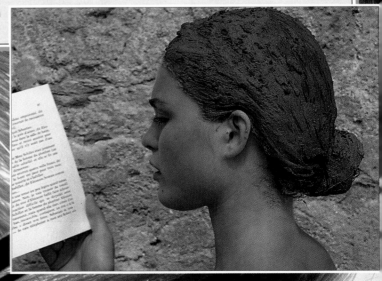

people with depression and other psychiatric problems, neglecting to cut, comb or even wash their hair may be an indication of how severe their condition is. It is often one of the first giveaway signs that the person is not coping and has stopped caring. Those suffering from poor self-image may be punishing themselves with neglect, or may simply despair of making any real improvement.

Encouraging depressed or ill people to experiment with new hairstyles may seem a frivolous form of therapy, but it can help them see themselves in new ways. If they can find a hairstyle they like and that is more compatible with a good self-image, they may come to feel more cared for in themselves and by others. Equally, it is important for everyone to find and maintain a look that makes them feel comfortable with themselves, confident of their appearance and happy about the image they project. An ugly hairstyle will not make you mentally ill, but it can make you unhappy, while an attractive hairstyle can do wonders for your self-confidence. **JAG**

Looking after your hair

Good haircare has an impact on the image we project to others and the image we have of ourselves. It can lift the spirits and raise the self-esteem of the clinically depressed. To gain these benefits, however, you have to know how to practice good haircare, be aware of the techniques that are available and decide what works best for you. Experts agree that the best way to keep hair beautiful is to be sure it is healthy. The formula for haircare is really very simple: wash it regularly, condition it often and avoid the things that can harm your hair.

Knowing a little about what hair is and how it grows will help you to care for it properly. Hair is a strong, tough outgrowth from the hair root or follicle. The clump of cells at the base of the follicle (the papillae) is fed by blood capillaries that stimulate it to produce hair cells. As these die and harden they form a long chain which protrudes through the skin – this is what we know as hair. The follicle will continue to produce hair cells, making the hair shaft grow, for between two and seven years. Hair will grow about half an inch (12 mm) a month. A sebaceous gland attached to the follicle produces a natural oil, sebum, which keeps the hair and scalp from becoming too dry. Each follicle eventually enters a fallow stage and its hair will fall out. Most people lose between 50 and 150 hairs a day.

Hair thickness, texture and curliness or straightness are determined by the size and shape of the follicle, which you have inherited along with your natural hair color. The amount of oil you produce, which may determine whether your hair is dry or oily, is also inherited. Nothing can be done to change the shape and size of the follicle or the activity of the sebaceous glands, but the right kind of haircare can modify many of the natural qualities of your hair.

Choosing the hairstyle that is right for you

Many of us want the sort of hair that we do not have. Those with thick curly hair often admire sleek bobs, while people with shiny, straight hair might prefer a mass of

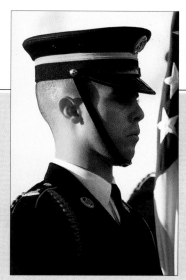

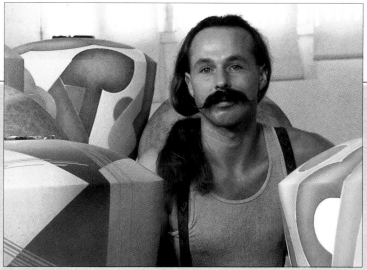

207

Men and the length of their hair

■ For modern men, hair length is probably the single most significant factor in projecting an image, though coloring and perms are becoming more popular. Since the 19th century long hair has been generally associated with alternative lifestyles, respectable or unrespectable. It is acceptable for university professors, men in "creative" professions, and musicians to have long hair – they are allowed to be dreamy, romantic, untidy and careless of their personal appearance. In less socially conventional men, such as hippies, street people, vegetarians and commune dwellers, we also expect long hair, but it is often associated with much more negative qualities including laziness, being dirty, fanaticism and naivety.

Notions about short hair differ, too. Extreme short cuts such as the skinhead look have connotations that are just as negative as the hippy look. The crew cut, when it was first introduced in the 1950s, was thought scandalous and was outlawed in most American high schools, though now it is perfectly respectable and even regarded as ultra-conservative. What counts as short hair also changes depending upon fashion. The Beatles' hair was thought to be extremely long in the early 1960s, though now it looks rather short compared to the excesses of later years.

unruly curls. Today you can change your hair drastically without doing it too much damage; but the style you admire may not be the right one for you. It might be wrong for your face shape and body type, or it may convey the wrong sort of image for the job and the social life that you have. A hairstyle that is attractive and well-maintained in itself might actually be a poor choice because it does not suit the person wearing it.

Often people admire a particular sort of hairstyle because it represents a fantasy of a very different sort of life. Many men adopt a tight, curly permed style, short in front and long at the back, known as "the sportsman's perm" because it was worn by many sporting figures in the 1970s (choosing the same hairstyle as a hero is one way of fulfilling fantasies or trying to realize an ambition). The style does not suit many men, however, and it now looks dated. If you have always longed for a style that is very different from your own, ask yourself what it represents for you. It may be a fantasy you would never really want to fulfill, or simply a desire for something different. But there may be qualities in it that you would like to imitate.

Exuberant curly styles are associated with a vivacious personality, and a woman who wants a long tousled mane of curls may wish to be more outgoing, for instance. She may not be able to maintain such a hairstyle or it may not be suitable for her physical type or her job, but she might be able to change her look in another way, by opting for a looser, more casual style, that would still express her desire to appear lively.

Think about your job and your social life. How do you usually spend your time? Are you trying to get ahead in a competitive business world, or are you working in a creative industry? Do you go hiking or dancing on the weekend? Your hairstyle has to be appropriate to the life you lead. If

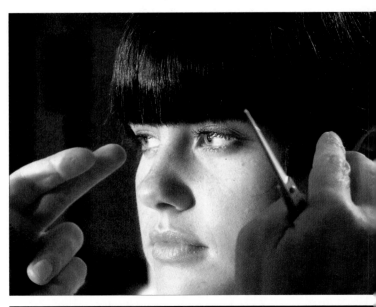

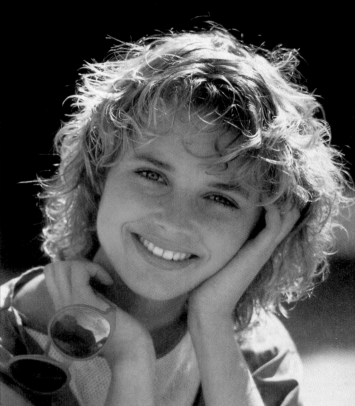

Face shapes and hairstyles

■ The shape of your face should influence your choice of hairstyle not just fashion:
Round face – avoid any style that mirrors the shape of your face, particularly jaw length styles with the fullness near your chin. Hair pulled severely off the face will also exaggerate full cheeks. Choose a slim, face-framing style with the fullness on top or at eye level.
Square face – geometric cuts and very short hair will only emphasize a square jaw. Go for softer, curly styles in longer lengths.
Long face and neck – bangs that cover the forehead and shorten and widen the face are a good option. Full, curled styles will also look good. Very short hair may make your head look too small, and should be avoided.
Short or thick neck – any short cut will elongate your neck. If your neck is thick, a style that is full around the ears will make it look more slender. Alternatively, a long sleek style may suit you as long as it avoids fullness at neck level.

■ **Maintenance and lifestyle** *are important factors in choosing a hairstyle. A blunt geometric cut* TOP *is not for everyone – if your hair is not naturally straight and smooth, it will take time to bring it under control, and the damage that can be done by overstyling may ruin the effect of the cut. Such styles also need trimming frequently, sometimes as often as every* two weeks. Those with naturally wavy or curly hair or who simply wish to spend less time taking care of it may opt for a casual tousled look ABOVE. This works successfully with many different kinds of hair and requires a minimum of styling - a wash-and-wear haircut.

your lifestyle has changed recently, take a good look at your hair. Many people make the mistake of keeping a hairstyle that was suitable when they were at school, but which is now too childlike and casual. Think about the qualities you want to convey and look for examples of hairstyles that might represent them.

The practical needs of your life also have to be taken into consideration. If you are very busy you may need a style that takes little maintenance. You may need to be able to keep your hair off your face, under a net or a hat for instance, particularly if you work with food or spend a great deal of time outdoors. The clothes you usually wear should also be taken into consideration. If you generally wear jeans, an elaborate hairstyle might look silly. What do attractive friends and colleagues do about their hair? Observing other people will often give you some good ideas.

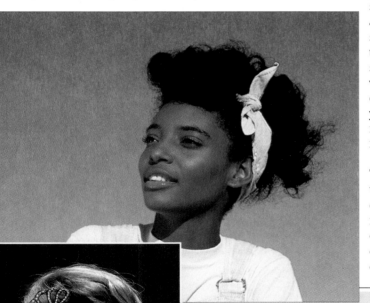

Matching a style to your hair and body type

You may know what image you want to convey and with which hairstyle, but you also need to match the style to your own physique. Straight bobs may be the executive look in your office, but if you have curly hair you will never be able to achieve this without a great deal of time, trouble and damage to your hair, and it may not look good on you. A neat, well-shaped style that makes the most of your curls but keeps them in control will be easier to look after and will probably suit you more. Perms and straighteners can modify your hair type for a while, but committing yourself to a style that is very different from the one that nature has given you may turn out to be a mistake and one that is, perhaps, difficult to rectify.

Besides your hair type, you will also need to consider your face and body. If you have a long face and neck, a long, straight, off-the-forehead style will exaggerate this. If you are very short, a curly, fluffy style may make you look even smaller. More and more salons are using computer imaging to help clients choose a suitable style (see *Ch27*). This system can reproduce an image of your face on screen, onto which different hairstyles can be superimposed, and by experimenting with looks on the computer instead of on your hair you can get an accurate picture of how well different styles will suit you without the disadvantage of making costly mistakes.

A change of hair color should match your skin and eyes. To avoid an unnatural effect, most hairdressers recommend that you do not go more than two or three shades lighter or darker than your own coloring. This should also be kept in mind if you are trying to camouflage gray hair. Skin and eyes change shades with age, and dyeing your hair its original color can look harsh and false. Graying hair should be camouflaged with lighter tones. **MK DC**

209

Styling for different hair types

■ Different hair types call for different styles and handling techniques. Fine hair requires a good accurate cut to hang well. Setting mousse, gel, perms, and color can give fine hair more body, but it is easily damaged and must be treated with care. Thick hair is usually quite strong, but it may be dry and lack elasticity. It will take a style more easily using wet styling methods like setting lotions and rollers. Curly hair is very elastic and strong. Damp and warmth can turn it into a frizzy mass. Mousse, gels, setting lotions and hair spray will help to establish a style and keep it in place.

Black people's hair has a lot of natural body, but it tends to be very dry and porous, and sometimes rather fragile. Chemical straighteners, if they are used at all, need to be applied carefully and are best done in a salon. Warm oil treatments and the use of a very wide-toothed comb, usually called an Afro comb, will prevent damage and improve hair condition. Corn row plaiting and other braiding methods look neat and tidy, and need little care. They should be unpicked and shampooed, and the scalp oiled, every seven to ten days. Black hair should be washed and dried with care.

Tease out tangles with the fingers. Use an Afro comb to style it when wet and dry the hair by covering it with a towel and squeezing the water out gently.

Children's hair is soft and needs gentle treatment. Its natural wave or curl can change frequently as the hair follicles enlarge and change shape. The color of a child's hair may also alter quite rapidly with age, usually becoming darker. It is best not to use perms or color on young hair until the hair type is well established. Use a shampoo that will not strip it of its natural oils and towel dry gently. **RR**

Why hair falls out

■ Hair has a powerful influence over self-image and the way others see us, and so hair loss has always been extremely distressing for both women and men. Balding, or fears about it, can cause people to feel inferior, inadequate, weak and unattractive.

Everyone loses hair every day, and though you may get a shock at the amount of hair you clean out of your brush or plughole remember that a loss of 50 to 150 hairs daily is quite normal. Many people have a seasonal pattern of hair loss, with follicles that have burgeoned in the summer entering a dormant period in the fall. Most haircare experts report an upsurge of worried patients at this time of year. If you are anxious about hair loss, look at the hair on your head, not at the hair that falls out. Is your overall hair distribution changing? Unless this happens, your hair loss is probably quite normal.

The search for a cure for hair loss can be traced back to the ancient Egyptian civilization, which devised cosmetic compounds to promote regrowth of lost hair. At the moment there is no certain cure or remedy, although experts are experimenting with a number of drugs that seem to be able to regenerate hair growth.

The first step in coping with hair loss is to determine what is causing it. Some forms of hair loss are strictly temporary; others are permanent.

In some cases only part of the hair is lost, while others involve loss of total head and body hair. Treatment is determined by the underlying cause.

Alopecia

Both men and women may develop a condition of partial or complete hair loss, known as alopecia, that leads to loss of both head and body hair. The cause is quite unknown and treatment has not been successful. People usually begin to develop severe alopecia during the teenage years, when the hair becomes gradually thinner and finer all over the head and body. Hair loss is evenly distributed and for this reason it may not become obvious for some time. In some people the condition is temporary or partial, but others lose all their hair permanently.

Stress, illness and hair loss

Stress and stress-related illnesses may involve hair loss. "My hair stood on end," we say when we have been frightened or angry, and that feeling is caused by a tightening of the scalp muscles in times of stress. It is possible that this reduces the supply of blood to the capillaries that feed the hair follicle, and that constant stress may eventually starve the follicles and cause them to die.

Some researchers report an increase in hair loss in women in high-stress jobs, and believe this may be caused by increased, stress-induced production of the male hormone testosterone. However, the evidence is not conclusive, and motherhood has, after all, never been a stress-free job. Such hair loss is often temporary and partial and responds well to anti-stress treatments.

Skin conditions that cause scales to build up on the scalp, like pityriasis, can lead to hair loss. Very poor nutrition causes the body to enter a starvation pattern, reserving nutrients for essential functions before supplying the hair follicles, which may result in hair falling out in handfuls. Exposure to X-rays and radiation, part of the treatment for some cancers, will cause the hair on both head and body to fall out. In all cases once the underlying cause is treated hair growth will begin anew.

Obsessive hair pulling (trichotillomania) is a form of self-abuse most common in teenage girls and often accompanies other psychological problems such as anorexia. It may begin as a nervous habit of twisting, tugging and biting the hair which escalates into more violent action, and can lead to large bald patches forming on the scalp. Continuous pulling can damage the follicles, but the hair will usually regrow once the habit is broken, usually as part of psychiatric counseling.

Hair loss with aging

As we get older, our hair gets thinner. The incidence of hair loss varies among races – Chinese people rarely go bald with age, while it is common in people of European descent. But everyone will find their hair getting thinner with age. The blood supply to the follicles slows, the hair itself

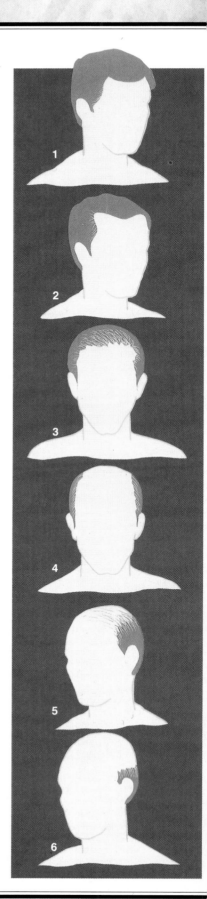

becomes more fine, and some follicles die off. The effects are seldom noticed until around the age of 50. Women may notice more rapid hair loss after the menopause; if it is severe it can be minimized by hormone replacement therapy. It does not usually lead to obvious baldness until a person is very elderly. JAG

Helpful treatments

Not all forms of hair loss can be treated effectively, despite continuous research. For cases of hair loss where the underlying cause cannot be removed or cured, anti-oxidant substances may slow down hair loss, and shampoos containing menthol and peppermint, natural antioxidants, are frequently prescribed. Scalp massage relaxes the muscles that may restrict the follicles and also stimulates scalp circu-lation, and has proved helpful in stress-related hair loss and some cases of alopecia and male pattern baldness. Drugs that cut down on male hormones are also being investigated for the prevention of hormone-related hair loss.

The drug Minoxidil (marketed as Rogaine) is the newest candidate in the campaign against hair loss. Minoxidil was first used to reduce high blood pressure, and balding male patients using it for this purpose began to report a resurgence of hair growth. It has recently been approved for use as a hair stimulant, though research into how it works is still continuing: 8 per-cent of users report dense hair growth, 31 percent moderate, but 61 percent little or none. It is most useful for male pattern baldness, but also helps some alopecia sufferers. MK DC

Hair transplants

When hair growth cannot be stimulated people often resort to hair transplants. This procedure involves taking a graft of skin from a site on the body, usually from the hairline along the base of the neck or over the ear, and transplanting it onto a balding part of the head. The operation is done under local anesthetic in several sessions; it can take two or three months to complete a transplant. Infection is a possible com-plication, and results are sometimes poor. The procedure works best on those who

have lost hair on the temples and forehead through male pattern baldness and who have relatively thick hair in other areas, that can be donated. Like all forms of cosmetic surgery, it is important for patients to have a realistic expectation of how the transplant might affect their lives. It cannot cure per-sonal or sexual inadequacies or deep-rooted psychological problems that are blamed on hair loss. Satisfaction tends to be greatest among those patients who have had the treatment to please them-selves not someone else.

Camouflaging hair loss

When other treatments are not effective, the psychological uplift of wearing a well designed hairpiece can be enormous, restoring confidence and self-esteem. Like hats and our own hair, they can also protect the head against the elements and prevent heat loss in cold weather. Modern hair-pieces are available in a wide variety of colors and styles, in human, animal or artificial fibers, and can look very natural.

People with alopecia treat wigs just like a natural head of hair. They may have wigs of differing lengths to give the impression of hair growth and cutting, and style them in many different ways. A hairdresser can cut the hair of the hairpiece while it is on the client's head to get the most suitable style. The wig can be kept firmly in place with special adhesives so a person can sleep or even swim in it. Cleaning, however, usually requires an organic solvent, and the hair may have to be sent to the drycleaners.

Toupees and partial hairpieces that have to blend with natural colors may be less successful, and if they are not well made, they can look unnatural and obviously false. Combing the hair over a bald area only works if the patch is small and the rest of the hair abundant. Long thin strands of hair combed over a large area of balding scalp do not usually work. After all, there is nothing wrong with being bald, whether you are male or female. Despite the stares of passers by, some female alopecia suffer-ers reject wigs and show their uncovered scalps with pride. As the range of accep-table hairstyles widens baldness is some-times used as a way of expressing individuality. JAG

◄ **Going bald**. *About 20 per-cent of all men eventually go bald, some beginning to notice hair loss in their early twenties. The gene is believed to be passed down from mother to son, but the pattern of hair loss in some men mimics that of their fathers, so exactly how male baldness is inherited is a mys-tery. The male pattern appears very rarely in women and is related to the effects of male hormones on hair follicles – this may be the reason why bald men are sometimes said to be especially virile.*

1 Typically, a balding man begins with a full head of hair.
2 Hair recedes first at the temples.
3 It thins out gradually on the crown.
4 Eventually there is a clear bald spot.
5 Hair is left in fringes at the sides and the back.
6 Very few reach the stage of almost complete baldness.

During pregnancy a woman's hormones will stimulate the activity of hair follicles, keeping more hairs in the active, growing phase than normal. After the baby is born, she will start to drop these extra hairs as well as those she would normally lose. Her hair may appear thinner for a while but quickly return to its pre-pregnancy state.

211

Men, women and body hair

Hair is distributed over every inch of the skin except the lips, the palms of the hands and the soles of the feet. Most of it is fine and downy. Women have as many follicles as men, but their downy hair is much finer, lighter in color, and softer. Downy body hair has little importance for social signaling, but it protects the skin from irritation and bacteria.

Pubic and underarm hair develops during puberty. It helps to prevent chafing and filters sweat through to the air. This hair growth signals sexual maturity.

Eyelashes, eyebrows, and hairs in the nose and ears are special fibers primarily designed to prevent dirt and germs from entering the eyes, nose and ears.

Though body hair serves many practical purposes, it is usually viewed as a social liability, and most people, especially women, spend time trying to reduce it.

Male body hair

Male body hair is considered a sign of virility, though many women do not find excessive amounts attractive. The amount of body hair a man has depends largely on heredity as well as hormone levels. If your father and uncles have little body hair you probably will not have much – this does not necessarily mean you have lower male hormone levels than very hairy men, and it certainly is no reflection on your virility.

Body hair is socially acceptable for men and they generally do not shave it, but underarm and pubic hair should be washed daily as odor-causing bacteria can be trapped in it. Men sometimes find that nose and ear hairs protrude and look untidy. They should not be plucked but trimmed with special scissors or electric clippers.

Beards and mustaches

Facial hair is a secondary sexual characteristic that appears in boys at puberty, like pubic and underarm hair. The texture and distribution of facial hair is inherited and varies considerably. Some men have very heavy beards while others have very fine, silky facial hair.

Beards and mustaches go through phases of popularity, and are most traditionally associated with naval officers, clergymen and college professors. Some research indicates that we associate beards with maturity, dominance, a liberal social and political stance, nonconformity and masculinity, but results are inconclusive – most of the research was done in colleges and universities, not among the general public.

If you do want to grow a beard or mustache, make sure it suits your face shape, and that the texture and distribution of your facial hair will allow for neat, even coverage. Thin, straggly facial hair will not usually make a successful beard, and the effect can be most unattractive. Crisp, curly facial hair usually makes the best beard. Take a good look at the color – if your facial hair is reddish and your hair is dark, as is often the case, the effect may be odd.

A beard will fill out a narrow chin and jaw, and a mustache will look best on a man with a long, full upper lip. Beards and mustaches are usually acceptable at work and on social occasions as long as they are short and neat. Special beard clippers and trimmers are now available which can be used like an electric razor to keep the beard at an even length. **MK DC**

Shaving male facial hair

Many men suffer unnecessarily from severe skin irritation and ingrown hair as a result of shaving badly. Shaving can actually be good for the skin if done well, because it removes layers of dead skin. Following a few simple rules will keep your face comfortable and in good condition. Unless you prefer an electric razor, remember to moisturize first, using warm water and then a good shaving foam or cream. This will keep the skin and beard soft, so the skin will be less likely to be stretched and scraped by the razor and the hair will cut easily. Use a sharp blade and shave in the direction of the hair. There is no need to use aftershave – most products contain alcohol which will sting and irritate the exposed skin. Aftershave balms and moisturizers are now available which comfort and soften facial skin.

Female body hair

Acceptance of female body hair has steadily increased since the 1950s but most women still remove hair from under

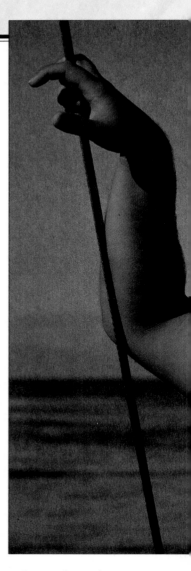

■ **Conventions of sex** *are particularly strong when it comes to body hair. The man who bares his hairy and muscular chest ABOVE displays raw masculinity – the male equivalent of the pin-up calendar girl. Both body and facial hair in men are associated with virility; the only places where they are considered unsightly are in the ears, nostrils and on the back. Women, on the other hand, convey femininity by their absence of body hair. Not every woman could pose for this photograph RIGHT – shaving may irritate the underarm skin, causing redness or bumps. Not shaving their underarms or legs has become more acceptable in the last few decades.*

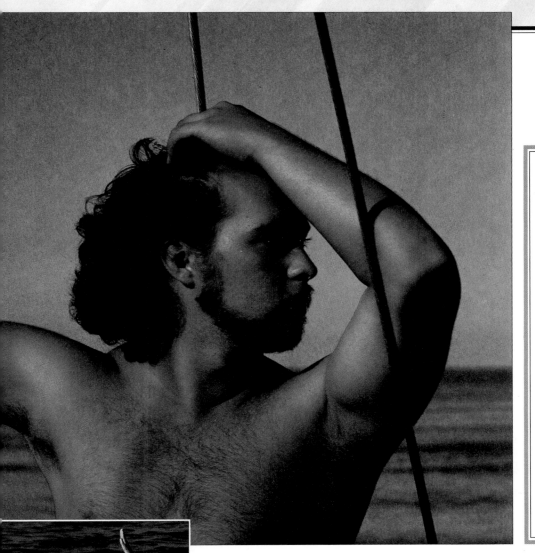

Ingrowing hair

■ Ingrown hairs can be caused by plucking, shaving, or pressure. Men commonly get them under the chin and on the back of the neck where it is hard to follow the direction of the hairs when shaving. Women who sit with their legs crossed may develop ingrown hairs on the back of the calf.

Men who are prone to ingrown hair on their face and back of the neck should be particularly careful when shaving, and should ask the barber to clip their neck hairs rather than shave them. Women who develop ingrown hairs on their calves should try to break the habit of sitting with the legs crossed. When shaving their legs they should make sure to shave in the direction of growth and always use a lubricating shaving foam.

their arms and from their legs, especially during the summer when these parts of the body are exposed. A number of methods are used, all having benefits and defects. Shaving is the most common, either with an electric or manual razor. It is quick, cheap, and works well, but you may cut yourself and your skin will feel stubbly after several days.

Abrasive mitts and pumice stones can be used to scrub away areas of unwanted hair, but these can irritate the skin and are ineffective if the hair is coarse or long. Tweezing is suitable for small areas like the eyebrows, but it can distort the hair follicle and it can be painful.

Waxing (see *Ch 32*) uses the application of warm liquid wax over the area to be treated. This is allowed to cool and solidify and is then stripped away, taking the hair with it. It removes the hair from below the skin so re-growth is slower, but some

people find it painful and it can irritate the skin. The only permanent method of hair removal is electrolysis (see *Ch 32*).

Facial hair in women

Women with facial hair, hair around the nipples, or around the bikini line often seek electrolysis treatment. Obvious facial hair on women is quite common but it is not socially acceptable and most women find it very distressing. It usually begins to appear around puberty. If you are worried about facial hair your doctor will be able to advise you. The cause may be a hormone imbalance which is creating not only facial hair but other physical problems. Many women with superfluous facial hair are perfectly normal hormonally, however, and what causes their condition is not clear. At the menopause women often develop coarse facial hair. Electrolysis or hormone replacement therapy can control this. **RR**

29

Beautiful Hands, Beautiful Feet

People notice hands, even feet ● *Looking after them properly is an essential part of creating a well-groomed impression* ● *Careful attention can also make a significant difference to your comfort and your good health.*

YOUR HANDS AND FEET work harder than any other parts of your body, but we seldom repay their labors with appropriate care and attention. Hands and feet are rarely short of exercise or prone to weight gain, and constant use keeps the joints and muscles fit well into old age. However, maintaining appearances is another matter, and many people fail to care for the skin and nails of the hands and feet properly. Nothing ruins the look of a well-dressed person so much as dirty, broken nails, rough skin on the hands or poorly maintained shoes. Conversely, your appearance can be enormously improved by some simple attention to the hands and feet. Though we may not consciously notice them, they have an enormous effect upon our first impressions of a person.

Your hands give you away

In folk tales the true identity of the hero or heroine is often discovered through their hands – not just the softness of their hands which indicates a life free of manual work, but also their shape and color, which were traditionally thought to indicate social status. Pale hands with long fingers, for example, were believed to be a sign of nobility. Palmistry, while it relies mainly on the lines of the palm of the hand to read a person's character and future, also suggests that a person's character and personality are indicated in part through the shape and condition of the hand. Square palms and short fingers with the nails cut short, for instance, are supposed to indicate a dynamic, high-achieving person with common sense.

Most of us would be wary of using this sort of character analysis as a basis for evaluating or understanding people, but nevertheless such "meanings" attached to hands are part of our culture and subconsciously we do tend to assess others on the basis of this kind of social signal.

Although there is not much research into the benefits of hand care compared with other types of cosmetic care, the same general principles that come into play with the use of facial cosmetics, hair care and fragrance seem to apply equally to hand care. In forming opinions about other people, all aspects of their appearance are important sources of information. The hands and fingernails and the care they receive are readily visible and so form a major part of any overall impression.

Aging and the hands

The hands are often the first sign of encroaching age, which shows up earlier and more decisively on the hands than on the face. The veins of the hand become more prominent, the skin thinner, dryer, and more wrinkled, and age spots or "liver spots" (dark brown irregular blotches like enlarged freckles) may appear on the backs of the hands. You can try to fade these spots using a special bleaching cream, but results vary and the creams may be harsh on the skin. Other treatments that we might use on the face to improve appearance, such as "lifts" and collagen injections, are not appropriate for the hands. The best way to keep the signs of age at bay on the hands is the frequent use of a

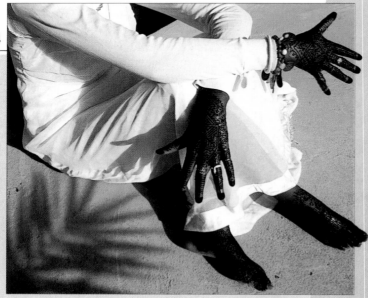

▲ **Intricate decoration** *is both highly visible and extremely eloquent on this Moroccan bride. How soon the mixture of* clay and pigment wears off will be some measure of her social status – of how much domestic work she has to do.

Cared for hands make an impression

■ A recent study on the psychological effects of handcare tried to measure how using a standard lotion on the hands and forearms affected other people's reactions to a group of volunteers.

The volunteers were hidden behind a screen with only their hands and forearms visible. A randomly selected group of people were then asked to rate them on aspects ranging from their personality (including sociability) to general appearance (including attractiveness) and on specific features such as the condition of their skin.

Those who examined the hands and forearms to which lotion had been applied tended to rate the subjects more highly, not just on skin condition, but also on personality and appearance. The study also found that if a fragrance was added to the hand lotion this prompted even more favorable impressions of the person. Remembering to take care of your hands does seem to influence other people's perceptions.

About 90 percent of women between the ages of 16 and 64 use hand cream or lotion of some kind, and three-quarters of these use the product at least once a day.

good skin lotion. Soft, resilient skin is less likely to wrinkle and dehydrate, and if the skin is plumped with moisture, raised veins will not be so prominent.

Aging is not the only factor that affects the appearance of your hands. Pigmentation disorders such as vitiligo (which causes large pale blotches on the hands due to a loss of pigment), nicotine stains in excessive smokers, chilblains, and excessively rough, cracked skin are unsightly and can be psychologically upsetting in varying degrees, as can nail irregularities including horizontal ridges, bumps, white spots, pitting and damaged cuticles. Extremely serious hand disfigurements such as missing or distorted fingers, swollen or damaged joints due to arthritis, and burn injuries are also likely to cause distress.

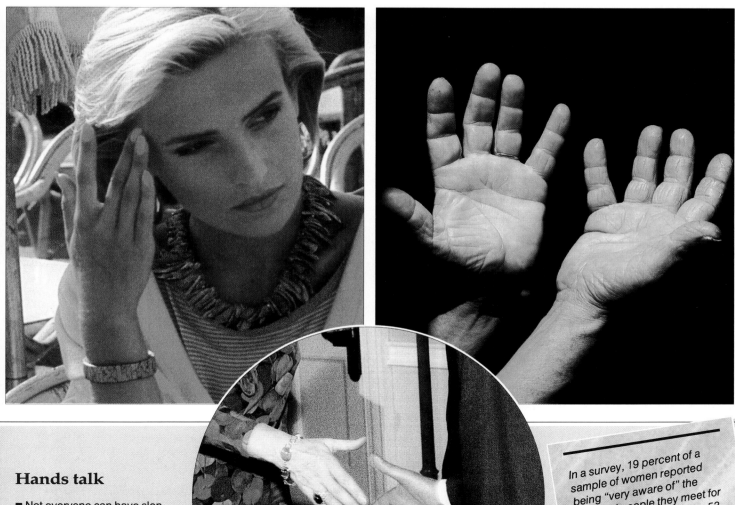

215

Hands talk

■ Not everyone can have slender, elegant hands. Even the most advanced plastic surgery cannot change short and stubby fingers or bony knuckles. But good grooming can make any hand look more distinguished, and with the right sort of cosmetic care you can make the most of your hands. Psychologically, the condition of the skin is an important aspect of the impression hands make.

■ *This fashion model TOP LEFT has a starting advantage, but given the care they deserve,* hands can be an essential component of an overall impression of elegance for almost anyone. These stone mason's hands TOP RIGHT may be excluded from the category of elegance, but they have character – fashioned by a lifetime's craft. The left hand has become enlarged from bearing the weight of stones hammered with the right. Hands are often the first point of contact when meeting people ABOVE. A handshake clinches the impact of these first few vital moments.

In a survey, 19 percent of a sample of women reported being "very aware of" the hands of people they meet for the first time, compared to 53 percent who were "very aware of" the faces of people they meet for the first time.

Healthy hands – healthy body

Your hands can give a doctor many clues about your health. Excessively curved nails are found in many patients with congenital heart conditions. Nails with a very round shape, called spoon nails, may indicate certain types of anemia. Fingers with flat, rounded, bulbous (spatulate) ends occur in patients with blood pressure problems. Nail irregularities such as ridges, spots, brittleness and flaking are often the result of poor nutrition. A tendency to fungal infections, marked by a dull yellow patch on the nails or by itching and flaking skin between the fingers, might cause a doctor to wonder about the state of the patient's immune system. Hand examinations can be a key to general health and nutrition and provide early warning of further problems.

Instruments of touch and caring

■ Although enhancing your appearance is the obvious, outward aim of any hand-care program, much of the benefit derived from it comes through the touch and care that is expressed through physical contact. In the "laying on of hands" power for healing is thought to be transmitted through direct contact between the healer and the person who needs healing. Certainly psychologists have found that touch itself can provide a feeling of well-being. Studies of deprived children have shown that touch is important for full, balanced emotional development.

If the touching hands themselves have not been cared for, and are dirty or rough, therapeutic contact is much less effective and is less comfortably received. Smooth, clean cared-for skin is of particularly vital importance for those who use their hands in caring work – nurses, doctors, masseurs and dentists, as well as manicurists. **JAG**

▶ **Hand-to-hand contact** *has profound emotional and spiritual connotations. It is particularly powerful when used by religious leaders such as this evangelist visiting a prison. On his part the hand clasp is a gesture of comfort in a harsh environment. For the prisoners it is a gesture of spiritual unity as they seek reconciliation with other people following their conviction.*

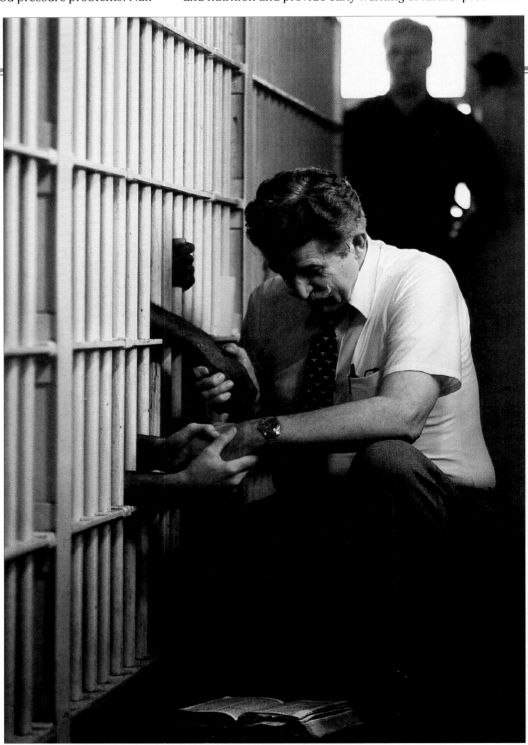

216

Camouflaging hand problems

There are many ways to improve the appearance of even the most damaged hands. In severe cases of discoloration, bleaching darker pigmentations can even out the skin color, though a perfect match is seldom attained. "Foundation" for the hands can also be used to mask discolored or blemished skin and give the hands a smooth, even appearance. Careful buffing and use of a pumice stone can reduce nail irregularities and remove calluses. Special nail products will strengthen and harden nails, making them less susceptible to unsightly damage.

Color in nail products can play an important role in camouflaging imperfect hands. If you have short, stubby fingers bright red nail polish will make them look even shorter; choose a pale skin-tone color that will extend their length. If your nails are stained or damaged, use an opaque color in several coats that will cover up any irregularities. Simply polishing your nails is not a substitute for good handcare, however.

The best camouflage for hand problems is clean, well-moisturized skin and neatly trimmed, clean nails. Good hand care can also eliminate many blemishes. Rough cracked skin can be combated by use of a moisturizer. Damage to the hands and nails is often caused by lack of care; chilblains, for example, are the result of letting the hands get too cold. Treat your hands well and they will repay you by looking good.

Regular treatment of the hands and nails is of benefit to everyone, sick and well – it improves self-image, makes us feel pampered and cared for, and has a positive effect on how others see us. Regular manicures by a professional are very enjoyable but they can be expensive and time-consuming. Fortunately it is easy to incorporate hand care into your daily routine. **JAG**

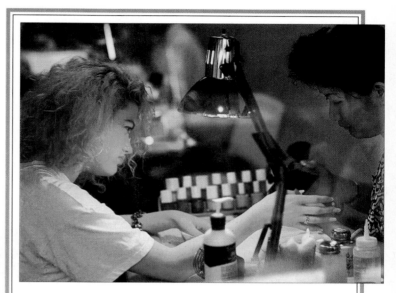

Helping you to like your hands

■ Manicurists often find they have to deal with people's feelings as well as their hand problems. The Jaques Dessange school in Paris incorporates a compulsory psychology course in its manicure training so that the students can help people come to terms with their hands, often a focus of dislike. Hand treatments seem to release stress in the whole body, and are useful in making people feel more relaxed and more comfortable about themselves.

Manicure as part of the service offered to hospitalized patients has proved to be of enormous psychological benefit. In Europe the Red Cross Volunteer Service regularly offers this treatment. Many American and Canadian hospitals offer general cosmetic services which often include manicure. For people who are not feeling very well, and who view their bodies as being endangered and "not right," manicure has a twofold value. It pays attention to appearance, something hospital patients often ignore, particularly when ill. It improves self-image and confidence and generates positive feedback from others to encourage the development of a positive psychological cycle. The experience of touch also promotes feelings of well-being and a sense of communication in people who feel ill and cut off from friends and family. Because our hands are so sensitive, and of prime importance to our sense of touch, generating a sense of well-being through them seems to be particularly effective. **JAG**

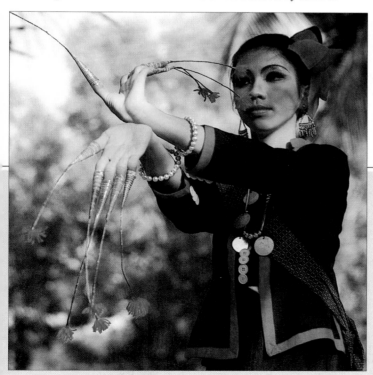

▲ **The subtleties of hand gesture** are amplified by the delicate finger-decorations worn by this dancer from Thailand. A complex system of joints and muscles gives the human hand a vast range of expressive possibilities. Art-forms as diverse as ballet and puppetry allow the hands to speak eloquently, and most of us use them in the course of almost all our everyday conversations.

Practicing perfect hand care

Caring for the hands often comes lowest in priority in a skin-care or grooming session, whether professional or amateur. Hands are often treated in a hurry, the nails cut badly and the cuticles pushed back harshly so that they become broken and inflamed. Yet hands are an important part of first impressions, and they work hard for us. They need proper care. A good hand-care routine need take only a few minutes each day, yet the benefits will last a lifetime. Hands that are cared for remain more supple, keep their good appearance longer, and are pleasant to touch and be touched by.

Daily hand care is very simple. First, keep your hands clean. Use a soft nail brush to remove dirt from underneath the nails and to remove stains such as ink and garden grime from the fingers. Use a moisturizer regularly – at least in the morning and evening, and whenever your hands feel dry or have been in water. If you work with paper, you may find your hands become very dry. This is because paper absorbs moisture from your hands. Typists, librarians, bookkeepers, and anyone who handles paper frequently should keep a moisturizer at work and use it regularly.

Hangnails are common problems. They are caused by rough treatment of the hands and are made worse by cold

Taking care of your hands

■ Care of the skin alone is not sufficient to make the hands attractive. Your fingernails also need to be kept clean and neat. Broken and bitten nails are often interpreted as the sign of a diffident, nervous or insecure person. Nails that are ragged or dirty could be seen as an indicator of a lazy or messy person who does not pay attention to details. Overdecorated nails might be thought to indicate frivolity. Tidy nails always give a good impression even if they are not specifically noticed.

■ Taking good care of your hands and nails helps create a good impression on others – and on yourself. After all, you look down at your hands as much as or more than others do. If your hands are not attractive to look at, they will not improve your self-image. Failing to take care of your hands properly may

indicate a lack of care about your whole self, whereas improving your hand care can be a step toward thinking more positively about yourself.

▼ **Finger tip information**. *Nails are produced by specific skin cells at the tips of your fingers. They protect the nail beds, which contain many sensitive nerve endings. The nail itself, the nail plate, is dead, horny tissue made of a material called keratin, which also makes up your hair. The whitish half-moon shaped area at the base of the nail is called the lunule. It is the bridge between the living cells under and around the nail and the dead nail plate. The cuticle is a thin membrane of skin at the base of the lunule overlying the area where new nail cells grow (the matrix), protecting the matrix and joining the nail plate to the nail bed.*

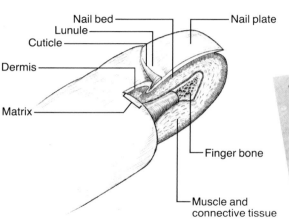

Nail bed
Lunule
Cuticle
Dermis
Matrix
Nail plate
Finger bone
Muscle and connective tissue

Most people's nails grow about 3mm (one eighth of an inch) per month. It takes from four to six months to produce a completely new fingernail. Nails grow faster in summer, and young people's nails grow faster than those of the elderly.

Give yourself a manicure

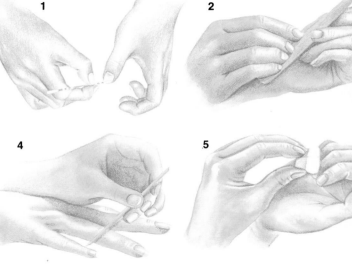

1
2
4
5

■ Every one or two weeks you will need to spend a little more time on your hands. Many people go to a professional manicurist but if you do not want to do that, you can still make an excellent job of your hands at home.

1 Remove any old nail polish using a cotton ball dampened with nail polish remover. Make a series of short strokes away from the base of the nail, otherwise you will push the polish and remover up under your cuticle. Use a cotton bud to remove polish from around the cuticles and under the nails.
2 When you are filing your nails always use an emery board, not a metal nail file – metal is too harsh and can make the nail split. File from the side of the nail up toward the center in long strokes going in one direction only. If you file back and forth you could damage the nail. Do not file deep into the edges, but leave some of the straight side intact, to prevent weakening.

weather, lack of moisture and general brittleness of the nails. A regular regime of good hand care and clipping away loose ends of any hangnails that do occur will soon improve the look of your hands.

Very dry nails often split and flake. This can be caused by poor nutrition, but is more usually due to poor filing of the nails, or overexposure to hot water and detergent. Using a moisturizer, learning good filing techniques and wearing rubber gloves to wash the dishes will help.

Protect your hands. Keep them dry and warm. Wear gloves when it is cold outside – if your hands get too cold they will dry out, become red and cracked, and possibly develop chilblains. If you are doing the dishes or cleaning the bathroom, wear cotton-lined rubber gloves to keep your hands from becoming too hot or damp. Wearing suitable gloves while gardening or doing any rough or dirty job guards against cuts and grazes, rough skin and chipped or broken nails.

File your nails whenever a rough place develops, and clip away any hangnails before they catch and tear. Always file the nails when they are dry, and cut them only when wet. Finally, use a cuticle cream regularly. Massage it into your cuticles and around the edge of the nail using the thumb and first finger of the opposite hand.

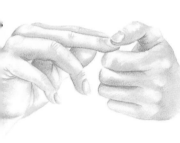

6

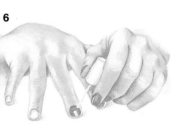

3 Massage cuticle cream or oil into the nails and soak them in a small bowl of warm soapy water for a few minutes.
4 Then apply cuticle remover to the base of the nails, using the hoof-shaped end of a plastic or wooden orange stick to lift the cuticle skin gently where it has grown onto the nail plate and carefully push it back into place. If necessary, use a cuticle knife or clippers to remove any over-hanging skin or rough edges. Wipe over each nail with polish remover, rinse the hands in clear water and pat them dry. Apply a moisturizing lotion and massage it in thoroughly.
5 You do not have to use nail polish to have attractive hands. Many people prefer simply to buff their nails, using a dry powder or paste and a nail buffer. Buff in even strokes from cuticle to tip. This strengthens nails by improving the circula-tion, removes some surface irregularities, and gives them a slight satiny sheen.
6 If you do want to use nail polish, always remember to apply a base coat to protect the nail from staining and to provide a smooth base. The nails must be dry. Hold the nail polish brush with the thumb and first finger. Do not overload the brush; remove excess polish on the edge of the bottle top. Paint the nail in four sections: the middle, the base, the right side, and the left side. You should apply one layer of base, one or two layers of enamel depending on the intensity of color you want and, if desirable, a top coat or fixative to seal the polish.

■ **How do I stop biting my nails?** Many people bite their nails as children or adolescents, but for some it becomes a habit that is hard to break. Bitten nails are unsightly and can even be painful if the free edge is bitten down to the nail bed, and infec-tions can result. One of the best methods of breaking the habit, though, is thorough hand care, including the application of nail polish. If the nails are smooth, free of rough edges, and look cared for there will be much less temptation to bite them.

Techniques for hand massage
■ Hand massage is best done by one person to another. It is a good way to release tension, particularly if you write or type a good deal, and keeps the hands supple. First, massage cuticle cream into the nail base using the thumb and first finger of the opposite hand. Warm hand cream, lotion or oil in the palm of your hand, and then spread it over the back and fingers of the opposite hand.
1 Massage the hand and wrist using the ball of the thumb in circular movements. Kneading movements of the thumb and the fingers relax the wrist and finger joints. Massage each finger gently from the knuckle to the tip.
2 Using only a very little pres-sure, pull each finger from the knuckle to relax the joint.
3 Take each finger and circle it clockwise several times. From the base of the fingers, mas-sage the hand with circular movements down to the wrist.
4 Put the palms of the hands together, entwine the fingers, and circle the wrist in a clock-wise movement. Finish with light stroking movements over the whole hand.

Hand-massage need only be an occasional part of your hand care. Regular all-round care will keep your hands looking good, improving your appearance, making you feel better, and favorably affecting the impress-ions others have of you.

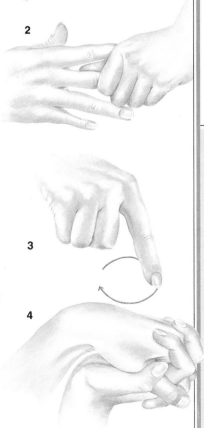

1

2

3

4

219

Putting your best foot forward

If any part of the body is more neglected than the hands, it must be the feet. They bear the weight of our whole body when we walk, and we walk a great deal more than we realize. The mother of a young family probably walks at least four miles a day. All adults seem to walk a minimum of a thousand miles a year, and by the age of 70 most people will have walked the equivalent of three times around the world. It is not surprising that our poor feet sometimes ache, especially if we have done much of that walking in badly-fitting shoes.

The feet are really very hardy parts of the body, however, and can take a great deal of the pressure and pounding which we subject them to each day. By following a few simple guidelines to protect and care for our feet, we can avoid most foot problems.

Caring for your natural shock absorbers

Even if your feet have been well cared for as a child, you can develop foot problems as an adult through poor foot care. Walking properly and having good quality, well-fitting shoes and hosiery can prevent most serious foot problems. When standing up, try to keep your weight evenly distributed on both feet. Shifting from one foot to the other can overstrain the muscles, bones and ligaments in the foot if you are standing for a long time.

As we walk, our weight is transferred alternately from one foot to the other and the foot acts as a kind of shock absorber, cushioning the impact of the ground. If you tend to walk on the outside or the inside of your foot, as many people do, your foot is not able to absorb the impact as effectively as it can through the sole, which is well cushioned. You can strain ligaments and tendons and your

Protecting tiny feet

■ Good foot-care should begin at birth. Children have soft bones, and if they are put into ill-fitting or tight shoes this can cause the shape of the foot to become distorted.

Babies should not be put into shoes until they are able to balance, support their own bodies and walk well. When a young child is just beginning to walk, bare feet are really the best, as this gives them a better grip on a flat surface. The feet can curl and flex.

A baby's first shoes should be chosen with care. Children grow very quickly, and most manufacturers and specialists recommend a minimum of 18mm (three quarters of an inch) extra growing space when a child is fitted with shoes. Young feet should be measured every three months up to the age of five, and width as well as length must be accounted for. Socks are also important; they can cramp if too tight.

The growth of the feet usually continues until between the ages of 16 and 20, when the soft growing cartilage is gradually replaced by hard bone. It is therefore just as important for teenagers to have well-fitted shoes as it is for younger children. **RR**

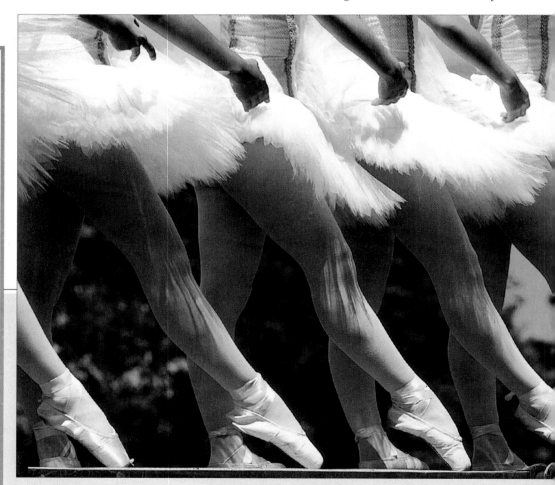

▲ **The feet of a dancer** *probably suffer more severely than those of any others. An exciting, athletic and finely-coordinated performance has its price – the foot is forced into unnatural positions, takes the impact of the body in shoes not* *designed to help absorb shock and on vulnerable parts of the foot, and is subjected to the constant pounding of practice and performance. Not surprisingly this can lead to dancers having serious foot injuries. If you or your child takes up* *dancing even on an amateur level, make sure that exercise shoes are properly cushioned and that young feet are not overstressed. Children should not be allowed to dance in point shoes for ballet until they are at least twelve.*

Looking after shoes

■ The editor of Vogue and major style arbiter, Diana Vreeland, once fired an assistant for having scuffed heels. Poorly maintained shoes can ruin your general appearance, making the most elegant outfit look sloppy. They can even hurt your feet if you let them deteriorate too far. Worn down soles do not provide enough support for the arch of your foot, and worn or broken heels can distort the way you walk. Use shoe trees to maintain the shape of the shoe, putting them in while the shoes are still warm from your feet. Polish your shoes frequently to protect the leather and keep it supple, and have the heels attended to regularly – they wear down rapidly and should be reheeled every six weeks or so.

All feet perspire, but this only leads to unpleasant foot odor when the perspiration reacts with bacteria on the feet. If you are prone to foot odor, wear cotton socks or tights, or cotton-soled nylons; stick to leather shoes which will not trap perspiration; and scrub your feet thoroughly and dust with talcum powder to remove bacteria and absorb perspiration.

feet will certainly hurt more after a long walk. Try walking toward your reflection in a full length mirror, and see if you really walk flat on the soles of your feet or on the sides. Practice walking correctly and your feet will feel better after a long day.

If the shoe fits...

Never rush into buying shoes. Many foot problems are the result of ill-fitting shoes and any purchase should be considered carefully. Bunions, corns and distortions of the big toe joint (hammer toe) are usually caused by badly-fitting shoes.

Shop in the afternoon – this is when your feet are at their most swollen, and will be sensitive to a bad fit. Walk up and down the store in the shoes several times. If the shoes are too slack they will not give you enough support. Stand on your toes – if the heels slip off they are not a good fit.

Shoes should have at least 1cm (about half an inch) of free space at the toe, and the width of the shoe should allow your foot to lie flat on the base. The arch of your foot should feel firmly supported. Rely on shoe fit rather than on sizing – sizes vary enormously between manufacturers and are only a rough guide to a good fit.

The type of shoe you buy is as important as the fit. Leather shoes are more comfortable to wear for long periods as the shoe "breathes" more freely and is more flexible than plastic. If you walk a great deal lace-up shoes are probably best, as they hold the shoe on the foot most securely and

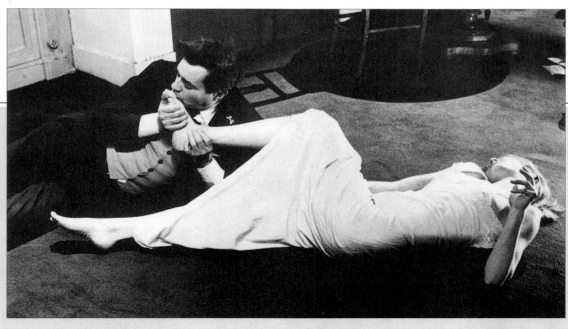

▲ **The allure of the foot** is not something that all of us would admit to recognizing – yet this sequence from the film "The Night Porter" strikingly demonstrates the erotic potential of removing no more than one's shoes. The kissing of feet is associated with submission to rulers. In ancient times, emperors were ritually kissed on the feet by their subjects. Lovers exploiting this association sometimes find by means of it an exciting expression of their submission to passion and the object of their love.

can be adjusted as the foot swells. High heels throw the weight of the body forward onto the balls of the feet and can put a strain on the spine because this changes the alignment of the pelvis. If you choose high heels try to wear them only for special occasions when you will not have to stand for a long time. Shoes with pointed toes can distort and restrict the toes unless they are quite a bit longer than the foot.

Shoes also restrict the foot's natural breathing and circulation, so it helps to change your shoes frequently. You will need various sorts of shoes for different activities. Different kinds will affect the feet differently, so changing the shoes will vary the stresses on your feet. Shoes also last longer if they are allowed to dry out between wearings. Treat your feet with care, and they will reward you with years of good service.

Pedicure and foot massage

You will occasionally need to cut your toenails and deal with hard skin on your feet. To really treat your feet, expand this routine to give yourself a pedicure and foot massage every few weeks or so. This treatment is available from beauticians, but you can carry it out easily at home.

A good regular pedicure will keep your feet looking and feeling wonderful. People are usually more concerned about the appearance of their feet during the summer months when they are on display more often; but keeping them well cared for throughout the year will remove the need for drastic treatments when you want to wear sandals. Most importantly, when your feet are relaxed and in good condition you will feel relaxed too, and you will feel much more comfortable in heavy winter shoes and boots if you pamper your feet. **RR**

Pampering your feet

■ **Walking properly** and wearing good shoes and hosiery should prevent serious damage to your feet. You can also improve the general condition and feeling of your feet with a little pampering.

One of the nicest things you can do for your feet is to take the weight off them. If it is appropriate at work, put your feet up. This will keep your feet from swelling by lessening the gravity-aided flow of blood to them. The feet are full of nerve endings which are connected to other parts of the body, and constant pressure on the feet does seem to trigger pain elsewhere. Sitting down and elevating the feet can relieve the pain of low backache or a headache.

When you are at home, wear slippers. Slippers allow your feet to breathe and flex more readily, reducing swelling and soreness. Slippers are usually lightweight. Removing the weight of a shoe from each foot will lessen the stress on your ankles and legs. The change will also give your shoes a break, allowing them to dry out.

■ **Relieve aches and pains with a foot bath.** If you are on your feet all day, even the best-tended feet may be sore and aching by the evening. A footbath is a quick way to make them feel better. Fill one large bowl with hot water and another with cold, and plunge your feet in each alternately for several minutes at a time. This will stimulate your circulation and reduce swelling. If you have to go out again in the evening this sort of water treatment will revive your feet for a night of dancing.

If you are staying at home, a longer relaxing soak may be best, followed by a gentle massage. Mustard added to a footbath of warm water warms and soothes the feet. Bicarbonate of soda will stimulate circulation and soften hard skin. There are also commercially made footbaths which use a vibrating base or bubbling water to massage the feet.

■ **Paraffin wax treatments** can be used on the feet to soften, cleanse and remoisturize skin. The wax used has a low melting point so that it is comfortably warm when it is applied. It is poured over the foot or hand or applied with a spatula until it is completely covered, and left

222

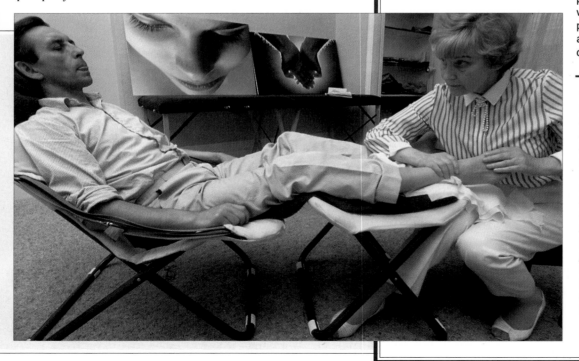

◄ **Foot massage.** *The nerve endings in the foot are connected to nerves all over the body, and pressure on the soles of the feet causes pain elsewhere. Foot massage is an extremely relaxing treatment which relieves tension and stress not just in the feet, but all over. It is said to help relieve many stress-related conditions from migraine to menstrual pain. It certainly improves the circulation and muscle-tone of the foot, and by alleviating stress it promotes a general feeling of well-being.*

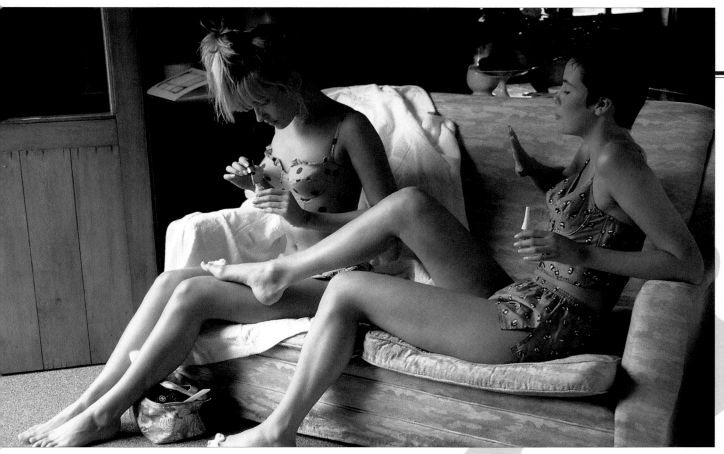

until it has hardened. Your feet will feel warm and moist. The wax then peels off easily. The treated area may be held under cold water for a minute or so, and then thoroughly moisturized. This treatment is offered by many beauty salons, or you can buy the wax and use it at home. Do not let it get too hot – you can easily burn yourself. It is a good idea to have this treatment at the beauty salon before trying to do it yourself.

■ **Foot exercises**. *Your feet contain 19 muscles, 115 ligaments and 26 bones. They get a great deal of exercise from walking, but they can also become stiff and sore. These simple exercises can keep them supple and strong. Seated, raise one foot from the floor, point your toes and write the alphabet in the air. Place a tennis ball on the floor and roll it round using the sole of your foot. Put a pencil on the floor and try to pick it up with your toes.*
Stand with your feet side by side. Rise slowly up on to your toes, count to ten and come down slowly. Repeat five times.

■ **Polishing your toenails**.
Many women enjoy painting their toenails, especially in the summer when they are visible in sandals. Remove any old nail polish from the toenails with polish remover, remembering to wipe away from the cuticle. Gently push back the cuticles, using cuticle remover and clippers if necessary. Separate the toes using cotton balls or wads of tissue (commercial toe separators of sponge rubber are widely available). This will prevent polish smudging against the skin and allow the polish to dry well. Use a base coat if the polish you are using is a vivid color. Apply polish just as you would to your fingernails – it is tempting to brush the color horizontally across the nail, but vertical strokes away from the cuticle are best. Let them dry thoroughly before putting on socks or shoes.

■ **Give yourself a pedicure**.
Bathe the feet in a large basin or bowl, brushing around the nails and between the toes with a soft nailbrush. Remove any hard skin with a pumice stone or file. Dry the feet thoroughly with a warm towel, especially between the toes.
Cut the nails of the toes straight across, and file them straight across with the strong side of an emery board. Nails should always be kept short, level with the top of the toes; otherwise they will cause pressure on the nail bed when wearing shoes. Do not shape the sides of the nail or it may become ingrown. Just take the point off the edge.

Apply cuticle cream or oil (almond or olive oil is excellent) to the cuticles of the toenails; these can grow quite far up the nail plate if not attended to regularly. Soak the feet in a fresh bowl of warm soapy water for a few minutes. Remove the feet from the bowl, rinse in clear water, and dry the feet carefully.
Apply cuticle remover and gently push back the cuticles with the hoof end of a plastic or wooden emery board, using a circular motion. Avoid using strong pressure as this can damage and inflame the cuticles.
Use a cuticle knife or clippers to remove any loose bits of skin. Apply more cuticle oil and foot lotion. Lightly massage the feet, using circular motions.
Liberally apply foot lotion and grasp the foot in both hands with the thumbs on top and the fingers beneath the sole, and work up and down the length of the foot, including the toes and the ankle.
Rotate the joints of the toes and the ankle. Finish with light strokes along the length of the whole foot.

223

30

Looking After Your Smile

Smiling is good for your mental and physical health ● *A happy, confident smile lets other people perceive you in a positive way* ● *Keeping your smile attractive means keeping your teeth and lips healthy.*

A SMILE is your most important nonverbal signal. It shows a strong response to another person, communicating pleasure, friendliness, enjoyment and a lack of hostility. People smile a great deal in the course of a day, in greetings, as part of conversation and discussion, and in parting from others. Our smiles make others feel welcome and appreciated, soothe anxiety and dampen aggression. Some psychologists even think that smiling stimulates our own sense of well-being. It is easier to use your smile if you are confident that it discloses good teeth, smooth lips and fresh breath.

What is a smile?

A true spontaneous smile involves pulling up the corners of the mouth and raising the cheek muscles. Lips may be parted to show the teeth. "Laughter lines" may crinkle around the eyes or run from the nose to the corners of the mouth. We all know when someone is smiling falsely as their eyes and cheeks do not change as they do in a natural smile.

Smiles are produced by the facial muscles, especially those known as zygomatic muscles that control the corners of the mouth. These muscles are all controlled by the facial nerve, which can be activated by two different parts of the brain. Spontaneous facial expressions come from the primitive lower brain; those which we control come from the motor cortex, the area of the brain dealing with conscious

movements. Facial expressions are a product of both spontaneous feelings and attempts to control them. The origins of these two neural systems are quite different: the lower brain is the result of evolutionary forces, while the motor cortex is controlled by what we have learned about what is proper and appropriate.

Does it come naturally?

People have more facial muscles than any other mammal, which allows us to convey more with our faces. Facial expressions probably evolved as social signals. Baring the teeth and frowning – the opposite of smiling – was originally part of attack behavior but later became just a signal of hostility. Monkeys, apes and dogs have a limited smile mechanism which they use to convey either fear (a smile of appeasement) or pleasure. A pure appeasement smile exists in some human cultures subject to social pressure. In

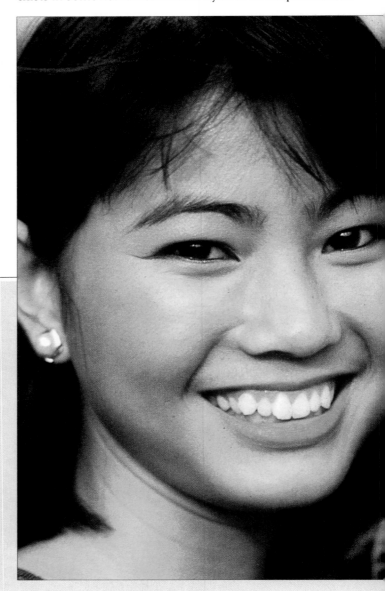

What does your smile say?

■ While they all indicate degrees of pleasure and lack of hostility, different types of smile can convey quite subtle meanings.

A spontaneous smile like that of the woman on the right involves every facial muscle, closing the eyes and causing distinct laughter lines around the eyes and mouth.

A smile intended to make an impression – a "social smile" – is more controlled, though still sincere. People who habitually smile in this way, like the woman on the left, are usually more self-conscious than unrestrained smilers.

A wide smile with wide-open eyes may indicate sexual attraction, and is highly favored for advertising. Open-mouthed, gaping smiles with the eyes almost closed usually indicate hilarity and mirth. Smiles with the lips drawn tight against the teeth and the brow wrinkled mean anxiety and the wish to appease. Close-mouthed smiles with the eyebrows elevated show a certain aloofness and perhaps snobbery. Open-mouthed smiles and raised eyebrows, on the other hand, indicate a query. Most of these social signals seem to be universal.

Japan, where people have to live in proximity within a rigid social structure, people smile a great deal, often to mask true feelings of anger, depression or disgust, and non-Japanese have to learn to interpret these smiles not as indicators of pleasure but as calming influences.

Children smile without being taught, and do so early in life. By the age of two and a half months they will smile at faces or masks that look like faces, even though infants are unable to recognize a familiar face until six or seven months. Children blind from birth will smile in response to a pleasant voice, though with a rather open-mouthed expression rather than a typical smile. Social training for the blind may involve the teaching of appropriate facial expressions, and very small blind children quickly pick up a natural smile.

Children learn the social rules about where and when to smile fairly quickly. In one experiment six-year-olds and ten-year-olds were given unsuitable toys which they might regard as babyish. The six-year-olds did not try to mask their disappointment, but almost all the ten-year-olds pretended to be happy with the toys.

Registering your emotions in a smile

Smiles are usually directed at someone. Researchers filmed groups of people at a bowling alley, and found that people rarely smiled at the pins – if they did it was usually a brief, tight smile of pleasure at a good score. They smiled a great deal at their friends, however, especially after knocking down most of the pins.

Observe people watching a film and you will see that they will show some spontaneous facial expression even when they think they are unobserved, particularly if they are watching a comedy. The strength of the expressions will increase enormously, however, if there are other people in the room who they know. They will also be likely to turn and look at each other, sharing smiles.

Because smiles are such an important part of our communication system, people are at a disadvantage if they have damaged facial muscles, poor teeth or bad breath that they wish to conceal. They are unable to smile naturally and spontaneously. Surgery can only occasionally restore full facial expressiveness if nerves and muscles have been damaged. No one, however, need suffer from self-consciousness about bad teeth or breath. Good hygiene, regular dental attention, and if necessary the formidable array of dental correcting techniques now available can help everyone to smile frequently and uninhibitedly. **MA**

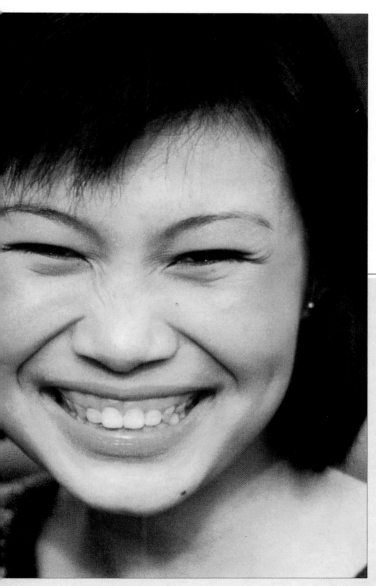

Smiling your way to good health?

■ We all feel better for a good laugh. But can a smile and a joke actually prevent or cure sickness? Many people think so. Norman Cousins, a New York newspaper editor, wrote a book and made a movie about his crippling, incurable illness which he claims was cured by watching Marx Brothers movies and telling jokes. Freud believed that humor relieved inhibitions and he used it to help his patients talk about repressed feelings and memories. Studies of personalities resistant to mental and physical illness show that a sense of humor is an important element. But what is the biological mechanism that operates in such situations?

We all know that laughter can release tension in a difficult situation. This may be because smiling and laughing send messages to the brain lowering levels of the stress hormone cortisol. The smile's origins as an aggression-appeasement expression make sense in relation to this. High levels of cortisol are known to inhibit the immune system, and there are many studies indicating that stress relief improves general health. Smiling will not stop you from contracting illnesses, but it just may be the first step towards stress reduction, which helps your body to handle sickness. Next time you feel tense or unwell, try smiling. **MA**

225

Preventing tooth decay

We often partly show the teeth when smiling and people who attempt to hide a bad set of teeth when smiling can look haughty, depressed or nervous – often exactly the opposite of the impression they are trying to convey. Attention to good dental hygiene can prevent many problems, and regular checkups will usually lead to successful treatment of those that develop.

Teeth usually fail us because of decay (caries). The same decay, untreated, is also usually the cause of chronic bad breath (halitosis). Particles of food lodge in the crevices between our teeth and just below the gum line. Bacteria interact with food, and together they can break down the hard enamel covering of the tooth and cause it to erode. Pits of decayed tooth matter, normally called cavities, develop and can eventually lead to the death of the tooth root. Bacteria may also build up into a hard ridge, known as plaque, at the base of the teeth. Plaque interacts with sugar in food to produce an acid which can dissolve the enamel of the tooth. Saliva contains powerful antibacterial agents which fight this decay process, but it cannot always kill all the bacteria lurking in the mouth.

Gum disease or periodontitis is also caused by decay, and is the major cause of tooth loss in middle-aged people. Decaying matter causes infection in the gums, which bleed easily when cleaned. The gums shrink away from the teeth, allowing them to loosen so much that eventually they have to be removed. Periodontal disease cannot always be cured,

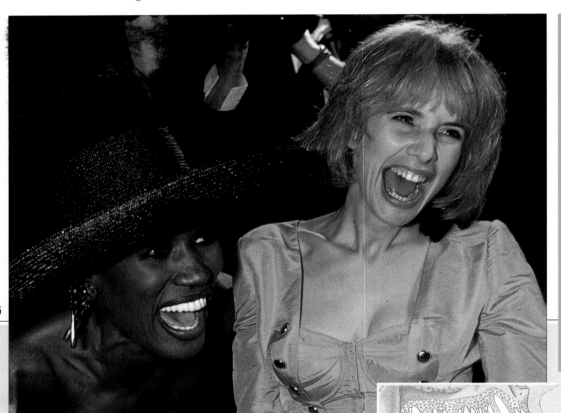

226

Smoking ruins your smile

■ Smoking damages your teeth and gums as well as your lungs. It dries the mouth, allowing plaque to build up around the teeth in the absence of anti-bacterial saliva. It also lowers the body's ability to metabolize vitamin C, essential to gum health and antibacterial activity. Heavy smokers can develop nicotine stains on the teeth which can be hard to remove with regular brushing. The combination of bacteria and stale nicotine deposits may lead to foul breath. Thorough brushing, regular checkups, and vitamin C supplements can improve the teeth of smokers, but giving up cigarettes is a healthier solution. **RR**

■ **Displaying a smile in public** is part of a day's work for well known figures like singer Grace Jones and movie star Rosanna Arquette ABOVE. But even if you are not a professional smiler, your smile is constantly on view and makes a big difference to how people respond to you. People with crooked or yellowing teeth either present an off-putting appearance, or else try to conceal their teeth by smiling only in a very restrained way, which may seem insincere.

The first step toward keeping your smile attractive is keeping your teeth healthy. Dental hygiene should concentrate on a few common trouble-spots RIGHT: between the gums and the teeth, and between the teeth themselves. These areas trap particles of food, providing a breeding-ground for the bacteria which cause tooth decay. Thorough brushing may be supplemented by the use of dental floss and dental sticks to minimize the risk of decay.

1 Third molars (wisdom teeth)
2 Second molars
3 First molars
4 Second premolars
5 First premolars
6 Canines
7 Lateral incisors
8 Central incisors

➡ Bacteria troublespots

though there are some surgical procedures for removing infected tissue which can help in severe cases. Good dental hygiene will keep gum disease under control in most cases.

Basic dental hygiene

Regular brushing twice a day – night and morning – removes food particles and bacteria. Cleaning the teeth after every meal is a good idea if at all possible; otherwise, try to eat cleansing foods such as apple or carrot – these have an acid content which will kill off some bacteria. Fluorides, which seem to retard tooth decay, are now often added to the water supply in many areas. Fluoride toothpastes and fluoride tablets are available as well. Too much fluoride can cause marks in teeth enamel, so do not supplement your diet with fluoride tablets if the water you drink is already treated.

Dental sticks, toothpicks and especially dental floss can be used to dislodge particles from between the teeth which the toothbrush cannot reach. These implements need to be used carefully or you can damage the gums and teeth and even force matter deeper below the gum line. Work the implement gently between the teeth and never push it too hard against the gums. Mouth rinses are useful if you are prone to periodontitis or bad breath, as they kill off bacteria on the flesh of the mouth and tongue as well as the teeth and gums.

Eating for healthy teeth

A good diet can also contribute to the health of your teeth. Sugar decays very rapidly in the mouth, and people with a high sugar content in their diet are more likely to get cavities. Sticky, sugary foods, soft drinks and hard candy or mints are particularly liable to contribute to tooth decay because they readily deposit a coating of sugar on the teeth.

Avoid these foods as part of your regular diet, and, when you do eat them, brush your teeth, rinse your mouth with water or eat some apple or carrot immediately afterwards.

A number of other conditions can increase the likelihood of caries and periodontitis. Inadequate levels of vitamin C can weaken gum tissue and lower the levels of anti-bacterial agents in saliva. Deficiency of folic acid (found in B complex vitamins) can also damage the gums. For some women, taking the contraceptive pill can lower resistance to tooth decay, because the pill may interfere with the body's absorption of B vitamins from food. They may be advised to take a B vitamin supplement.

Calcium and phosphorus are essential building blocks for strong teeth, and people deficient in these minerals often have bad teeth. Osteoporosis or brittle bone disease can affect the bony tooth sockets, leading to tooth loss. Sinus problems can also lead to tooth decay, as breathing through the mouth dries up the saliva that fights bacteria. Finally, some people are simply genetically predisposed to tooth decay and especially gum disease. If there is a history of tooth and gum disease in your family, let your dentist know so that preventive measures can be taken before any actual damage occurs.

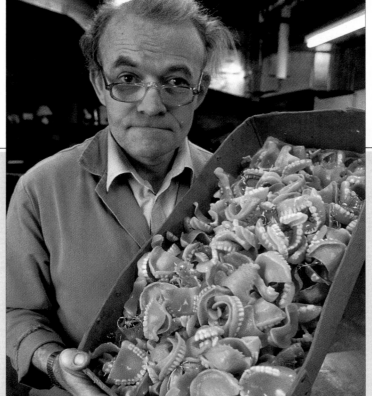

An apple a day...

■ Does an apple a day keep the dentist away? Apples are a naturally cleansing food. The rough surface of the apple scrapes away food particles, and its acid juice will dissolve and wash away particles lodged between the teeth. However, that same acid will linger in the mouth for a while and, if you brush your teeth after eating an apple, can soften the enamel, which can damage the tooth. If you have eaten an apple and want to brush your teeth, it is better to wait for half an hour or to rinse the mouth thoroughly with clear water before brushing.

▶ **Lost property**. *Losing your teeth was once a fact of adult life, even when dental care was reasonably good. People were resigned to the fact that they would not keep their natural teeth into old age, to the extent that in parts of French Canada and Scotland a set of dentures used to be a prized part of a woman's bridal trousseau. With improved hygienic practice, fluoride supplementation, and regular checkups, most people under 50 have only one or two cavities and can expect to keep their teeth throughout life.*

Reconstructing a smile

Dental surgery was once only a matter of pulling out rotten teeth. It was frequently carried out by barbers. Not until the 19th century did professional associations of dentists arise. With the increasing availability of reliable anesthetics dentists found themselves able to do more for their clients, and around the turn of the century some dentists began to pioneer cosmetic treatments to straighten teeth. Dental surgeons now have at their disposal a range of techniques for improving a smile. Crooked teeth may appear unattractive, and they have the added disadvantage of providing more crevices to trap food particles. It is now common for children to receive corrective dental, or orthodontic, treatment once their adult teeth have all appeared (usually starting between the ages of ten and fourteen). Bands of metal or plastic are fitted around the teeth and connected to each other by a wire that can be tightened. The pressure created this way pulls the teeth gradually into alignment. Improvements have made braces less obvious and more comfortable, and results are generally excellent.

Replacement of decayed or damaged teeth is another aid to health and appearance. If a damaged tooth is not completely removed, a crown or cap made of porcelain or metal can be fitted over the stump. A bridge consists of a porcelain tooth or teeth with wires to fasten over the adjoining natural teeth; it is useful if only one or a few teeth are missing. If many teeth are gone or are in poor condition, a set of false teeth or dentures may be the best solution. Fitting them securely and comfortably takes time and patience, and gum shrinkage and jawbone loss as a result of tooth removal may cause false teeth to become loose, especially if the wearer takes them out for long periods. Implants may eventually replace dentures, though the technology is still in its infancy. Some dental pioneers

have used the ceramic hydroxyapatite to create false roots planted in the gums, and in Sweden a process called osseo-integration implants small screws in the jawbone to which false teeth can later be permanently attached. Implants prevent bone loss after tooth removal, and as techniques improve implants may well replace dentures and bridges, especially in people under 60.

Cosmetic camouflage for teeth

Teeth sometimes become pitted and discolored, especially with age, illness and damaging practices like poor hygiene and smoking. Some people are simply born with weak enamel. If the teeth are not too badly damaged already, the application of a thin plastic coating, lasting three to four years, can protect vulnerable teeth from bacteria. Otherwise, dentists will try bonding or porcelain

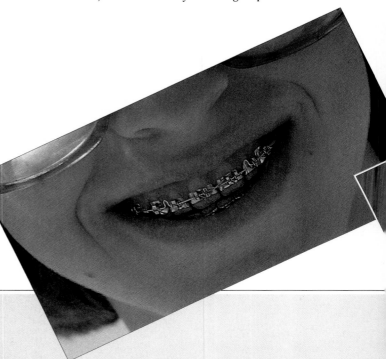

Designer smiles

■ *The right smile on the right face can make a big difference, compensating for and even camouflaging other less attractive features.*

◆ **Dental embellishment** *reaches the point of eccentricity with tattooed teeth TOP RIGHT, an idea from which most dentists would dissociate themselves.*

The phrase "long in the tooth" is inaccurate. Human adult teeth do not grow after they have come in, and can wear down considerably, ground by our eating processes. In the elderly, gum shrinkage may give the appearance of long

teeth, but in reality the teeth are much shorter than they were when they first developed. Older teeth also tend to become smooth from the friction of talking and eating. Certain cosmetic dental treatments can make teeth look younger. Dentists can mimic the effect of younger teeth by creating ridges (using laminates or bonding), and may also lengthen the teeth, using crowns or laminates. "Bulking out" the teeth in this way also gives more support to the muscle and skin between the nose and mouth, making the whole face look younger.

◆ **Adjusting natural defects** *may begin in childhood or adolescence with the application of braces TOP LEFT. Straightening the teeth is more than a matter of cosmetic surgery – crooked teeth work less efficiently and are hard to keep clean, which makes them liable to decay. Cosmetic dental surgeons can use crowns or contouring to make a round face look longer and narrower by lengthening the front teeth or a long face appear shorter by creating a horizontal line with the top teeth.*

◆ **The character** *of the patient is also important. Sporty or casual types may choose bonding – the application of a compound which strengthens the tooth enamel while still looking natural. A glamorous character might prefer the shinier effect of laminates TOP CENTER. Newscasters, actors, and models often ask for absolutely even teeth, while people who pride themselves on their individuality might ask a dentist to retain a gap or slightly protruding teeth which they feel is part of their character.*

laminate veneering. In bonding the dentist applies a liquid ceramic compound to the teeth which binds with the natural enamel, producing a stronger, whiter tooth. A laminate is better for more severely damaged teeth. This is a thin porcelain or plastic shell bonded to the tooth, which can also be structured to improve the shape of the teeth.

Bleaching removes plaque and improves tooth appearance. The dentist applies a special peroxide solution over a series of visits. A new procedure involves using a clear plastic mold over each tooth which is regularly filled with a mild bleach; this is much faster and can be done by the patient under medical supervision. Bleaching can be very successful at removing nicotine stains or "lifting" a naturally dark tooth color.

As the search for the perfect smile intensifies, dentists develop new techniques, and improve on old ones. Tooth filing is in fact a very old custom; some African peoples still regularly file their teeth into points, which they think very attractive. Dentists in the industrialized world can contour teeth into more desirable shapes using the same sort of methods. Dr Jeff Golub, clinical assistant professor at New York University, has found that contouring the teeth so that they become shorter towards the back of the mouth makes the teeth themselves "smile," mimicking the curve of the lower lip and producing a permanent smiling effect.

Many people, including some dentists, balk at the very idea of cosmetic surgery. After all, teeth are important functioning structures, helping us to talk and eat, and the first consideration has to be supporting and strengthening them for these tasks. But the smile is also a major focus of our social interaction. The better it looks and the prouder we are of it, the more it will work in our favor. **RR**

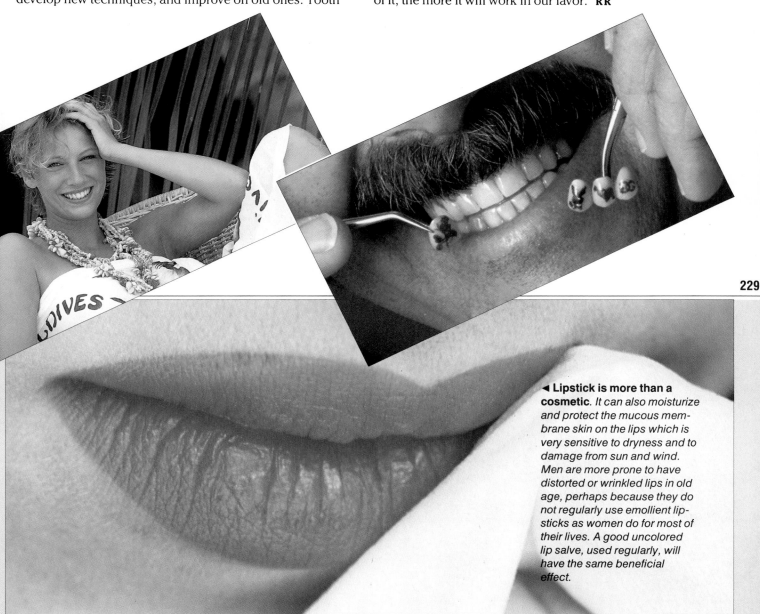

◄ **Lipstick is more than a cosmetic.** *It can also moisturize and protect the mucous membrane skin on the lips which is very sensitive to dryness and to damage from sun and wind. Men are more prone to have distorted or wrinkled lips in old age, perhaps because they do not regularly use emollient lipsticks as women do for most of their lives. A good uncolored lip salve, used regularly, will have the same beneficial effect.*

31

Fragrance and Aromatherapy

*For thousands of years, the power of fragrance
has been used to heal, and to enchant the senses*
● *Do we really respond physically to the power
of scent, or is the effect mostly psychological?*
● *Aromatherapy combines both.*

AS INFANTS, it is our sense of smell that provides us with most of the information we need about the world, since our eyes cannot focus and sounds do not make sense. As adults, vision and hearing are the senses that may come to mind as being most important in social interaction but our sense of smell is an equally powerful channel of communication. Researchers have estimated that humans are capable of distinguishing more than 5,000 different odors but they often go unnoticed unless they are particularly strong or unpleasant. Nevertheless, odors that may not be consciously perceived seem to have an impact on our physical functioning, sexuality and attraction, our identification of others and our state of mind.

A personal aroma

We each have a personal scent which is unique to us. It can even play a part in helping us to identify others. In one study, volunteers were asked to refrain from using deodorants and perfumes for a week and then to come into the laboratory for recognition tests. Researchers found that, in general, people were able to identify their own clothing and distinguish between the clothing of male and female strangers purely on the basis of odor. Half of the volunteers could correctly identify a partner's clothing, and parents could usually pick out their children's.

Another study looked at the relationship between odor and physical functioning in a group of women undergraduates at the University of Chicago over the course of two semesters. Researchers established a tendency for the menstrual cycles of friends and roommates to move from an average of 8.5 days apart to an average of less than 5 days apart. A follow-up study in San Francisco tried to discover if odor was the synchronizing factor. By placing the odor of

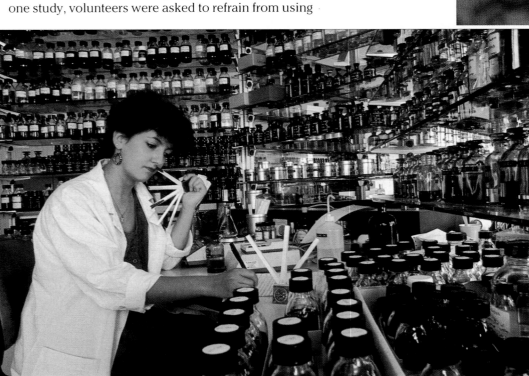

▲ **Artist and scientist**. *Master perfumers are called noses because their sense of smell is so crucial to their profession. In addition to being trained* chemists, *they are also artists with highly developed natural talent. Perfumery began in ancient Egyptian civilization with the use of flowers and* plants *for cosmetic and medicinal purposes. The modern industry developed in France in the 1700s, and France remains the international center*.

■ **Flowers and fragrance**. *Flowers have been used for three thousand years in the production of perfumes and essences. We now have floral scents (a single fragrance such as lily of the valley), bouquets (a combination of several flowers' essences) and sweet scents (usually based on jasmine, tuberosis and gardenia). Layer-*

A wardrobe of fragrances

■ There was a time when a woman's perfume was her signature. She would be faithful to the same scent all her life; it was a part of getting dressed – she would never go out without it.

Now fragrance is less formal, a woman feels freer to choose a scent that suits her mood. She pleases herself rather than using perfume to attract a man, and as her roles have multiplied so have her fragrances.

Some women use the same perfume all the time; others have a selection of scents to choose from to suit the situation or mood; yet others "layer" their scents, wearing more than one at a time.

Your choice of fragrance should vary to suit different situations and show different sides of your character. A change of scent refreshes you and is good for you.

one subject who had a regular 28-day cycle and did not use perfume or deodorant on the upper lips of female volunteers three times a week for four months, the researchers succeeded in moving the cycles of the volunteers from an average of 9.3 days apart to 3.4 days from the cycle of the subject with the regular cycle. Four of the women synchronized to within a day and a control group who had alcohol placed on their lips instead did not change at all.

Sexual attractiveness is strongly affected by some natural scents. Research suggests that the presence of the hormone androstenol may have significant effects on our perceptions of others. In controlled studies, ratings of female sexual attractiveness and male friendliness increased in the presence of androstenol. And yet, each year in the United States, men and women spend millions of dollars on soaps,

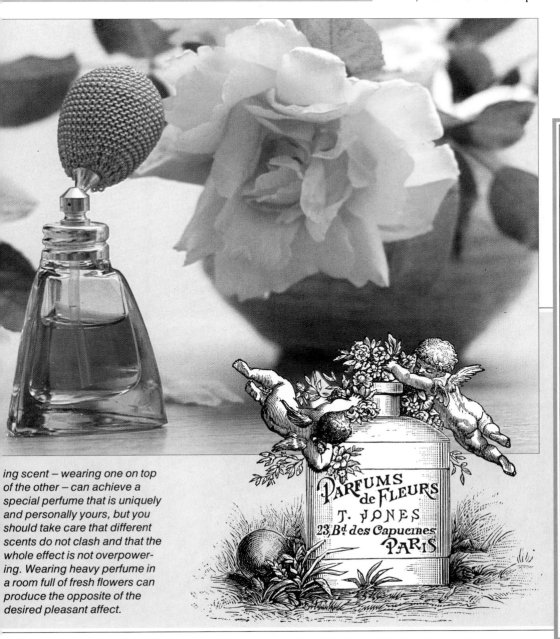

ing scent – wearing one on top of the other – can achieve a special perfume that is uniquely and personally yours, but you should take care that different scents do not clash and that the whole effect is not overpowering. Wearing heavy perfume in a room full of fresh flowers can produce the opposite of the desired pleasant affect.

Osmotherapy

■ Osmotherapy is purely connected with the sense of smell. The term refers to the beneficial effects of inhaling fragrance on an emotionally disturbed state and was coined by the Olfaction Research Group at Warwick University in England.

The Warwick group has demonstrated that an odor can be paired with an emotional state, re-evoking it when the same odor is experienced later. They are exploring the hypothesis that fragrance can produce a measurable change in relaxation levels in patients suffering from anxiety-related disorders.

Osmotherapy has been used as part of enhanced relaxation therapy where patients listen to relaxing sounds through headphones in a darkened room: first, a piece of electronic music composed for the film of the Apollo space missions to convey weightlessness, then the sound of the sea accompanied by a stream of sea fragrance. It is believed that the fragrance, which is the most novel feature of the therapy, makes a powerful contribution.

deodorants, perfumes and mouth washes. At the same time we seem to show particular enthusiasm about products which promise to make us smell "natural and sexy."

The power of familiar smells

Each of us makes strong associations between particular odors and places or events – the smell of fresh-cut grass, a hotdog eaten in a ballpark, a hospital corridor or a bakery early in the morning may all bring back memories with startling clarity and evoke strong emotional responses. There are even millions of dollars spent on "odor delivery systems" that can fill a room with the odor of fresh popcorn, roasted coffee or burning cedar in order to create pleasant, relaxing or nostalgic moods.

Researchers currently investigating the possibility that odors can affect our moods for its potential health benefits, are pursuing the idea that stress-related disorders such as hypertension, anxiety, phobias and irritability may respond to aromatherapy. In a recent study, a researcher exposed a group of people to various fragrances and then had them answer questions designed to induce stress. Those volunteers who had been exposed to the fragrances showed less stress than those who had not. **MK DC**

Fragrant influences

Stress seems to be an inescapable aspect of the fast pace of life in today's society, and the need to relax is more important than ever before. Fragrance may play a central role in reducing stress and lifting your mood.

Is there any concrete evidence for this? In one study a group of multiply handicapped and severely retarded children with a mental age of less than one year were given fruit-scented soaps and lip balms to play with. Whereas normally these children were almost incapable of a response of any kind, they began to smile, make eye contact and grasp objects. The fruit fragrance appeared to be the crucial component that awakened their senses and, at the same time, provided an enjoyable learning experience.

Just as the children were attracted to and benefited from the fruit scents, so we as adults can look for fragrances that appeal to our senses, uplift our moods and make us feel good.

Fragrant attraction

If scents can affect the way we feel about ourselves, what sort of effect do they have on the image we project and on how attractive we are to other people? One study showed that fragrance in a skin care product such as hand cream favorably influences perceptions of both the product and the personality of the user. Another study which looked at the use of perfumes and colognes found that wearing a pleasant fragrance increased the attractiveness of the person wearing it in an informal dress situation, but had the opposite effect in a formal dress situation.

◄ **The well-dressed man never leaves home without it.** *Men's fragrance has become as personal – and as commercially lucrative – as women's. Scents vary from rich musks to fresh crisp fragrances associated with the outdoor or sportsman's life, and the subtle sophistication of some of the classic colognes. Men must be particularly careful to adapt their choice of fragrance to the occasion. A heavy musk worn to a business meeting may create the wrong impression, but would be perfectly appropriate for a romantic evening.*

Male interviewers rate female applicants lower when they wear scent, but female interviewers do the opposite. Fragrance used by females has, however, been shown to be popular among teenagers. From a range of cosmetics, boys rated perfume the most attractive item used by the girls in their age group, particularly when used at night.

To maximize the potential beneficial effects of a fragranced product, it is necessary to use an amount of the product that is appropriate to the situation and that you feel comfortable with in that particular context. For example, the sort of cologne that might be appropriate for a man to wear on a romantic dinner date might not be the right one for him to wear to work. The choice of cologne or fragrance you use can help to put you in the right frame of mind to meet the demands of the situation you are in. Also worth considering is the environment around you – will your perfume be overpowering in a confined space?

Researchers have found that different perfumes each convey their own mood or image for a specific situation, moods including feminine and romantic, cheerful and extroverted, refined and delicate. This research has also established that consumers tend to describe them in terms of different moods (cheerful), the situation they might be suitable for (daytime or nighttime) and personality types (lively, subdued).

This information, together with the likes and dislikes of the consumer, can be relayed back to the fragrance industry and used to find marketing concepts to develop new products that will be appropriate for different places, situations or moods and perhaps even prove that a certain kind of mood really can be projected by a particular fragrance. **JAG**

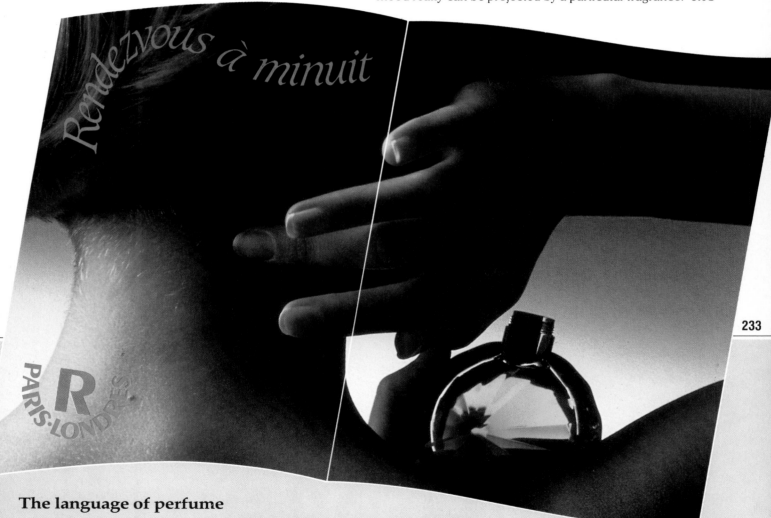

The language of perfume

■ The people who market perfume tend to classify it as either romantic or sexy. The marketing of scents with overtly sexual names, such as Passion and Obsession, relies on shock value, often employing scenes of lovemaking, nude or partially clad models. Making the connection between perfume and sexuality is an effective way of reaching into our secret fantasy lives and also underlining the possibility that scent may actually have an erotic effect, stimulating that part of the brain that generates sensations of excitement and pleasure.

Marketing of other perfumes, such as florals or contemporary scents, still tends to lean heavily toward portraying scenes of romantic excitement, such as candlelit dinners or masquerade balls.

The older, more classic scents like Shalimar, Joy and Miss Dior are more subtle and tend to be fresher. The great classics reflect the feeling that the traditional, durable things in life may also be the best – real leather, antique furniture and Chanel No 5, the 1921 original.

Aromatherapy

■ Fragrance works directly on the limbic system, the part of the brain most closely bound up with emotion and memory. The sensation of a smell reaches the brain more quickly than a sensation of pain. Scent can also bring back vivid memories. It may not always recreate a scene from the past, but it can revive the emotion you felt when you encountered the scent before.

This is one of the ways in which fragrance can create a sense of well-being. Another way is by appealing directly to our emotions, simply by smelling attractive. When everything seems to be going wrong, the right scent may bring contentment, and restore a positive attitude to life.

Aromatherapy is a treatment that attempts to harness these benefits of fragrances. It is also concerned with other beneficial effects of the fragrant oils – called essences – that it employs.

Essential oils

One aspect of aromatherapy is "essential oil therapy" or "plant essence therapy." All essential oils come from plants and are the organic substances that give plants their scent. They may be extracted from leaves, flowers, bark, fruit, herbs, spices and resins by distillation. Once captured, the substance is known as an essential oil but in this form it is highly

▶ **Jasmine blossoms** *provide what is sometimes considered to be the best of the flower oils. The blooms are often picked at night when the fragrance is at its most powerful, and the process of distillation – a delicate one requiring great skill – makes jasmine oil one of the most expensive essences. With its exotic perfume it makes a luxurious massage oil. It is also used to alleviate depression and is reputed to have aphrodisiac qualities.*

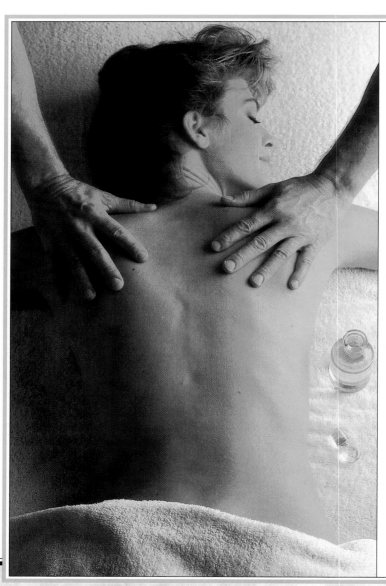

Using essential oils

■ Aromatherapy can be used in a variety of different ways, imparting a special quality to some of the everyday things we do to improve our health, appearance and well-being.

● **Massage**. Essential oils should never be applied neat to the skin and must be suspended in a "carrier" oil such as almond or avocado.

● **In the bath**. Sprinkle a few drops into the water before getting in. For babies and young children, dilute the essence in a carrier oil first.

● **Inhalations**. Essential oils are very good for colds and flu. A few drops added to a bowl of steaming water will clear a blocked-up nose; sprinkled on your pillow, they will help you sleep.

● **Compresses**. Essential oils can be used to make hot or cold compresses. Add a few drops to either very hot or ice-cold water. A piece of cotton laid on the surface will soak up the oils and should be wrung out and applied to the area requiring treatment.

● **Room fresheners**. Essential oils are perfect for this because they evaporate easily and many are antiseptic. Add a few drops to a bowl of water placed on a

source of heat such as a radiator.

● **Perfumes**. Oils may be used individually or in combination to make your own personal fragrances.

Essential oils are usually too strong to use in cooking, but peppermint and aniseed make good flavorings. Rosemary oil and basil may be diluted in vinegar and used in salads.

■ **Essential oils** are highly concentrated and should never be taken internally or applied directly to the skin, but always diluted in water or in natural oil. Here is a selection of oils often used for medicinal and cosmetic purposes.

Basil. Thought to be a nerve tonic that is also refreshing to the skin and can help you sleep.

Bergamot. Refreshing and uplifting, bergamot is thought to have the power to relieve depression and anxiety.

Camomile. The soothing, calming properties of camomile make it an excellent oil for skin problems. It may also have a sedative effect on the nervous system.

Eucalyptus. Effective as an inhalant for colds and flu and as a chest rub, it contains a power

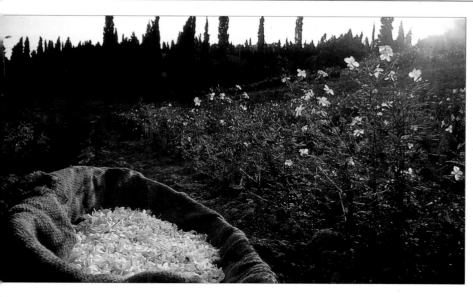

concentrated and should not be applied neat to the skin. In massage, for example, a few drops of essential oil would be suspended in a carrier oil such as avocado or nut oil.

The skills of using essential oils for the skin and for minor ailments have been taught in India and other countries for hundreds of years but it is only in comparatively recent years that these treatments have become available in the West.

The term "aromatherapy," which first appeared in the 1920s, means far more than simply inhaling vapors. It is the art of harnessing the benefits of essential oils extracted from aromatic plants to improve and enhance health and beauty. However, it is probably our sense of smell, linked so strongly with emotion, that is the most important factor in our appreciation of aromatherapy.

There are many ways in which essential oils can be used: a few drops on a tissue may be inhaled to alleviate the symptoms of a cold; an aromatic bath can be created by adding a few drops to the water; essences may be added to vegetable oils and massaged into the skin; or the oils can simply be used as perfume.

Because of their affinity with sebum, the body's own natural oil, it is believed that essential oils can enter the body through the skin's sebaceous glands and hair follicles and enter the bloodstream. As you breathe in the aroma, your lungs also ingest particles of oil.

Plant power

You can try some simple aromatherapy techniques on yourself. Revive aching feet after a shopping trip by soaking them in a bowl of water into which you have sprinkled six drops of peppermint oil, and follow this with a gentle foot massage. Inhaling the vapors of lavender oil from a bowl of steaming water may alleviate the symptoms of colds and flu. Soak away tension and fatigue at the end of the day in a relaxing geranium or ylang-ylang bath. In the morning, a few drops of rosemary or clary sage in your bath may refresh you and help you face the day. **RR**

235

ful antiseptic and is an excellent way of freshening the room during illness.

Geranium. Also known as rose geranium, it is believed to stimulate the lymphatic system and is good for most skin types.

Lavender. Of all the oils, this is the most versatile and the only one that may be used directly on the skin. It is particularly effective in relieving insect bites and burns. A lavender bath will relax and refresh you; a massage with lavender oil will ease muscular and rheumatic aches.

Melissa. Also known as lemon balm, this oil is particularly effective for allergies and acts as a gentle tonic.

Neroli. With its beautiful fragrance and powerful effect on stress, neroli makes the perfect relaxing bath oil.

Peppermint. A very important and versatile oil, it has powerful digestive and antiseptic properties. Added to a bowl of water it makes a refreshing footbath and, mixed with rosemary and juniper, an invigorating bath.

Pine. A good inhalant for colds, bronchitis and flu. It is powerfully antiseptic and makes a stimulating bath, particularly for relieving muscular aches.

Rosemary. Good for the hair and scalp, this stimulating oil is also helpful for headaches and depression. A few drops on the pillow at night will help to ease the symptoms of a cold.

Sage. The relaxing properties of sage make it ideal for the bath. Also good for mouth and throat infections, it is an effective ingredient in gargles and mouthwashes.

Sandalwood. A very mild oil, excellent for all types of skin, it also makes an exotic and lasting perfume and is often used as a fixative for other oils.

Thyme. A good room freshener, it is also very useful for sore throats and bad breath. As an inhalant, it will bring relief to a blocked nose, and it will also make a stimulating bath oil.

Ylang-ylang. With its heavy and exotic perfume, this oil may have a sedative effect. Equally soothing to the skin, it makes a sensuous massage oil.

Sage

Lavender

Thyme

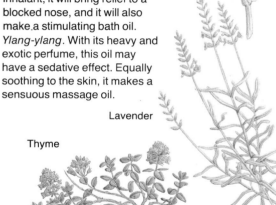

32

Professional Beautycare

What can professional treatments do for us that we cannot do for ourselves? ● *Many people seek them when poor self-image leads them to feel unattractive* ● *The physical benefits are often complemented by a psychological boost.*

MOST BEAUTY treatments can be carried out at home, using readily available tools and easily purchased substances. Why waste money on professional treatment? On a day to day basis, it is certainly easier and quicker to do things for yourself. However, professional help can make a huge difference for certain treatments or on particular occasions. For weddings, important interviews or big parties – when you want something other than your normal look – you may need someone to cut or put up your hair, to help you choose your clothes or to do a really good makeup.

In addition to the wide range of beauty treatments available in salons, a number of techniques have been developed by medical science, that can help to improve and rejuvenate the appearance of your face or body. These treatments are carried out by dermatologists or plastic surgeons. Some of the more commonly used treatments for different areas of the body as well as for the face are set out here. In addition to physical alteration, the treatments usually have a psychological component. Poor self-image or a general feeling of being unattractive are often what prompt people to seek out treatment in the first place. In turn, many of the benefits of the treatments are psychological and social – not just looking better but feeling better about yourself too.

Getting beautifully away from it all

Spas and health farms offer a period of complete relaxation combined with a series of professional health and beauty treatments. Usually situated in the country (though more and more are cropping up in large city hotels), they will have a range of programs from one day to a week, and will tailor a course of treatments to your needs and desires.

American style spas tend to concentrate on physical fitness and detoxification, giving the chance to build up good, new habits of exercise and eating. The gym will be well-equipped and many different sports may be taught. European style spas lay more stress on passive beauty and health treatments such as mud baths, massage and saunas. More and more health farms are beginning to combine these two aspects of health and beauty care, and most establishments now tend to offer a comprehensive range of activities to suit everyone.

Diet remains an important part of spa life, but spas are not the "fat farms" they used to be. Very few offer or even allow starvation diets; the emphasis is on learning healthy eating habits and most have both a diet and a nondiet dining room to cater for those who are trying to lose weight and those who may be simply trying to wean themselves from a diet that consists mainly of junk food.

Spas have become a popular form of vacation, particularly for those leading busy and stressful lives. They offer the chance to wind down, give the body a rest from unhealthy lifestyles, and break bad habits. As well as developing exercise programs, many spas run treatment courses for people wanting to stop smoking. The key word for spas today is "detoxification" – freeing the body and mind of harmful processes and providing new strategies for living in a stressful world.

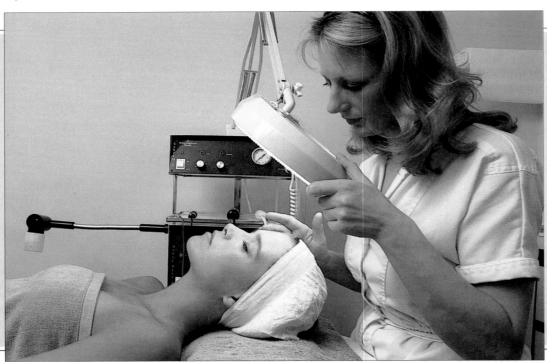

◄ **A professional assessment** is a sound starting point for a program to improve your looks. It is true that for most people beauty treatment happens at their own dressing table with commercially available products – but with the help of an expert you can ensure that your treatment is therapeutic rather than just cosmetic. A beautician can advise you on such matters as your skin and hair type and which beauty products are best suited to you. Few of us can afford professional treatment every week, but one course of professional treatment can change your entire outlook on beauty care and will help you to establish new and beneficial habits.

Hydrotherapy — water treatments

Ever since the first person experienced the pleasure of a hot spring, relaxing in water has been a favorite form of physical and mental therapy. Some researchers theorize that the feelings of peace and well-being that people normally experience in water are due to subconscious memories of floating in the womb or to an ancestral attachment to our origins in the sea. In any case, nothing soothes the spirit and refreshes the body like a long hot bath or shower, and most hydrotherapies are rather more elaborate versions of

the treatments that we give ourselves at home every day.

The jacuzzi has become a fixture of gyms and health clubs as well as spas, and you can even purchase jacuzzi attachments for your bath at home. Warm water is circulated rapidly around the pool or bath with an admixture of air bubbles, massaging the body. Still-water bathing in mineral springs or sequences of cool, warm and hot pools offers the same relaxation, skin stimulation and muscular relief. In many spas, marine algae, peat or mud are added to baths, usually to improve skin condition.

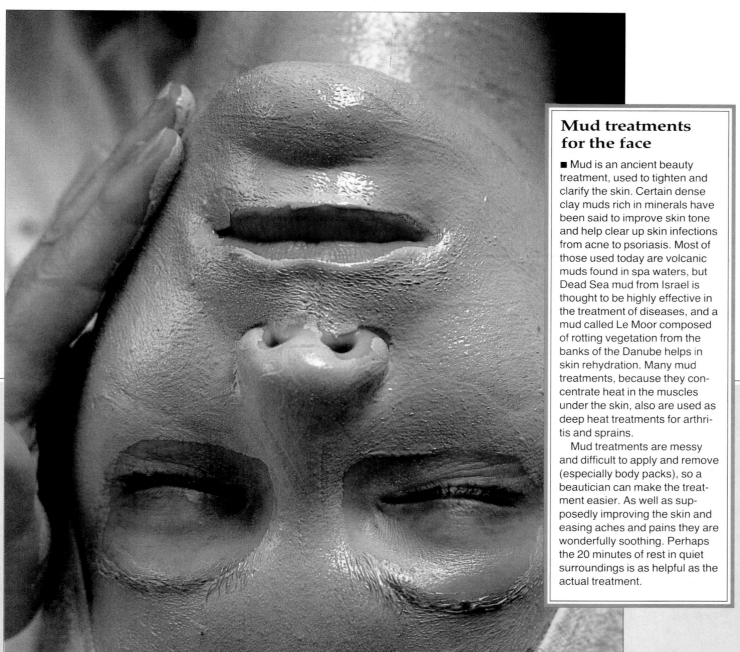

Mud treatments for the face

■ Mud is an ancient beauty treatment, used to tighten and clarify the skin. Certain dense clay muds rich in minerals have been said to improve skin tone and help clear up skin infections from acne to psoriasis. Most of those used today are volcanic muds found in spa waters, but Dead Sea mud from Israel is thought to be highly effective in the treatment of diseases, and a mud called Le Moor composed of rotting vegetation from the banks of the Danube helps in skin rehydration. Many mud treatments, because they concentrate heat in the muscles under the skin, also are used as deep heat treatments for arthritis and sprains.

Mud treatments are messy and difficult to apply and remove (especially body packs), so a beautician can make the treatment easier. As well as supposedly improving the skin and easing aches and pains they are wonderfully soothing. Perhaps the 20 minutes of rest in quiet surroundings is as helpful as the actual treatment.

237

French spas offer a water massage treatment, consisting of alternate jets of cold and warm water which both soothe and stimulate skin and muscles. American spas too are beginning to explore water massage and many luxury bathrooms are fitted with shower heads which deliver a strong pulsating beat of water.

Hydrotherapy is good for the skin and muscles alike. Exercise in water takes the weight off damaged limbs while still providing good strengthening exercise for the muscles. Elderly people, pregnant women or anyone recovering from injury will find that taking exercise in water is particularly beneficial.

Some mineral waters appear to have an impressive record of results in improving skin complaints and speeding recovery from muscular injury. Even racehorses are given water therapy now, which allows them to use an injured leg without putting any weight on it. Even if you are not seeking a cure for a specific problem, water treatments can be extremely relaxing and enjoyable.

Heat treatments

Treatments using heat (dry or damp) have been a popular form of beauty and health therapy since the Romans invented their elaborate bathing complexes. Many are available at beauty salons, spas and health clubs. The sauna and the Turkish bath are probably the best known. The sauna is a Scandinavian invention, and consists of a room or room-sized cabinet heated to produce a hot, dry atmosphere. Users sit in it naked or draped only in a towel until they begin to sweat; the Finnish form includes a massage with birch twigs, now generally simulated by a good stiff brush. A sauna cleanses the skin, bringing up dirt and sebum from the depths of the skin, and soothes aching limbs – that is why it is so popular in gyms.

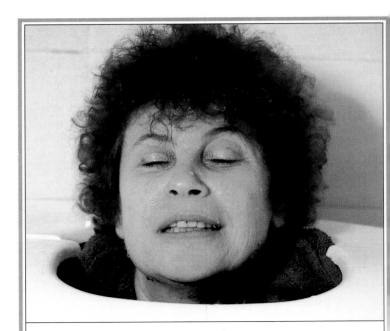

Turkish baths and heat wraps

■ Turkish baths or steam cabinets use damp heat. A room or cabinet (where you sit with only your head protruding) is filled with circulating steam. Like the sauna, it deepcleanses the skin, and eases painful joints and muscles. Turkish baths and cabinets are generally only found at spas now, though some older cities still have municipal Turkish baths. Spas and beauty salons sometimes offer various forms of heat wrapping, in which the body is covered in essential oils or marine gels and wrapped in an insulated or electrically heated cover. Heat wrapping is supposed to be good for eliminating cellulite, improving circulation, and losing weight, though most of the weight you lose is water (through sweating) and the inches are quickly regained. Another drawback is that many people find wrapping claustrophobic and boring.

Removing hair with wax

■ The ancient Egyptians were the first people to use strips of wax to remove unwanted hair from the body as part of a cosmetic treatment.

Today it is still a preferred method of eliminating body hair from the legs and bikini line. The development of cold wax applications in the late 1970s revolutionized home waxing, but more efficient and comfortable waxing takes place in the salon, where warm wax is usually used. The beautician coats an area of hair with melted beeswax, covers it with a piece of felt which adheres to the wax, and removes hair, wax and felt in

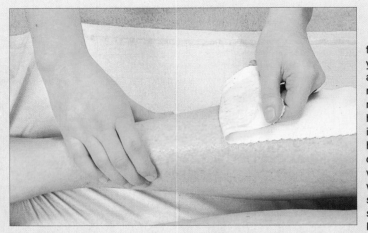

one swift movement. Whole leg treatments usually take about half an hour, a job that might take an hour to do by yourself at home.

■ **Other wax treatments**. Ordinary low-melting-point paraffin wax is an excellent way to cleanse, soften and moisturize your skin. You can buy the wax from a pharmacist and treat yourself at home, but melting and applying the wax can be messy and hard to do, so it is more relaxing and rewarding to have it done by a beautician. It is normally used to treat the hands or feet, but some salons offer full-body wax baths. The wax melts at a comfortably warm temperature, and is spread evenly with a wooden spatula. The beautician will then leave the wax to cool for fifteen or twenty minutes. It peels off easily without pulling at hairs. The hot wax draws out embedded skin impurities and moisturizes the skin.

Breast treatments – French style

Breast treatments are common in France, where women treat the skin of the breasts as carefully as the skin of the face. No such treatment is able to do anything about sagging breasts or breast size – this is a result of the fat and muscle composition of the bust – but they can improve the tone and tightness of the skin which is rather delicate and thin.

Bust treatments are usually offered as a course of four to six sessions once a year or so. The beauty therapist massages the breasts with a special milk or serum, often specifically intended for dry or oily skin. The process is designed to strengthen, firm, and tighten breast skin. A cold bust tonic finishes the treatments; alternatively, the beautician will hold cups over each breast which douse them with alternative bursts of cold and warm water. French women swear by these treatments, although medical experts are doubtful if they produce any real effects. Most women do agree, however, that they are relaxing and refreshing.

Hair treatments

Many people have coloring and perming done in a hair salon, especially if they are planning anything elaborate. Home perms and colorants are fairly safe to use but inexperienced handling can lead to a less than satisfactory effect. Salon perms and color treatments, on the other hand, have a high satisfaction rate.

Few people are aware of the many other special treatments hair salons now offer. Next time you go to have your hair cut, take a good look at your salon's price list. There will probably be a range of treatments, including deep moisturizing, anti-dandruff and itchy scalp applications and head massage. Especially in midwinter when the hair and scalp are in delicate condition, a special salon treatment can make a great deal of difference to the state of your hair.

Hairdressers are usually eager and willing to tell you all about these treatments and how they can help you – they do not have to be expensive.

Minor surgery for cosmetic reasons

Among the medical treatments for the face or body, one of the least drastic is for broken capillaries or spider veins. These are small blue or purple veins that appear on the legs, for example. They do not protrude like varicose veins but they may make you embarrassed to show your legs uncovered. This is a common complaint in women and can even cause psychological distress, but it can be treated quite simply by injecting a solution into the blood vessels. Initially this causes some irritation and swelling, but ultimately it causes the vessels to disappear gradually over a 3-6 week period.

Many people investigate minor surgery as a means of getting rid of small blemishes on their skin. Before the removal of warts, moles or skin tags from the face or body, you will need to have a consultation with your doctor or a dermatologist. Although often quite small in size, blemishes of this kind can cause self-consciousness, embarrassment and lack of confidence. A medical consultation will establish whether they may be safely treated, and effective and hygienic removal can then be undertaken with fairly minimal discomfort.

Small skin tags (which are usually benign and may be numerous) are cauterized (a simple surgical procedure which destroys tissue) for which a local anesthetic is not necessarily required. Larger raised moles, often brownish or pink in color, and protruding from the surface, are usually removed under local anesthetic. The procedure does leave a scar, of course, but for moles on the face, where a "good cosmetic job" is of particular concern, a range of techniques

239

Removing hair by electrolysis

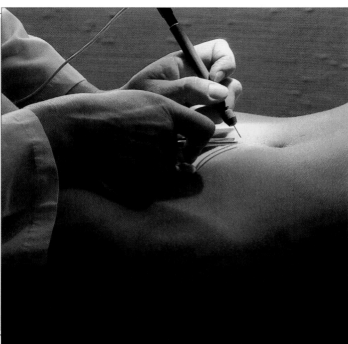

■ The only permanent method of removing body hair is electrolysis. A fine needle is inserted along the hair shaft and the follicle is treated either with a galvanic chemical reaction or, more commonly, an electrical current which deadens it. The hair may grow again, but more finely, and after several treatments the follicle will eventually die. Electrolysis is slow, can be painful, and really must be done in a salon. Inserting the needle in the wrong way can lead to scarring, and inadequately sterilized needles can cause infections, so avoid home electrolysis kits and only go to an

accredited practitioner. It is not a suitable form of general hair removal, and is commonly used only for small areas of superfluous or excessive hair growth.

■ **Most people know** that electrolysis uses electrical currents to permanently remove unwanted hair; but the same process is also used to treat thread veins, especially on the face and legs. Thread veins or broken veins are small surface skin capillaries that have burst, leaving a red blotch or line on the skin. Electrolysis dries up the blood deposit and seals the capillary, leaving no scar.

have been developed and each should be considered according to the size, shape and location of the mole and the types of scar they might leave.

For example, a raised mole on the eyebrow might be removed by cutting an ellipse of skin around the mole, leaving an elongated scar which might blend fairly easily with the eyebrow line. The alternative procedure (straight excision across the base of the growth) could leave a round pockmark-shaped scar possibly with a slight indentation, which might be more noticeable in that region of the face. However, scars on the face do heal more readily than scars on the body.

Finally, it should be remembered that, although it may seem quick and easy, removal of blemishes is a surgical procedure and the body needs to adjust to it. You will need appropriate and sensible care for a few days after surgery.

Skin resurfacing

If the facial skin is badly damaged (by aging or too much sun) or if it is disfigured, there are medical techniques for resurfacing the damaged area. This normally affects the epidermis, and selected parts of the dermis (see *Ch 25*). Some involve the use of chemicals to kill superficial layers of the skin producing a smoother look. This procedure is particularly effective for the fine lines and wrinkles around the eyes and mouth. Peels can also be used to remove brown age spots on the skin, or dark areas under the eyes. Dermabrasion (planing the skin by mechanical means using motorized wire brushes and other mechanisms) is

used for controlled removal of the upper layers of skin that may have been damaged by aging, photo-aging (see *Ch 25*), or perhaps a skin disease such as acne. Dermabrasion requires use of a local anesthetic.

The skin will take on a red appearance for some 7-10 days after surgery whilst the dermis regenerates, and regrowth of the epithelial tissue occurs. Ultimately the procedure produces a younger, smoother and firmer skin.

Tissue replacement techniques

There are also techniques for replacing tissue in damaged areas, that may have been lost through disease, injury or aging. Injectable collagen can be used for deeper frown

Eyebrow and eyelash tinting

■ Changing the look or shape of your eyes need not involve surgery. People who change their hair color often have their brows done to match; others have mismatched hair and brow color naturally, or very fair brows that would probably look better with a darker tint.

Tinting the eyelashes makes them look darker, longer and thicker, doing away with the need for mascara. It is particularly suitable for people who play sports, those with sensitive eyes, and for contact lens wearers, who find that mascara fibers can irritate their eyes.

Professionals are trained to apply the dye so that the chem-

icals do not endanger your eyes. They apply vaseline around the eye area, and paint on the dye (usually black, brown, or blue is available) with a small wand or cotton bud.

They can get much closer to the root with the dye than you could if you were applying it yourself, and a skilled person can even outline the eye with dye like an eyeliner. It takes five or ten minutes resting with cotton pads over the eyes for the dye to set, and lasts about six weeks (until the lashes begin to drop out naturally or pale roots show). The results are often subtle but can be very attractive.

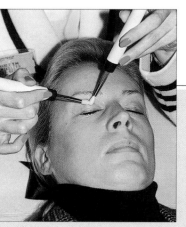

▲ **High-tech beauty treatment.** *This electronic technique supposedly eliminates wrinkles to provide a more youthful appearance. The treatment has none of the hazards of surgery, and claims to be far more effective than cosmetic creams – hence the high prices which people have been prepared to pay. A weak electric current is applied to the skin, causing a* pleasant sensation with no pain involved, and the electrical stimulation improves the tone of the skin and muscles. The treatment need not be confined to the face – it works equally well on all regions of the body.

▶ **For a permanent eyeliner effect,** *a beautician applies a tattooed line to a client's eyelids – this will have the same effect as makeup without the need to apply it every morning, and without the problems of it becoming smudged during the course of the day.*

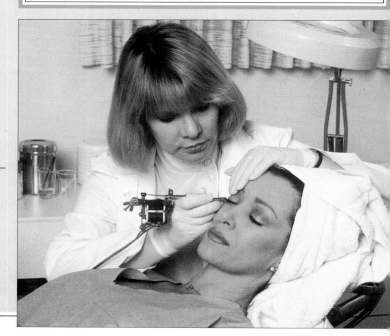

lines on the forehead, smile lines, folds around the nose and mouth or depressed corners of the mouth. It is also used to treat fine lines around the lips (often accentuated in women when lipstick "bleeds" into them) or to change the shape of the lips – to make them fuller, for example. Collagen implants can also be used to treat scars and the pockmarks left by acne, but the implants seem to work best for vertical forehead frown lines or vertical lines between the eyebrows, and less well on the skin around the eyes.

Collagen is originally taken from cattle, then purified and processed with water and an anesthetic, to produce a solution that can be injected easily under the skin. Anyone beginning collagen implant therapy should be screened for allergic reactions. In the screening process a small amount of collagen is injected into the skin of the forearm and the area is evaluated after about a month. A positive allergic reaction would be redness, swelling or itching. Even when treatment is successful, the injections need to be repeated to maintain an acceptable result.

Much media attention has been given to the use of silicone to enlarge or restructure areas of the face or body. Available as a fluid or semi-solid gel, it may be used for breast enlargement, or for the treatment of hemiatrophy where one side of the face is sunken and needs rebuilding. Fluid silicone is injected in very small amounts, to augment the soft tissue. As with collagen, allergies may occur.

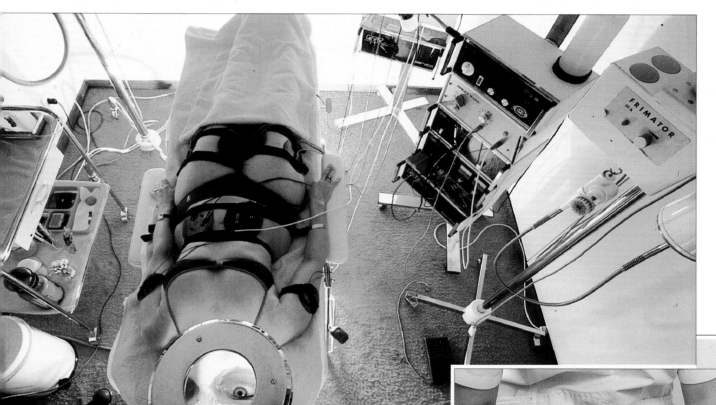

■ **The war on fat**. *Vacuum suction RIGHT is intended to help eliminate flabby subcutaneous fat. The machine is like a vacuum cleaner with soft cups attached to the nozzle. The cup is run around the area of fat to be treated then guided toward the nearest lymphatic glands and the suction is released. This treatment is supposed to encourage the drainage of fat "toxins" through the lymphatic system. In fact the massage element may be what produces results, along with the diet and exercise that are usually recommended to accompany the treatment. Slendertone treatment ABOVE comprises a system of pads which convey gentle electric shocks to the musles, supposedly exercising them while you lie still. Specialists are doubtful about the value of this treatment, and it can be uncomfortable and boring.*

Cosmetic plastic surgery

Attitudes to cosmetic plastic surgery are changing rapidly. A few decades ago it used to be practiced quietly and was not entirely acceptable to academic surgeons. In the main, it was the province of the rich, the neurotic, the vain and those who wanted to change their identity. Now it is more readily available for anyone who feels a real need to improve any particular aspect of their face or body. Increasingly, cosmetic surgery is an accepted, respectable and thriving medical concern. This is particularly true in the United States, and for men as well as women (although women are still more likely to have plastic surgery).

Among the most common cosmetic operations are the face-lift (including incision under the chin to remove excess fat), altering the upper and lower eye lids (blepharoplasty) and nose reconstruction (rhinoplasty). Other fairly common procedures are chin implant (mentoplasty) for a receding chin, jaw reconstruction, forehead-lift, ear pinning (for protruding ears), augmentation, reconstruction or reduction of the breasts (mammoplasty), buttock lift, thigh lift, abdominal lift and arm lift. There are also several redraping techniques to remove the excess skin and sagging that can come with aging, and sometimes to remove underlying fat as well by liposuction (a technique using a machine to suck out fat from any particular area).

People considering these options often forget that plastic surgery is not just a cosmetic treatment; it is surgery and should be treated with the respect it deserves. It involves

Is plastic surgery the answer?

■ "If only I could change this one thing, everything would be perfect." Many of us have looked into the mirror at some time with this thought in mind. Modern body consciousness has made us enormously critical of the way we look, and the flawless models shown in advertising and magazines have raised our standards of attractiveness far beyond the average person's reach. Exercise, diet and cosmetics can make great improvements to our appearance, but basic structures cannot be altered in this way. At the same time, restructuring techniques in cosmetic plastic surgery have been developed in the past 20 years, and these have been widely advertised in the faces of famous people. The cost of plastic surgery has also dropped. While still expensive, it is within the range of ordinary salaries should people choose to save up for it. It has also become much more socially acceptable. But is it right for you?

Cosmetic surgeons often find that the greatest obstacle to successful surgery is the patient's own perceptions of what surgery will do. Unrealistic expectations include the belief that the physical change will have a disproportionate effect upon the client's emotional and social life, and disillusion follows quickly if this does not happen. Even the physical results are often not what was expected. People may fail to realize the importance of proportion in the face and body, and locate their "faults" in the wrong place. If you think your nose is "wrong," look carefully at your face from all angles. You may find that the real problem is to do with the proportions of your chin or neck. Cosmetic surgeons are skilled at diagnosing precisely what can and should be done. It is also vital to remember that, although plastic surgery is amazingly sophisticated now, it is still a surgical procedure that will involve bruising, swelling, discoloration, scarring and all the risks that any operation involving anesthetics brings. Also, the results cannot always be guaranteed to be perfect. Doctors can make mistakes, and flesh cannot be carved as easily as marble.

Nevertheless, surgeon Frank Kamer says that "cosmetic surgery is quick and cheap psychotherapy, cheap when you compare it to years and years on the couch." For people who have reasonable expectations about what cosmetic surgery can do, even minor changes that are hardly noticeable to other

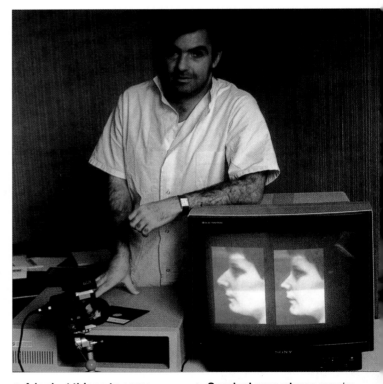

▲ **A look at things to come.** *A problem with cosmetic surgery is not knowing how your new nose or jawline will alter the look of your face. Computer graphics provide a solution – the technician creates on a computer screen an image of a face as it is at present, and how it will look with selected alterations. Clients can redesign their faces to their own tastes.*

▶ **Surgical procedures** *require a full complement of medical personnel even when their purpose is no more than cosmetic, such as the reshaping of breast tissue. When considering measures like this remember that their cosmetic aims do not make them any less serious than any other surgery, with all its risks, discomfort and possible side effects.*

scars, anesthesia, and – as with any surgical procedure – there may be complications. You also need to choose a reputable surgeon who inspires confidence in you.

Cosmetic therapy

Less drastic than surgery, cosmetic therapy (see *Ch 26*) is the skillful application of cosmetic treatments to people in need of a physical and psychological boost. Cosmetic therapy can also serve as a bridge to link a person undergoing surgical change back into successful social rehabilitation – teaching them new makeup or camouflage techniques, for example. Many of these techniques are used to minimize embarrassment or self-consciousness during the healing after surgery. They may also involve the right choice of

clothes to conceal the "offending areas." Scarves or high-necked sweaters can conceal neck or chin surgery, dark glasses hide eye bruising, and so on. Cosmetic therapy can provide the necessary short term "hiding place" needed until the obvious scars or redness disappear and the skin resumes its normal appearance.

After blepharoplasty, for example, the person may need to be encouraged to adopt a new style of eye makeup. For victims of accidents and burns, where reconstructive as well as cosmetic surgery may be required, cosmetic therapy can also provide psychological support after (especially facial) surgery. It can improve self-image and enhance the results of the surgery as well, making it easier to return to a normal social and working life. **JAG**

people can bring a fresh sense of confidence. This is very true for people having age-related cosmetic surgery – face lifts, collagen injections to fill in wrinkles or blepharoplasty (eyelid reconstruction). Should you decide to seek surgical assistance to improve your appearance, think very carefully about what you expect to gain.

Face-lift
Aim: remove wrinkles
Side effects: temporary numbness, swelling
Complications: nerve injury
Malar augmentation
Aim: increase prominence of cheekbones
Side effects: swelling
Complications: infection; extrusion of implant

Blepharoplasty
Aim: remove heavy folds from drooping eyelids
Side effects: prolonged bruising
Complications: scarring; poor result (no major difference or wide-eyed look)
Brow lift
Aim: remove brow wrinkles
Side effects: prolonged numbness

Complications: raised hairline; surprised look
Rhinoplasty
Aim: nose reconstruction
Side effects: swelling
Complications: scarring, poor aesthetic result
Chin implant
Aims: improve jaw line, remove double chin
Side effects: swelling
Complications: infection, extrusion of implant
Collagen injections
Aims: fill in wrinkles, increase lip size
Side effects: swelling
Complications: allergic reaction; results are not permanent; may need to be repeated.
Breast augmentation
Aims: increase breast size, improve shape
Side effects: swelling
Complications: hardening of breast around implant
Breast reduction
Aims: reduce breast size, improve shape
Side effects: bad scarring and bleeding
Complications: inability to breastfeed, loss of sensitivity
Liposuction
Aim: remove body fat resistant to diet and exercise
Side effects: swelling, bruising, skin discoloration
Complications: uneven results, infection.

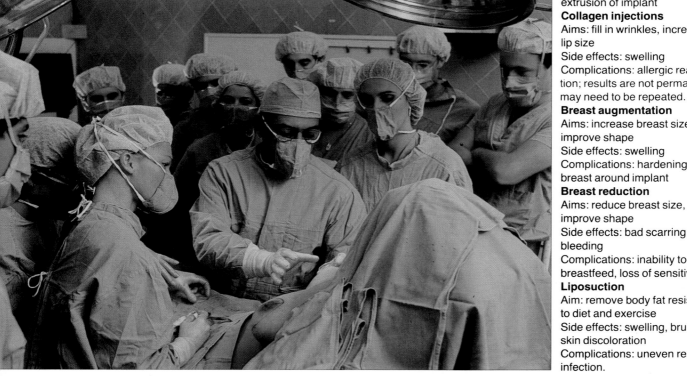

33

Looking Good, Feeling Great

It may be time for a change in your image
● *Is your life at one of its many turning points –*
getting married, taking a new job, moving to a
new neighborhood? ● *How should you look in*
your new surroundings?

HOW YOU LOOK, how you feel and how others feel about you are three inseparable keys to the rewards you are looking for in social interactions. If you look right for the situation you are in – the way you present yourself creates the right mood – people will react favorably, and sensing this or even anticipating it, your own mood will be the right one for the occasion. Most important of all, the fact that you feel right – because you know you have taken the trouble to create the right impression – will make you confident, and this more than anything else will create a favorable impression.

Making these three elements – appearance, impression, mood – work together successfully means balancing what is possible with what is desirable, and what is personal – the real you – with what is easy for others to relate to. It also means backing up the first impressions you create with a long-term truth – there is little to gain from pretending to be someone other than yourself.

Changing your personal style

Most of us have a vague idea of what sort of changes we would like to make or should put into practice to make a better impression. But somehow the day never comes when we really get to grips with changing; or within a few weeks we begin to backslide into our old habits. Lifelong habits are truly difficult to break, and it is important to realize this from the outset. The task is made harder by the fact that we may have unrealistic expectations about how a new image and lifestyle might work for or against us.

Adopting a businesslike image at work, for example, undoubtedly gives you a leading edge, but only an edge. A group of businesswomen, given a cosmetic make-over (see *Ch27*), were estimated to expect a salary level 12 percent higher than that calculated before their make-overs when

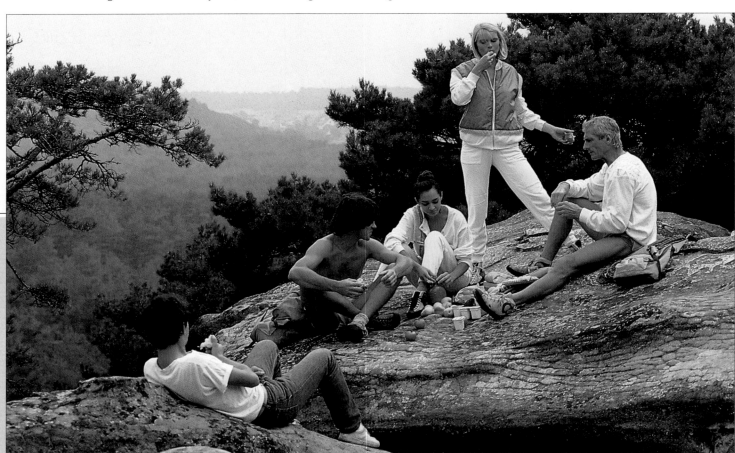

▲ **A day in the great outdoors** brings a glow of health. The feelings of relaxation produced by enjoying exercise and fresh air benefit us individually and enhance our relationships with one another. The psychological and physical benefits reinforce each other. Combined with a good diet, this is a recipe for feeling – and looking – great.

judged by employment agencies and the personnel directors of large corporations in the United States. But this was only an estimate, not a reality. Really getting ahead in business requires good skills for the job and the dedication to do well. The right image will gain you respect and give you confidence, but it cannot do the job for you, any more than losing weight will immediately make you sexually desirable (though it may help).

Unfortunately many people do expect that a major change will produce immediate, dramatic results. When they find that this does not happen they may either intensify the pressure on themselves, or they may give up altogether.

Other people seem to fear the pressures of an improved lifestyle, and talk for the rest of their lives about what they will do when they lose weight. By never acting on their bad habits, the habits become an excuse for what they do not achieve.

A common fear that prevents people from making changes is worry about appearing frivolous and projecting a false image. Concern with appearance is associated with empty-headedness, particularly in women, and if you are trying to improve your image you might fear that a major transformation will mark you out as all style and no content.

Defining aims and strategies

The problem behind all these failures to change our lives for the better is the lack of a clear aim or goal. If you think carefully about your goals you can avoid adopting unreal expectations and creating unfavorable impressions. You have to separate your fantasies ("I want to be Marilyn Monroe") from your real strengths and possibilities ("I am good at managing sales and would like to run my own shop one day"). Once you get this clear in your mind, you can

begin to map out what needs changing to achieve these goals, and how far you are prepared to go to drop bad habits and develop good ones.

Mood management is a key to the effective pursuit of your aims. If you feel happy and comfortable with yourself, your mood will be picked up by other people, and will have a positive effect on the way they treat you and in turn how you react to them. Taking control of your life allows you to dictate your moods to some extent, rather than allowing them to rule you. Looking after yourself will have a beneficial effect on your mood and therefore your behavior.

There are many ways in which choice of cosmetics, hair-care, fragrance and fashion can be geared to conveying a mood for a particular situation. Mood is the psychological factor that links color, makeup, fragrance and behavior.

Creating the right mood

Most of us have a general idea of what sort of image we might like to convey most of the time, but we can also *modify* that image or change it quite dramatically to serve particular purposes. For the full psychological effect to

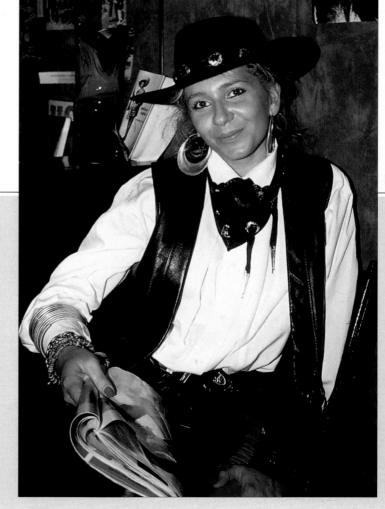

245

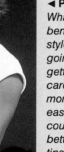

◄ **Put some lift in your life.** *What is the secret of making a beneficial change in your lifestyle? Major life changes like going to work for the first time, getting married, making a career move – provide moments when new goals are easier to accommodate. What could you do to look and feel better? How could a new routine fit into this stage of your life, or the next?*

► **When you feel good, you look good**. *Being comfortable with your whole self is a worthwhile life goal. Good looks complement each other, producing confidence.*

Making an impact

■ First impressions last, but perhaps not for as long as you imagine. Research shows that the initial impact that you make with your appearance has the most effect in the first five minutes; after that appearance becomes less important in the evaluations people make of us. A really successful image has to relate to your personality and abilities in order to prevent that crucial first appearance generating disappointment. In certain situations, first impressions have a disproportionate effect. In job interviews, public speaking events and parties, where people make decisions about you based on relatively small amounts of information, appearance may tip the balance one way or another if all other factors are equal.

occur, both the image-maker and the observers should believe in and expect to experience a relationship between image and mood, even if not thinking consciously "red makes me happy" or "dresses are romantic." We are all inculcated with the social meanings of styles, colors, smells, etc from childhood, so changes in our appearance can modulate moods in quite sophisticated ways.

Color is one of the clearest indicators of mood and expectation though we are not always consciously aware of how it affects us. A study asking participants to choose lipstick and eyeshadow colors appropriate to general daytime wear, work situations, and evening or celebratory events showed a clear breakdown in color preference for type of event. Soft, rich pinks and purples were associated with evening. For casual daytime the participants preferred ordinary blues, greens, browns and peach colors. They chose subdued browns and grays for work situations.

Probably more important than the actual colors, though, are the qualities of the colors – rich, ordinary, subdued. This is true of clothes and hair colorants as well as makeup. You may want to wear green a great deal because it suits you, but different shades of green will still reflect quite different moods. Other aspects of our appearance that are under our control (especially hairstyles and fashions) carry the same range of meanings as color and can be manipulated just as successfully.

Integrating different aspects of image

Most of us like to vary our moods and the image we project depending on what we are doing, and changes in personal style allow us to do that. Because the range of meaning in appearance is so extensive and subtle, it is important to try to achieve a consistent image within each variation. It can be very disconcerting to see a woman in a

▲ **Creating a mood** *is the art that ties together all our self-presentation. Are your colors bright or subtle? Do you like classic styles or something unusual? How you behave is also part of the mood. Is your body language flamboyant or restrained? Do you speak loudly and colorfully or simply and clearly? Signals like these combine to create a mood, which must have some consistency if it is to be convincing – though surprises are always welcome.*

The real you is what matters

■ Many people who avidly read about self-improvement end up feeling inadequate. Women, in particular, are persuaded by the media that physical perfection is necessary and that it is also natural and effortless.

The inevitable failure to live up to the glossy images that are thrown at us can lead to an obsession with health and lifestyle in a frantic effort to "get it right" or a complete rejection of self-improvement.

It may help to remember that the point of changing your image and improving your health is to help you, to make you feel better because you are worth taking trouble over. If your attempts to change make you feel unhappy and inadequate, the problem lies in the nature of the change or the way you have gone about it, not in you.

Looking good will only help you feel better if you have a positive sense of self-worth that recognizes human variety (including your own idiosyncrasies) and acknowledges the impossibility of perfection.

smart, tailored business suit and with an outrageous hair-style. What is she trying to say about herself? She may be confused about her own image, or she may be combining favorite aspects of her daytime and nighttime self.

Image makes its greatest impact in the first few minutes, and clear, unambiguous statements appear to get a message across most effectively. It is a good idea to take a hard look at any transformation of yourself to see whether the image you are conveying is clear and consistent – otherwise your efforts may simply cancel themselves out.

Cosmetic changes can go some way to helping us achieve higher standards of health and beauty. They provide us with

a vehicle to help build confidence as we project a more positive image. Paying attention to good health practices is equally beneficial in making us feel good and look better. Taking healthy living and cosmetic care more seriously and building them into everyday lifestyles sets in motion positive psychological processes that encourage our health and happiness. The point of looking after your body, outside and inside, is to promote total well-being. If we neglect personal relationships or intellectual development at the expense of an obsessive pursuit of the perfect body, we will not achieve real psychological health, and we will probably not be very happy. **JAG**

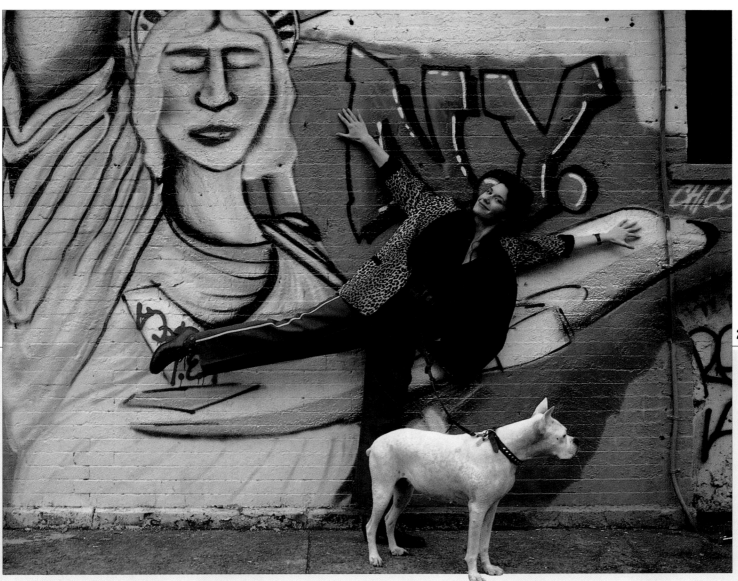

▲ **Your image must fit in** with what you want to be and do, and it has to have some genuine content behind it. What is important is to look comfor- table and confident with the image you project – this will enable an attractive, open per- sonality to shine through. If your image is not in line with your abilities or aims, you need to reassess what you are trying to project. The secret may be to aim for simplicity rather than sophistication.

READERS may want information about other aspects of a subject, or details on particular topics that have aroused their interest. Some generally available books and periodicals suggested for further reading are listed below. The main published sources consulted by the contributors to this book follow the further reading suggestions.

1 Good Health From Birth
Cousins, N 1981 *Anatomy of an Illness as Perceived by the Patient* Bantam Books, London; Lederman, F K 1989 *Your Health in Your Hands* Green Books, Bideford, Devon; Patel, C 1987 *Fighting Heart Disease* British Holistic Medical Association/Dorling Kindersley, London; Whiteside, M and Whiteside, T 1989 *Staying Healthy* Cassell, London.

2 Your Sex and Your Health
Clay, J 1989 *Men at Midlife* Sidgwick and Jackson, London; Phillips, A and Rakuson, J 1989 *The New Our Bodies, Ourselves* Penguin, London; Stoppard, M 1982 *Every Woman's Health Guide* Macdonald and Co, London.

3 The Rhythms of Life
Ayensu, E S and Whitfield, P (eds) 1982 *The Rhythms of Life* Book Club Associates, London; Bromley, D B 1988 *Human Ageing: An Introduction to Gerontology* Penguin, London; Conroy, R and Mills, J 1971 *Human Circadian Rhythms* Williams and Wilkins, Baltimore, MD; Luce, G G 1973 *Body Time: The Natural Rhythms of the Body* Paladin, London; Minors, D and Waterhouse, J M 1981 *Circadian Rhythms and the Human* Wright, London; Rodin, J 1983 *Will This Hurt?* Royal College of Nursing, London; Stott, M 1981 *Ageing for Beginners* Blackwell, Oxford; Twining, T C 1988 *Helping Older People: a Psychological Approach* Wiley, Chichester.

4 Stress
Blackburn, I M 1987 *Coping With Depression* Chambers, Edinburgh; Burns, D D 1980 *Feeling Good: The New Mood Therapy* Signet, New American Library, New York; Rowe, D 1983 *Depression: the Way Out of Your Prison* Routledge and Kegan Paul, London.

5 Learn to Relax
Cooper, C L, Cooper, R D and Eaker, L H 1988 *Living With Stress* Penguin, London.

6 The Healing Power of Sleep
Coates, T and Thoresen, C 1977 *How To Sleep Better: A Drug Free Program For Overcoming Insomnia* Prentice Hall, Englewood Cliffs, NJ; Dement, W C 1972 *Some Must Watch While Some Must Sleep* Norton and Co, New York; Lambley, P 1982 *Insomnia and Other Sleeping Problems* Windsor Publishing Corp, New York.

7 Sexuality
Barbach, L G 1976 *For Yourself: The Fulfillment of Female Sexuality* Anchor, Garden City, NY; Comfort, A 1972 *Joy of Sex* Quartet, New York; Cox, G and Darrow, S 1988 *Making the Most of Loving* Sheldon Press, London; Griffith, N 1987 *My Secret Garden* Penguin, Harmondsworth; Rice, E P 1988 *Human Sexuality* Brown, Boston, MA; Zilbergeld, B 1978 *Male Sexuality* Little, Brown and Co, Boston, MA.

8 Good Nutrition
Brody, J 1987 *Jane Brody's Nutrition Book* Bantam, New York; Guthrie, H A 1986 *Introductory Nutri-* tion Times Mirror/Mosby College Publishing, St Louis, MI; Yetiv, J Z 1986 *Popular Nutritional Practices: A Scientific Appraisal* Popular Medicine Press, Toledo, OH.

9 The Diet Dilemma
Boskind-White, M and White, W C Jr 1987 *Bulimarexia: The Binge/Purge Cycle* Norton, New York; Gamman, L and Marshment, M (eds): 1988 *The Female Gaze: Women as Viewers of Popular Culture* Women's Press, London; Katahn, M R 1989 *The T-Factor Diet* Norton, New York; Logue, A W 1986 *The Psychology of Eating and Drinking* Freeman, New York.

10 Weight Control and Self-Image
Bennett, W and Gurin, J 1982 *The Dieter's Dilemma* Basic Books, New York; Polivy, J and Herman, C P 1983 *Breaking the Diet Habit* Basic Books, New York; Seid, R P 1989 *Never Too Thin: Why Women are at War with Their Bodies* Prentice-Hall, New York; Solomon, H A 1984 *The Exercise Myth* Harcourt Brace Jovanovich, New York.

11 Exercise and Physical Fitness
Kavanagh, T 1985 *The Healthy Heart Program* Key Porter Books, Canada; Editors of Prevention Magazine 1986 *The Master Plan*, Rodale Press, Emmaus, PA.

12 Making Exercise Part Of Your Life
Martin, J and Dubbert, P 1987 "Exercise Promotion" in Blumenthal, J and McKee, D (eds): *Applications in Behavioral Medicine and Health Psychology: A Clinician's Source Book* Professional Resource Exchange, PA.

13 Are Sports Good For You?
Read, M and Wade, P 1984 *Sports Injuries* Breslich and Foss, London; Schurman, D 1975 *Athletic Fitness* Atheneum, New York.

14 Smoking
Carr, A 1987 *The Easy Way to Stop Smoking*, Penguin, London; Casey, K 1987 *If Only I Could Quit* Hazelden, Center City, MN; Ernester, V L 1985 "Mixed Messages for Women: A Social History of Cigarette Smoking and Advertising" *New York State Journal of Medicine* 85, pp335-40; Warner, K E 1986 *Selling Smoke: Cigarette Advertising and Public Health* American Public Health Association, Washington, DC.

15 The Effects of Alcohol
Gwinner, P and Grant, M 1979 *What's Your Poison?* British Broadcasting Corporation, London; Robertson, I and Heather, N 1986 *Let's Drink to your Health: a Self-Help Guide to Sensible Drinking* British Psychological Society, Leicester, England.

16 Drugs, Pills and Painkillers
Curran, V and Golombok, S 1985 *Bottling It Up* Faber and Faber, London; Goscop, M 1987 *Living with Drugs* Institute for Study of Drug Dependence, London; Edwards, A and Jaffe, J (eds) 1983 *Drug Use and Misuse Cultural Perspectives* Croom Helm, London; Gossop, M 1987 *Living With Drugs* Wildwood House, London; Plant, M 1978 *Drugs in Perspective* Hodder and Stoughton, London; Strait, T 1987 *The Heroin Users* Pandora, London; Tyler, A 1987 *Street Drugs* New English Library, Sevenoaks.

17 Illness and Disability
Fox, D 1986 *Health Policies, Health Politics* Princeton University, NJ; Lansdown, R 1980 *More Than Sympathy: The Everyday Needs of Sick and* *Handicapped Children* Tavistock, London; Larson, G (ed): 1986 *Managing the School-Age Child With a Chronic Health Condition* Diabetes Centre, Minnesota; Sarton, M 1988 *After the Stroke* Women's Press, London.

18 Hospital Care
Alman, B M and Lambrou, R T 1984 *Self-Hypnosis: A Complete Manual for Health and Self-Change* International health Publications, San Diego, CA; Broome, A K and Wallace, L M (eds) 1984 *Psychology and Gynaecological Problems* Tavistock Press, London; Health Education Authority 1989 *Birth to Five: A Guide to the First Five Years of Being a Parent* London; Johnston, M and Wallace, L M (eds) 1990 *Stressful Medical Procedures* Oxford University Press, Oxford; Russell, L B 1986 *Is Prevention Better than Cure?* Brookings Institute, Washington, DC; Shaper, A G 1988 *Coronary Heart Disease, Risks and Reasons* London Current Medical Literature; Soskis, D A 1986 *Teaching Self-Hypnosis: An Introductory Guide for Clinicians* Norton Press, New York; Wallace, L M and Bundy, E C 1990 *Living with Angina* Thorsons, Wellingborough, England.

19 Do Looks Matter?
Bull, R and Rumsey, N 1989 *The Social Psychology of Facial Appearance* Springer-Verlag, London; Graham, J A and Kligman, A M 1985 *The Psychology of Cosmetic Treatments* Praeger, New York; Hatfield, E and Sprecher, S 1986 *Mirror, Mirror: The Importance of Looks in Everyday Life* State University of New York Press, Albany, NY; Morris, D 1985 *Bodywatching: A Field Guide to the Human Species* Crown, New York.

20 Your Bodyshape
Hatfield, E and Sprecher, S 1986 *Mirror, Mirror: The Importance of Looks in Everyday Life* State University of New York Press, Albany, NY; Knapp, M L 1978 *Nonverbal Communication in Human Interaction* Holt, Rinehart and Winston, New York; Morris, D 1985 *Bodywatching: A Field Guide to the Human Species* Crown, New York.

21 What Clothes Say
Argyle, M 1988 (2nd edn) *Bodily Communication* Methuen, London; Hatfield, E and Sprecher, S 1986 *Mirror, Mirror: The Importance of Looks in Everyday Life* State University of New York, Albany, NY; Knapp, M L 1978 *Nonverbal Communication in Human Interaction* Holt, Rinehart and Winston, New York; Morris, D 1985 *Bodywatching: A Field Guide to the Human Species* Crown, New York.

22 Bodytalk
Argyle, M 1988 (2nd edn) *Bodily Communication* Methuen, London.

23 Personal Style
Begoun, P 1989 *Blue Eyeshadow Should be Illegal* Arlington Books, London; Morris, D 1977 *Manwatching* Cape, London.

24 Looking Better With Age
Graham, J and Kligman, A (eds) 1985 *The Psychology of Cosmetic Treatments* Praeger, New York, pp77-92; Hatfield, E and Sprecher, S 1986 *Mirror, Mirror: The Importance of Looks in Everyday Life* State University of New York Press, Albany, NY.

25 Skincare
Coleman, V 1984 *Taking Care of Your Skin* Sheldon, London; Marks, R 1988 *The Sun and Your Skin* Macdonald Optima, London; McKie, R *Eczema and Dermatitis* Macdonald Optima, London.

26 Putting Cosmetics to Work
Margrove, C 1985 *Cosmetic Surgery* Penguin, Harmondsworth; Partridge, J 1990 *Changing Faces* Penguin, London; Piff, C 1985 *Let's Face It* Gollancz, London; Trust, D 1986 *Overcoming Disfigurement* Thorsons, London.

27 Being Made Over
Graham, J A and Kligman, M A 1984 "Cosmetic Therapy for the Elderly" *Journal of the Society of Cosmetic Chemists*, 35, pp133-45; Graham, J A and Kligman A M (eds) 1985 *The Psychology of Cosmetic Treatments* Praeger, New York.

28 Hairstyle and Haircare
Cooper, W 1971 *Hair: Sex, Society, Symbolism* Stein and Day, New York; Graham, J A and Kligman A M 1985 *The Psychology of Cosmetic Treatments* Praeger, New York; Harkavi, I 1987 *I'll Make You Beautiful* New American Library, New York; Knapp, M L 1978 *Nonverbal Communication in Human Interaction* Holt, Rinehart and Winston, New York; Powlis, L V 1988 *Beauty From The Inside Out: A Guide For Black Women* Doubleday, New York.

29 Beautiful Hands, Beautiful Feet
Hagman, A 1981 *The Aestheticienne: Simple Theory and Practice* Stanley Thorness, London; Hutton, D 1982 *The Vogue Health and Beauty Book: Complete Beauty* Octopus, London; Zeff, L 1988 *The Beauty Treatment Handbook* Piatkus, London.

30 Looking After Your Smile
Argyle, M 1988 *Bodily Communication* Methuen, London; Beresford, J 1986 *Good Mouthkeeping* Oxford University Press, Oxford.

31 Fragrance and Aromatherapy
Cunningham, S 1989 *Magical Aromatherapy* Llewellyn, St Paul, MN; Davis, P 1988 *Aromatherapy A-Z* C W Daniel, London; Jackson, J 1987 *Aromatherapy* Dorling Kindersley, London; Labows, J N Jr 1985 "Social-Sexual Effects of Pheromones" in Graham, J A and Kligman, A M (eds) *The Psychology of Cosmetic Treatments* Praeger, New York; Mensing, J 1985 *The Psychology of Fragrance Selection: Feminine Notes* Haarmann and Reimer; Tisserand, R 1988 *Aromatherapy for Everyone* Penguin, London.

32 Professional Beautycare
Goin, J M and Goin, M K 1981 *Changing the Body: Psychological Effects of Plastic Surgery* Williams and Wilkins, Baltimore, London.

33 Looking Good, Feeling Great
Comfort, A 1990 *A Good Age* Pan Books, London; Juhan, D 1987 *Job's Body* Station Hill Press, Barrytown, NY; Marshall, C 1986 *Prime Time Woman* Sidgwick and Jackson, London; Shapiro, J (ed) 1987 *Ourselves Growing Older* Fontana, London.

CONTRIBUTORS' SOURCES

1 Good Health From Birth Becker, M H 1974 *The Health Belief Model and Personal Health Behavior* Slack, Thorogare, NJ; Herzlich, C 1973 *Health and Illness: A Socio-Psychological Analysis* Academic Press, London; King, 1983 "Attribution Theory and the Health Belief Model" in Hewstone, M (ed): *Attribution Theory: Social and Functional Extensions* Blackwell, Oxford; Rodin, J and Langer, E J 1977 "Long-Term Effects of a Control-Relevant Intervention With the Institutionalized Aged" *Journal of Personality and Social Psychology*, 35, pp897-902; Rosser, R and Kind, P 1978 "A Scale of Valuations of States of Health: Is There a Social Consensus?" *International Journal of Epidemiology*, 7, pp347-57; Weinstein, N D 1984 "Why It Won't Happen to Me: Perceptions of Risk Factors in Illness Susceptibility" *Health Psychology*, 3, pp431-57; Williams, R G A 1983 "Concepts of Health: An Analysis of Lay Logic" *Sociology*, 17, pp185-205; Wright, S J 1989 "Health Status Measurement: Review and Prospects" in Bennett, P, Spurgeon, P and Weinman, J (eds): *Current Advances in Health Psychology* Harwood, London.

2 Your Sex and Your Health Barnett, R C, Biener, L and Baruch, G E 1987 *Gender and Stress* (The Groundbreaking Investigation of How Stress is Caused and Experienced – Differently – in the Lives of Women and Men) Free Press, New York; Blechman, E A and Brownell, K D 1988 *Handbook of Behavioral Medicine for Women* Pergamon, New York; Falk B and Blackwood, R 1987 *Why Kill Yourself?* Gollancz, London; Gold, M 1988 *Living Without Cruelty* Green Print, London; Locke, S and Colligan, D 1986 *The Healer Within* (The New Medicine of Mind and Body) Dutton, New York; Matarazzo, J D, Weiss, S M, Herb, J A, Miller N E, Weiss, S M 1984 *Behavioral Health* (A Handbook of Health Enhancement and Disease Prevention) Wiley, New York; O'Mullane, J and Muir, C 1986 *The Fat Factor* Thorsons, Wellingborough; 1987 *Oxford Textbook of Medicine* (2nd edn) Oxford University Press, Oxford; Rodwell, L 1988 *Women and Medical Care* Allen and Unwin, London; Saab, P G, Matthews, K A, Stoney, C M and McDonald, R H 1989 "Premenopausal and Postmenopausal Women Differ in Their Cardiovascular and Neuroendocrine Responses to Behavioral Stressors" *Psychophysiology*, 26, pp270-280; Stoppard, M 1983 *50 plus Lifeguide* Dorling Kindersley, London.

3 The Rhythms of Life Arendt, J and Broadway, J 1987 "Light and Melatonia as Zeitgebers in Man" *Chronobiology International*, Vol 4 (2), pp273-82; Armstrong-Esther, C A, Bonner, A B, Browne, K D and Hawkins, L 1989 "Cognitive Impairment in the Elderly and Its Relationship to Their Circadian Rhythms" in Morgan, E (ed): *Chronobiology and Chronomedicine: Basic Research and Applications*, Lang, London; Czeisler, C A, Allan, J S, Strogatz, S H, Ronda, J M, Sarchez, R, Rios, C D, Freitag, W O, Richardson, G S and Kronauer, R E 1986 "Bright Lights Reset the Human Circadian Pacemaker Independent of the Timing of the Sleep-Wake Cycle *Science*, 233, pp667-71; Eiser, C 1985 *The Psychology of Childhood Illness* Springer, New York; Maddux, J E, Roberts, M C, Sleddon, E A and Wright, L 1986 "Developmental Issues in Child Health Psychology" *American Psychologist*, 41, pp25-34; Moore-Ede, M C, Sulzman, F M and Fuller, C A 1982 *The Clocks That Time Us* Harvard University Press, Cambridge, MA; Rosenthal, N, Sack, D, Gillin, J, Lewy, J, Goodwin, F, Davenport, Y, Mueller, P, Newsome, D and Wehr, T 1984 "Seasonal Affective Disorder: A Description of the Syndrome and Preliminary Findings With Light Therapy" *Archives of General Psychiatry*, 41, pp72-80; Wehr, T A, Wirz-Justice, A, Goodwin, F K, Duncan, W and Gillin, J C 1979

"Phase Advance of the Circadian Sleep-Wake Cycle as An Anti-Depressant" *Science*, 206, pp710-13.

4 Stress Barefoot, J C, Dahlstrom, W G and Williams, R B Jr 1983 "Hostility, CHD Incidence, and Total Mortality: A 25-Year Follow-Up Study of 255 Physicians" *Psychosomatic Medicine*, 45, pp59-63; Chesney, M A and Rosenman, R H (eds): 1985 *Anger and Hostility in Cardiovascular and Behavioral Disorders* Hemisphere, New York; Cooper, G L , Cooper, R D and Eaker, L H 1988 *Living With Stress* Penguin Health, Harmondsworth; Graham, J 1984 *Evening Primrose Oil* Thorsons, Wellingborough, Northants; Greenblatt, R G, Mahesh, V B and Gambrell, R D 1985 *Unwanted Hair. Its Cause and Treatment* Parthenon Press, Lanforth, Lancs; Harry, R G, Wilkinson, J B and Moore, R J (eds): 1982 *Harrys Cosmeticology* Godwin, London; Hepper, C 1987 *Herbal Cosmetics* Thorsons, Wellingborough, Northants; Moon, J R and Cisler, R M 1983 "Anger Control: An Experimental Comparison of Three Behavioral Treatments" *Behavior Therapy*, 14, pp493-505; Siegman, A W and Dembroski, T M (eds) 1989 *In Search of Coronary-Prone Behavior: Beyond Type A* Erlbaum, Hillsdale, NJ; Smith, T W and Assrd, K D 1989 "Blood Pressure Responses During Social Interaction in High and Low-Cynically Hostile Males" *Journal of Behavioral Medicine*, 12, pp135-43; Smith, T W, Pope, M K, Sanders, J D, Allred, K D and O'Keeffe, J L 1988 "Cynical Hostility at Home and Work: Psychosocial Vulnerability Across Domains" *Journal of Research in Personality*, 22, pp525-48.

5 Learn to Relax Lavey, R S and Taylor C B 1985 "The Nature of Relaxation Therapy" in Burchfield, R S (ed): *Stress: Psychological and Physiological Interaction* Hemisphere, Washington, DC; Nigl, A J 1984 *Biofeedback and Behavioral Strategies in Pain Management*, Medical and Scientific Books, New York; Shapiro, D H 1985 "Meditation and Behavioral Medicine: Application of a Self Regulation Strategy to the Clinical Management of Stress" in Burchfield, S R (ed): *Stress: Psychological and Physiological Interactions* Hemisphere, Washington, DC.

6 The Healing Power of Sleep Hartmann, E, Baekeland, F and Zwilling, G R 1972 "Psychological Differences Between Long and Short Sleepers" *Archives of General Psychiatry*, 26, pp463-8; Hauri, P 1982 *The Sleep Disorders* Upjohn, Kalamazoo, Michigan; Kryger, M H, Roth, T and Dement, W C 1989 *Principles and practice of Sleep Medicine* Saunders, London; Mendelson, W B 1987 *Human Sleep: Research and Clinical Care* Plenum, New York; Moldofsky, H and Scarisbrick, P 1976 "Induction of Neurasthenic Musculoskeletal Pain Syndrome by Selective Sleep Stage Deprivation" *Psychosomatic Medicine*, 38, pp35-44; Parkes, J D 1985 *Sleep and Its Disorders* Saunders, London.

7 Sexuality Bancroft, J 1983 *Human Sexuality and its Problems* Churchill Livingstone, Edinburgh; Kaplan, H S 1978 *The New Sex Therapy: Active Treatment of Sexual Dysfunctions* Peregrine, New York; Leiblum, S, Bachmann, E, Kemmann, E, Colburn, D and Swartzman, L 1983 "Vaginal Atrophy in the Postmenopausal Woman" *JAMA*, 249, pp2195-8; Leiblum, S R and Rosen R C 1989 *Principles and Practices of Sex Therapy: Update for the 1990s* Guildford Press, New York; Masters, W H and Johnson, V E 1966 *Human Sexual Response* Little, Brown and Co, Boston, MA; Masters W H and Johnson, V E 1970 *Human Sexual Inadequacy* Little, Brown and Co, Boston, MA; Sherwin, B B and Gelfand M M 1987 "The Role of Androgen in the Maintenance of Sexual Functioning in Oophorectomized Women" in *Psychosomatic Medicine*, 49, pp397-409.

8 Good Nutrition Brody, J 1987 *Jane Brody's Nutrition Book* Bantam, New York; Guthrie, H A 1986 *Introductory Nutrition* Times Mirror/Mosby College

CONTRIBUTORS' SOURCES CONTINUED

Publishing, St Louis, MI; Katahn, M and Pope-Cordle, J 1989 *The T-Factor Diet and the T-Factor Fat Gram Counter* Norton, New York; Mervyn, L 1989 *Thorsons Complete Guide to Vitamins and Minerals* Thorsons, Wellingborough, Northants; Pope, J 1987 "Nutrition in the Golden Years" in *Old Age is Not for Sissies*, Art Linkletter, Viking, New York; Yetiv, J Z 1986 *Popular Nutritional Practices: A Scientific Appraisal* Popular Medicine Press, Toledo, OH.

9 The Diet Dilemma Abraham, S, Carroll, M D, Najjar, M F and Fulwood, R 1983 "Obese and Overweight Adults in the United States" *Vital and Health Statistics, Series 11*, Vol 230, DHHS pub no (PHS) 83-1680, Public Health Service, U S Government Printing Office, Washington, DC; Millar, W J and Stephens, T 1987 "The Prevalence of Overweight and Obesity in Britain, Canada and the United States" *American Journal of Public Health*, 42, pp38-41; Negri, E, Pagano, R, Decarli, A and La Vecchia, C 1988 "Body Weight and the Prevalence of Chronic Disease" *Journal of Epidemiology and Community Health*, 42, pp24-9; Schlundt, D G and Johnson, W G 1990 *Eating Disorders: Assessment and Treatment* Allyn and Bacon, Boston, MA.

10 Weight Control and Self-Image Bennett, W 1987 "Dietary Treatments of Obesity" *Annals of the New York Academy of Sciences*, 499, pp250-63; Epstein, L H and Wing, R R 1980 "Aerobic Exercise and Weight" *Addictive Behaviors*, 5, pp371-88; Ernsberger, P and Haskew, P 1987 "Rethinking Obesity: An Alternative View of its Health Implications" in a Special Monograph Issue of *The Journal of Obesity and Weight Reduction*, 6, 1(57)-81(137); Fisher, M C and Lachance, P A 1985 "Nutrition Evaluation of Published Weight-Reducing Diets" *The American Dietetic Association*, 85, pp450-4; Folkins, C H and Sime, W E 1981 "Physical Fitness Training and Mental Health" *American Psychologist*, 36, pp373-89; Gordon, L 1984 "33,000 Women Tell How They Really Feel About Their Bodies" *Glamour* February, 1984; Gurin, J 1989 "Leaner, not Lighter" *Psychology Today*, June, 1989, pp32-6; Gwinup, G 1975 "Effect of Exercise Alone on the Weight of Obese Women" *Archives of Internal Medicine*, 135, pp676-80; Keys, A 1980 *Seven Countries: A Multivariate Analysis of Death and Coronary Disease* Harvard University Press, Cambridge, MA and London; Rock, C L and Coulston, A W 1988 "Weight-Control Approaches: A Review by the California Dietetic Association" *Journal of the American Dietetic Association*, 88, pp44-8; Weinsier, R L, Wadden, T A, Ritenbaugh, C, Harrison, G G, Johnson, F S and Wilmore, J H 1984 "Recommended Therapeutic Guidelines for Professional Weight-Control Programs" *The American Journal of Clinical Nutrition*, 40, pp865-72.

11 Exercise and Physical Fitness American College of Sports Medicine 1978 "Position Statement on the Recommended Quantity and Quality of Exercise for Developing and Maintaining Fitness in Healthy Adults" *Med Sci Sports*, 10, pp7-10; American College of Sports Medicine 1986 (3rd edn) *Guidelines for Exercise Testing and Prescription* Lea and Febiger, Philadelphia, PA; Blumenthal, J A, Williams, R S, Needles, T L and Wallace, A G 1982 "Psychological Changes Accompany Aerobic Exercise in Healthy Middle-Aged Adults" *Psychosomatic Medicine*, 44, pp529-36; Blumenthal, J A, Emery, C F, Walsh, M A, Cox, D R, Kuhn, C M, Williams, R B and Williams, R S 1988 "Exercise Training in Healthy Type A Middle-Aged Men: Effects on Behavioral and Cardiovascular Responses" *Psychosomatic Medicine*, 50, pp418-33; Folkins, C H and Sime W F 1981 "Physical Fitness Training and Mental Health" *American Psychologist*, 35, pp373-89; Hughes, J R 1984 "Psychological Effects of Habitual Aerobic Exercise: A Critical View" *Prevent Med*, 13, pp66-78; Paffenbarger, R S Jr, Laughlin, M E,

Gima, A S et al 1970 "Work Activity of Longshoremen as Related to Death from Coronary Heart Disease and Stroke" *New England Journal of Medicine*, 282, pp1109-14; Paffenbarger, R S, Jr, Wing, A L and Hyde, R T 1978 "Physical Activity as an Index of Heart Attack in College Alumni" *American Journal of Epidemiology*, 108, pp161-75; Paffenbarger, R S, Jr, Hyde, R T, Wing, A L and Hsieh, C-C 1986 "Physical Activity, All Cause Mortality, and Longevity of College Alumni" *New England Journal of Medicine*, 314, pp605-13.

12 Making Exercise Part Of Your Life American College of Sports Medicine 1978 "Position Statement on the Recommended Quantity and Quality of Exercise for Developing and Maintaining Fitness in Healthy Adults" *Med Sci Sports*, 10, pp7-10; Borg, C V 1970 "Perceived Exertion as an Indicator of Somatic Stress" *Scandinavian Journal of Rehabilitation Medicine*, 2, pp92-8; Brownell, K 1987 *The LEARN Program for Weight Control* University of Pennsylvania, Philadelphia; Dishman, R D 1982 "Compliance/Adherence in Health-Related Exercise" *Health Psychology*, 1, pp237-67; Leon et al 198 "Leisure-time Physical Activity Levels and Risk of Coronary Heart Disease and Death" *JAMA*, 258, pp2388-95; Marlatt, G A and Gordon, J R 1980 "Determinants of Relapse: Implications for the Maintenance of Behavior Change" in Davidson, P and Davidson, S (eds): *Behavioral Medicine: Changing Health Lifestyles* Brunner/Mazel, New York; Martin, J E, Dubbert P M et al 1984 "Behavioral Control of Exercise in Sedentary Adults: Studies 1 through 6" *JCCP*, 52, pp795-811; Oldridge, N B 1983 "Predictors of dropout" *American Journal of Cardiology*, 51, pp70-4; Paffenbarger, R S et al 1986 "Physical Activity, All-Cause Mortality, and Longevity of College Alumni" *New England Journal of Medicine*, 314, pp605- 13; Walsh-Riddle, M 1989 "How to Beat the Heat" *The Lean Times*, 7.

13 Are Sports Good For You? Bredemeier, B 1985 "Moral Reasoning and the Perceived Legitimacy of Intentionally Injurious Sports Acts" *Journal of Sport Psychology*, 2, pp110-20; Bredemeier, B, Weiss, M, Shields, D and Cooper, B 1986 "The Relationship of Sport Involvement with Children's Moral Reasoning and Aggression Tendencies" *Journal of Sport Psychology*, 4, pp304-18; Raglin, J and Morgan, W 1985 "Influence of Vigorous Exercise on Mood State" *Behavior Therapist*, 9, pp179-83; Raglin, J and Morgan, W 1987 "Influence of Exercise and Quiet Rest on State Anxiety and Blood Pressure" *Medicine and Science in Sports and Medicine*, 4, pp456-63; Scanlan, T, Stein, G and Ravizza, K 1989 "An In-depth Study of Former Elite Figure Skaters: Sources of Enjoyment" *Journal of Sport and Exercise Psychology*, 1, pp65-83; Smith, R, Smoll, F and Ptacek, J 1990 "Conjunctive Moderator Variables in Vulnerability and Resiliency Research – Life Stress, Social Support and Coping Skills, and Adolescent Sport Injuries" *Journal of Personality and Social Psychology*, 2, pp360-70.

14 Smoking Ernster, V L 1985 "Mixed Messages for Women: A Social History of Cigarette Smoking and Advertising" *New York State Journal of Medicine*, 85, pp335-40; Fielding, J E 1986 "Smoking: Health Effects and Control" in Last, J M (ed): *Maxcy-Rosenau Public Health and Preventive Medicine* 12th ed, Appleton-Century-Crofts, Norwalk, CT; Jacobson, B 1982 *The ladykillers: Why Smoking is a Feminist Issue* Continuum, New York; U S Department of Health and Human Services 1988 *The Health Consequences of Smoking – Nicotine Addiction*, USDHHS, Rockville, MD; U S Department of Health and Human Services 1989 *Reducing the Health Consequences of Smoking – 25 Years of Progress: A Report of the Surgeon General* USDHHS, Rockville, MD; Warner, K E 1986 *Selling Smoke: Cigarette Advertising and Public Health* American Public Health Association, Washington, DC.

15 The Effects of Alcohol Hore, B and Ritson B 1983 *Alcohol and Health* Medical Council on Alcoholism, London; Robertson I and Heather N 1986 *Let's Drink to Your Health* British Psychological Society, Leicester, England.

16 Drugs, Pills and Painkillers Alexander B and Hathaway P 1982 "Opiate Addiction: The Case for an Adaptive Orientation" *Psychological Bulletin* Vol 92 (2), pp367-81; Coleman, V 1989 *The Home Pharmacy* Macmillan, London; Curran, V and Golombok, S 1985 *Bottling It Up* Faber and Faber, London; Diclemente C 1986 "Self-Efficacy and the Addictive Behaviours" *Journal of Social and Clinical Psychology*, Vol 4 (3), pp302-15; Gossop, M 1987 *Living With Drugs* Wildwood House, London; Hurley, D 1989 "Cycles of Craving" in *Psychology Today*, July/August 1989; Hutton, D 1983 *Vogue Complete Beauty* Octopus Books, London; Institute for the Study of Drug Dependence 1988 *Drug Abuse Briefing: A Guide to the Effects of Drugs and to the Social and Legal Facts About Their Non Medical Use in Britain* 3rd edn, Institute for the Study of Drug Dependence, London; Lord, R 1984 *Controlled Drugs: Law and Practice* Butterworth, Sevenoaks; Marlatt, A and George, W 1984 "Relapse Prevention, Introduction and Overview of the Model" *British Journal of Addiction*, Vol 79, pp261-73; Miller W and Pechacheck T 1987 "New Roads: Assessing and Treating Psychological Dependence" *Journal of Substance Abuse Treatment*, 4, pp73-7; Pietroni, P, Foreword in *Bloomsbury Good Health Guide* 1987 edn, Bloomsbury, London.

17 Illness and Disability Burish, T G and Bradley, L A 1983 *Coping With Chronic Disease* Academic Press, London; Kaptchuk, T and Croucher, M 1986 *The Healing Arts* BBC Publications, London; Robinson, I 1988 *Multiple Sclerosis: The Experience of Illness* Routledge, London; Russell, M (ed) 1988 *Stress Management for Chronic Disease* Pergamon, Oxford.

18 Hospital Care Ashcroft, J, Owens, G and Leinster, S J 1985 "Informal Decision Analysis and Treatment Choice by Breast Cancer Patients" *Bulletin of the British Psychological Society*, 38, A53-A54; Crown, J 1982 "Screening in Disease Prevention" *British Journal of Hospital Medicine*, June 1982, pp577-9; Faculty of Community Medicine 1989 "Child Health Surveillance: A Time for Change" *Guideline for Health Promotion*, 16, Royal College of Physicians, London; Knox, E G 1974 "Multiphasic Screening" *Lancet*, Dec 14 1974, pp1434-6; Wallace, L M 1984 "Psychological Preparation as a Method of Reducing the Stress of Surgery" *Journal of Human Stress*, 3, pp62-77; Wallace, L M 1985 "Informed Consent to Elective Surgery: the 'Therapeutic' Value?" *Social Science and Medicine*, 22, (1), pp29-33; Wallace, L M 1986 "Day-Care Laparoscopy: Patient Preferences, Adjustment and Management" *Journal of Psychosomatic Obstetrics and Gynaecology*, 5, 207-16; Wakeman, R J and Kaplan, J Z 1978 "An Experimental Study of Hypnosis in Painful Burns" *American Journal of Clinical Hypnosis*, 21, pp3-11.

19 Do Looks Matter? Banner, L W 1983 *American Beauty* University of Chicago Press, Chicago, IL; Bull, R and Rumsey, N 1989 *The Social Psychology of Facial Appearance* Springer-Verlag, London; Coopersmith, S 1967 *The Antecedents of Self-Esteem* Freeman, San Francisco, CA; Graham, J A and Kligman A M 1985 *The Psychology of Cosmetic Treatments* Praeger, New York; Hatfield, E and Sprecher, S 1986 *Mirror, Mirror: The Importance of Looks in Everyday Life* State University of New York Press, Albany, NY; Wright, B A 1960 *Physical Disability – a Psychological Approach* Harper and Row, New York.

20 Your Bodyshape Cahnman, W J 1968 "The Stigma of Obesity" *Sociological Quarterly*, 9, pp283-99; Comfort, A 1971 "Likelihood of Human Pheromones" *Nature*, 230, pp432-3; Ehrlichman, H and Halpern, J N 1988 "Affect and Memory: Effects of Pleasant and Unpleasant Odors on Retrieval of Happy and Unhappy Memories" *Journal of Personality and Social Psychology*, 55, pp769-79; Ekman, P 1969 "Facial Signs: Facts, Fantasies, and Possibilities" in Sebeok, T (ed): *Sight, Sound, and Sense* Indiana University Press, Bloomington, IN, pp124-56; Garner, D M, Garfinkel, P E, Schwartz, D and Thompson, M 1980 "Cultural Expectations of Thinness in Women" *Psychological Reports*, 47, 483-91; Kirk-Smith, M, Booth, D, Carroll, D and Davies, P 1978 "Human Social Attitudes Affected by Androstenol" *Psychiatry and Behavior*, 3, pp379-84; Lavrakas, P J 1975 "Female Preferences for Male Physiques" *Journal of Research in Personality*, 9, pp324-34; Peck, H and Peck, S 1970 "A Concept of Facial Aesthetics" *Angle Orthodontist*, 40, pp284-317; Porter, R H, Balogh, R D, Carnoch, J M and Franchi, C 1986 "Recognition of Kin Through Characteristic Body Odors" *Chemical Senses*, 11, pp389-95; Wells, B W P 1983 *Body and Personality* Longman Group, Harlow, Essex; Wells, W and Siegel, B 1961 "Stereotyped Somatypes" *Psychological Reports*, 8, pp77-8.

21 What Clothes Say Argyle, M and McHenry, R 1971 "Do Spectacles Really Affect Judgments of Intelligence?" *British Journal of Social and Clinical Psychology*, 10, pp27-9; Bardack, N R and McAndrew, F T 1985 "The Influence of Physical Attractiveness and Manner of Dress on Success in a Simulated Personnel Decision" *Journal of Social Psychology*, 125, pp777-8; Bickman, L 1974 "The Social Power of a Uniform" *Journal of Applied Social Psychology*, 4, pp47-61; Bushman, B J 1984 "Perceived Symbols of Authority and Their Influence on Compliance" *Journal of Applied Social Psychology*, 14, pp501-8; Faux, S 1988 *Wardrobe* Piatkus, London; Goffman, E 1956 *The Presentation of Self in Everyday Life* Edinburgh University Press, Edinburgh; Gostelow, M 1985 *Dress Sense* Batsford, London; Harris, M B, James, J, Chavez, J, Fuller, M L, Kent, S, Massanari, C, Moore, C and Walsh, F 1983 "Clothing: Communication, Compliance and Choice" *Journal of Applied Social Psychology*, 13, pp88-97; Hensley, W E 1981 "The Effects of Attire, Location, and Sex on Aiding Behavior: A Similarity Explanation" *Journal of Nonverbal Behavior*, 6, pp3-11; Hoult, R 1954 "Experimental Measurement of Clothing as a Factor in Some Social Ratings of Selected American Men" *American Sociological Review*, 19, pp324-8; Kaiser, S B 1985 *The Social Psychology of Clothing and Personal Adornment* Collier Macmillan, London; McKelvie, S J 1988 "The Role of Spectacles in Facial Memory: A Replication and Extension" *Perceptual and Motor Skills*, 66, pp651-8; Polhemus, T 1978 *Social Aspects of the Human Body* Penguin, Harmondsworth; Samuel, K 1986 *Lifestyles, Fashionstyles* Orbis; Solomon, M R 1986 "Dress for Effect" *Psychology Today*, 20, 20-22, pp26-9; Thornton, G 1944 "The Effect of Wearing Glasses Upon Judgments of Personality Traits of Persons Seen Briefly" *Journal of Applied Psychology*, 28, pp203-7.

22 Bodytalk Ekman, P 1982 *Emotion in the Human Face*, 2nd edn, Cambridge University Press, Cambridge; Hall, J A 1984 *Nonverbal Sex Differences* John Hopkins University Press, Baltimore, MD; Scherer, K R 1986 "Vocal Affect Expression: A Review and Model for Further Research" *Psychological Bulletin*, 99, pp143-65.

23 Personal Style Argyle, M 1988 *Bodily Communication*, 2nd edn, Methuen, London; Argyle, M, Furnham, A and Graham, J A 1981 *Social Situations* Cambridge University Press, Cambridge; Graham, J A 1989 "New Directions in the Psychology of Cosmetics and Fragrance" *Invited address (unpublished) Society of Cosmetic Scientists' Northern Lecture*; Roach, M E

and Eicher, J B (eds): *Dress, Adornment, and the Social Order* Wiley, New York.

24 Looking Better With Age Fogel, R, Hatfield, E, Kiesler, S and Shanas, E (eds) 1981 *Aging: Stability and Change in the Family* Academic Press, New York; Penny, A (ed) 1981 *Vogue Stay Young* Macmillan, London; Wylie, R 1961 *The Self-Concept*, Vol 1 and 2, University of Nebraska Press, Lincoln, NA.

25 Skincare Basra, D 1986 *The Ageing Skin* Diva, London. Colman, V 1984 *Taking Care of Your Skin* Sheldon, London; Justice, B 1988 *Think Yourself Healthy* Thorsons, London; Marks, R 1986 *The Sun and Your Skin* Macdonald, London; Ornstein, R and Sobel D 1989 *The Healing Brain* Macmillan, London.

26 Putting Cosmetics to Work Bernstein, N R, Breslau, A J and Graham J A (eds) 1988 *Coping Strategies for Burn Survivors and Their Families* Praegar, New York; MacDonald, E E 1959 "The Hospital Beauty Scheme" *Journal of the Society of Cosmetic Chemists*, 10, pp246-57; Roberts, R 1986 "Cosmetic Camouflage" *Nursing*, 5, Bailliere Tindall, London, pp190-5. Roberts, R 1989 "Cosmetic Camouflage" *Physician* Mark Allen, London, pp192-3.

27 Being Made Over Collins, S 1979 *Beauty* St Michael, London; Daly, B 1980 *Daly Beauty* Macdonald Educational and Thames Television, London; Daly, B 1984 *Makeup Made Easy* St Michael, London; Hutton, B 1984 *Vogue Complete Beauty* St Michael, London; McKnight, G 1989 *The Skin Game: The Beauty Business Brutally Exposed* Sidgwick and Jackson, London; Miller, D 1985 *Let's Makeup* Piatkus, London; Winter, R 1984 *A Consuer's Dictionary of Cosmetic Ingredients* Crown, New York.

28 Hairstyle and Haircare Batterberry, M and Batterberry A 1982 *Fashion: The Mirror of History* 2nd edn, Greenwich House, New York; Bernstein, N, Breslau, A and Graham, J A (eds) 1988 *Coping Strategies for Burn Survivors and Their Families* Praeger, New York; Gosselin, C 1984 "Hair Loss, Personality, and Attitudes" *Personality and Individual Differences*, 5, pp365-9; Graham, J A 1982 "Looking at Hair from the Inside Out" *The Psychology of Hair* The Silkience Seminar, September, (audiotranscript); Graham, J A and Jouhar, A J 1981 "The Effects of Cosmetics on Person Perception" *International Journal of Cosmetic Science*, 3, pp199-210; Kilgour, O F G and McGarry 1989 *Complete Hairdressing Science* Heinemann Professional, Oxford; Kleinsmith, D and Perricone, N V 1989 "Common Skin Problems in the Elderly" in Gilchrest, B (ed): *Clinics in Geriatric Medicine* 5, *Geriatric Dermatology* Saunders, Philadelphia, PA, pp189-211; Lurie, A 1981 *The Language of Clothes* Random House, New York; Orentreich, N and Durr, N P 1985 "The Four R's of Skin Rehabilitation" in Graham, J A and Kligman, A M (eds): *The Psychology of Cosmetic Treatments* Praeger, New York, pp227-37; Resnik, H L 1980 "Psychiatric Observations on Patients Who Seek and Undergo Hair Transplantation" *Journal of Dermatology, Surgical Oncology*, 6, pp1023-5; Rhodes, R L 1974 *Man at His Best: How to be More Youthful, Virile, Healthy, and Handsome* Doubleday, Garden City NY; Staff August 29 1988 "Hair from a Tube Gets Nod (Minoxidil is Approved by the Food and Drug Administration)" *US News and World Report* p15; Starr, C 1987 "Beauty by Prescription: A Dream Coming True" *Drug Topics*, 131, pp34-44; Uzuka, M 1988 "Topical Treatment Agents (Trichogens) for Hair Loss and Baldness" in Kligman, A M and Takase, Y (eds): *Cutaneous Aging* University of Tokyo Press, Tokyo; Weiss, G 30 December 1985 "The Bald Facts – Is Minoxidil All that It's Cracked Up To Be?" *Barrons* pp32-4.

29 Beautiful Hands, Beautiful Feet Bahr, R 1984 *Good Hands* Thorsons, Wellingborough, Northants; Hagman, A 1981 *The Aestheticienne: Simple Theory and Practice* Stanley Thornes, London; Hutton D 1982 *The Vogue Health and Beauty Book: Complete Beauty*, Octopus, London; Samman, P D and Fenton, D A 1986 *The Nails in Disease* Heinemann Medical Books, London; Zeff, L 1988 *The Beauty Treatment Handbook* Piatkus, London.

30 Looking After Your Smile Ekman, P (ed) 1982 *Emotion in the Human Face* Cambridge University Press, Cambridge; Ekman, P and Friesen, W V 1975 *Unmasking the Face* Prentice-Hall, Englewood Cliffs, NJ.

31 Fragrance and Aromatherapy Baron, R A 1981 "Olfaction and Human Social Behaviour: Effects of a Pleasant Scent on Attraction and Social Perception" *Personal Social Psychology Bulletin*, 7, pp611-616; Baron, R A 1983 "Sweet Smell of Success? The Impact of Pleasant Artificial Scents on Evaluations of Job Applicants" *Journal of Applied Psychology*, 68, pp709-13; Graham, J A and Furnham, A F 1981 "Sexual Differences in Attractiveness Ratings of Day/Night Cosmetic Use" *Cosmetic Technology*, 3, pp36-42; Jouhar, A J, Louden, M, Graham, J A and Bergamini, N 1986 "Psychological Effects of Fragrance" *Soaps, Perfumery, Cosmetics*, 59, pp209-11; Knapp, M L 1978 *Nonverbal Communications in Human Behavior* Holt, Rinehart and Winston, New York; Labows, J N Jr 1985 "Social-Sexual Effects of Pheromones" in Graham, J A and Kligman, A M (eds) *The Psychology of Cosmetic Treatments* Praegar, New York; Mensing, J 1985 *The Psychology of Fragrance Selection: Feminine Notes* Haarmann and Reimer; Nemy, E 1982 "A Futuristic World of Scents" *New York Times*, April 17, 1982.

32 Professional Beauty Care 1983 "Collagen Implants May Cause Allergic Reactions" *Dermatology Times* May, p22; Goin, J M and Goin, M K 1981 *Changing the Body: Psychological Effects of Plastic Surgery* Williams and Wilkins, Baltimore, London; Graham, J A 1985 "Overview of Psychology of Cosmetics" in Graham, J A and Kligman, A M *The Psychology of Cosmetic Treatments* Praeger, New York, p33; Kleinsmith, D 1989 (Paper presented at Shiseido International Forum) *The Graying of America: A Dermatologist's Perspective* West Bloomfield, MN; McConnell, S 1981 "A Thinking Woman's Guide to Cosmetic Surgery" *Town and Country*, January 1981, pp88-91; Orentreich, N and Durr, N P 1985 "The Four R's of Skin Rehabilitation" in Graham, J A and Kligman, A M (eds): *The Psychology of Cosmetic Treatments*, Praeger, New York, pp227-37.

33 Looking Good, Feeling Great Avon 1981 *Looking Good Feeling Better* Simon and Schuster, New York; Castleton, V 1975 *The Handbook of Natural Beauty* Rodale Press, Emmaus, Pennsylvania; Clayton, L 1985 *Modelling and Beauty Care* Heinemann, London; Graham, J A and Kligman, A M 1984 "Cosmetic Therapy for the Elderly" *Journal of the Society of Cosmetic Chemists*, 35, pp133-45; Hunnicutt, G 1984 *Health and Beauty in Motherhood* Viking, Penguin, Harmondsworth; Kenton, L 1983 *The Joy of Beauty* Century, London; Molloy, J T 1977 *The Woman's Dress for Success Book* Follett, Chicago, IL; Wates, J 1985 "Cosmetics and the Job Market" in Graham, J A and Kligman, A M (eds): *The Psychology of Cosmetic Treatments* Praeger, New York.

251

ACKNOWLEDGMENTS

PICTURE AGENCIES/SOURCES

ASp Allsport UK Ltd.
B/C Blackstar/Colorific.
C Colorific Photo Library Ltd, London, New York.
C/C Colorific/Contact Press.
C/PG Colorific/Picture Group.
C/V Colorific/Visages.
EW Elizabeth Whiting.
F/L/FSP Ferry/Liaison/Frank Spooner Pictures, London.
FSP Frank Spooner Pictures, London.
G/FSP Gamma/Frank Spooner Pictures, London.
G/L/FSP Gamma/Liaison/Frank Spooner Pictures, London.
H The Hutchison Library, London.
I Impact Photos, London.
KC The Kobal Collection, London.
L/FSP Liaison/Frank Spooner Pictures, London.
ME Mary Evans Picture Library, London.
MG Magnum Photos Ltd, London, Paris, New York.
MPA Mashed Potato Archive, Oxford.
N Network Photographers, London.
PFL Popperfoto, London.
R Rex Features Ltd, London.
R/S Rex/Sipa, London.
SPL Science Photo Library, London.
SRG Sally and Richard Greenhill, London.
TCL Telegraph Colour Library, London.
TIB The Image Bank, London.
TIB/G+J The Image Bank/G and J Images, London.
TSW Tony Stone Photo Library, London.
TW Transworld Features, London.
V Viewfinder, Colour Photo Library, Bristol.
WP/C Wheeler Pictures/Colorific, London.
Z Zefa, London.

KEY TO PHOTOGRAPHERS

A Abbas. **AA** Albert Allard. **ADu** Alexis Duclos. **AGe** Alfred Gescheidt. **AK** Art Kane. **AlS** Al Satterwhite. **AR** Alon Reininger. **AS** Anthea Sieveking. **ASc** A Schumacher. **ATs** Alexander Tsiaras. **AV** A Venzago. **AU** Alvis Upitis. **AWe** Alex Webb. **BD** Bruce Davidson. **BDo** Bill Dobbans. **BEd** Boleshlan Edelhaift. **BGl** Burt Glinn. **BH** Brian Harris. **BL** Barry Lewis. **BMa** Butch Martin. **BR** Bernard Reca 'gent. **BRy** Brian Rybolt. **BS** Blair Seitz. **CBn** Cecil Beaton. **CEd** Charles Edwards. **ChM** Chris Morris. **CMa** Charles Mahaux. **CVd** Christian Vioujard. **CW** Cary Wolinsky. **DB** David Burnett. **DBk** Dennis Black. **DBr** David Brownell. **DHa** David Hamilton. **DHl** Daniel Hummel. **DKi** Douglas Kirkland. **DL** David Levenson. **DS** Dennis Stock. **EA** Eve Arnold. **EAd** Eddie Adams. **EE** Elliott Erwitt. **EF** Enrico Ferorelli. **EH** Erich Hartmann. **EHa** Ernst Haas. **ER** Eli Reed. **ERi** Eugene Richards. **ESa** Eric Sander. **FHr** Frank Herrmann. **GBc** Gilles Bassignac. **GCl** Geoffrey Clifford. **GPe** Gilles Peress. **HG** Harry Gruyaert. **HMo** Hank Morgan. **HS** Homer Sykes. **I** Illhami. **IB** Ian Berry. **JCob** J Cob. **JCo** John Cole. **JDr** John Drysdale. **JGu** J Guichard. **JLa** John Laurois. **JMcH** Jim McHugh. **JMcN** Joe McNally. **JNa** James Nachtwey. **JRa** Jake Rajs. **JRu** John Running. **JWa** John Walmsley. **LBa** Linda Bartlett. **LD** Larry Dale Gordon. **LS** Laurie Sparham. **LT** Liba Taylor. **MAn** Martin Anderson. **MBl** Martin Black. **MG** Mike Goldwater. **MGl** Mike Greenlar. **MMe** Michael Melford. **MMn** Miguel Martin. **MMl** Michael MacIntyre. **MN** Michael Nichols. **MPo** Mike Powell. **MY** Mike Yamashita. **NB** Nancy Brown. **NDMcK** Nancy Durrell-McKenna. **OA** O Abolafia. **OB** Omar Bradley. **PAr** Peter Arkell. **PaC** Paolo Curlo. **PCp** Peter Cooper. **PFo** Paul Forster. **PFu** Paul Fusco. **PH** Phillip Hayson. **PJG** Philip Jones Griffiths. **PT** Penny Tweedie. **RCh** Russell Cheyne. **RNe** Robert Nelson. **RPl** Robin Platzer. **SBo** Steve Benbow. **SFe** Sally Fear. **SGr** Susan Greenwood. **SHa** Sean Haffey. **SMcC** Steve McCurry. **SMe** Susan Meiselas. **SPo** Steve Powell. **SSm** Steve Smith. **TD** Tony Duffy. **TL** Tom Levy. **TSa** Tobey Sanford. **VL** Vladimir Lange. **ZG** Zao Grimberg. **ZK** Zigy Kaluzney.

PICTURE LIST

Page number in **bold** type. Photographers initials in parenthesis.

Frontmatter
2 Woman with red gloves, TW. **3** Jogger, ASp. **11** Woman leaping (PaC) TIB. **13** Women on beach, TW.

Part One Your Health
14-15 Swimmers (EHa) MG.

1 Good Health from Birth
16 Mother and baby (PAr) I. Girl on treadmill (TSa) C. **17** Doctor and boy, Z. **18** Jumping in river, H. **18-19** Couple on beach, TW. **19** Doctor, Z. Patient, Z. **20** Sunbathing on deck (SGr) FSP. **21** Adults exercising, TW. **22** Couples dancing (ZK) FSP. **23** At computer (JMcN) C. **24** Overweight men (AWe) MG. **24-25** Woman smoking (ZK) FSP.

2 Your Sex and Your Health
26 Couple cycling (PFu) MG. **27** Monitoring newborn baby (BGl) MG. Blast furnace (CEd) V. **28** Arterial damage, SPL. Heart attack at home, SPL. **29** Working over lunch (CW) C. Medical check-up, SPL. **31** Breast examination by kind permission of the Woman's National Cancer Control Campaign. **32-33** Doctor and patient (HS) I. **33** Girls at table (JWa) I.

3 The Rhythms of Life
34 Clock (AGe) TIB. **36** Sunset (PH) C. **39** Winter's night (DHa) TIB. Daydreaming, TW.

4 Stress
40 Man and riot police (ChM) C. **40-41** Mexican/USA border (SMe) MG. **41** Man at computer (MG) N. **42** Corrections officer (MGl) C. **43** Checking blood pressure (GPe) MG. **44** Wedding (EF) C. **45** Tending grave (AU) TIB. **46** Stunt artist (JDr) C. **46-47** Reading (BGl) MG.

5 Learn to Relax
48 Family by pool (EF) C. **49** Relaxing on porch (LT) H. **50** Massage, R. **52-53** Stress at work (EF) C. **53** River Scene (MAn) MPA. "Relaxman," R.

6 The Healing Power of Sleep
55 Children asleep (AK) TIB. **57** Sunrise (ESa) FSP. **58** Man sleeping (JMcN) C.

7 Sexuality
60-61 Couple, TW. **64-65** Couple in bed, TW. **65** Couple close up, TW.

8 Good Nutrition
66-67 Round table with food, TW. **68** Children's party, TCL. **70** Fruit stall (PFo) I.

9 The Diet Dilemma
72 Night snack (MMe) TIB. **73** Supermarket weigh-in (TSa) C. **74** At beach (HG) MG. Jane Fonda (DKi) C. **76** Man pinching waist, Andromeda. **77** Baby on scales, SRG. **78** Joanne Carson (SSm) C. **79** Eating ice cream (PFu) MG.

10 Weight Control and Self-Image
80 Group of ladies (EH) MG. **81** Girl on scales, TW. **83** Anorexic girl, R.

11 Exercise and Physical Fitness
84 Marines in training (JNa) MG. **84-85** Jogging, ASp. **86** Aerobic dancing (MN) MG. **87** Treadmills (ESa) FSP. Pulsometer (BR) ASp. **88** Man and woman in gym (BR) ASp. Stretching (NB) TIB. **89** Yoga, TW. Aerobics (MPo) ASp. **90** Hikers, TCL.

12 Making Exercise Part of Your Life
92 Dance therapy (JWa) I. **93** Family with weights (PJG) MG. **94** Woman and dog (DBr) TIB. **95** Laundromat, L/FSP. **96** American football (SHa) ASp. **97** Athletes on track (SPo) ASp.

13 Are Sports Good For You?
98 Gymnast (TD) ASp. **98-99** Rugby (RCh) ASp. **99** Weight-lifting (BDo) ASp. **100** Marathon, TW. **101** Racing crowd (HS) I.

14 Smoking
102 Girl smoking, Z. Thermograms of arms, SPL. **103** Healthy lung, SPL. Smoker's lung, SPL. **104** Pregnant woman smoking (BL) N. Sonic aerosol treatment (I) R. **105** Young people (LS) N.

15 The Effects of Alcohol
106 Alcoholics Anonymous (ESa) FSP. **107** Teenagers at party (ER) MG. **108** Woman drinking, Z. **109** Water bar (ADu) FSP.

16 Drugs, Pills and Painkillers
110 Drinking coffee, TW. **111** Crack den, Brooklyn (ERi) MG. **112** Pills, Z. **114** Cannabis, R/S. Smoking crack (OB) C/PG. **115** Ecstasy drug (MMe) C. **116** Drug rehabilitation clinic (ESa) L/FSP. **117** Narcotics department, R.

17 Illness and Disability
118 Painting with mouth (RNe) C/PG. **119** Stevie Wonder (RPl) R. Peter Werner in wheelchair (TL) G/L/FSP. **120** Ultra sonography (ATs) SPL. **121** Ear examination (BS) SPL. **123** Handicapped child (LBa) C.

18 Hospital Care
124 Boy waiting to be X-rayed (ATs) SPl. **124-125** Hospital, Germany, Z. **125** Intensive care (PFu) MG. **126** Heart surgery (AU) TIB. **127** Orthapedic nurse and patient (PFu) MG. **128-129** Hospital volunteer with children (AU) TIB. **129** Cancer patient (DBk) B/C. **130** "Tens" (HMo) SPL. **131** Patient in wheelchair (VL) TIB.

Part Two Your Appearance
132-133 Model, Japan, TW.

19 Do Looks Matter?
134 Man looking in mirror, TW. **135** Putting on lipstick (ASc) TIB. **136-137** Photographers (EE) MG. **138** Couple (BRy) I. **139** Couple dancing (AWe) MG. **140** Woman in floral dress, PFL. Woman in red sweater, TW. **141** Japanese woman wearing Western clothes, TW. Japanese women wearing traditional kimono (BGl) MG. **143** Marilyn Monroe (EA) MG.

20 Your Bodyshape
144 Man and woman exercising (JCob) TIB. **145** Woman in exercise suit, TW. **145** Twiggy, R. Woman on phone (A) MG. **146-147** 6. Female model (BMa) TIB. 5. Mr Weinfeld, R. 3. Robin Wright (JCo) I. 4. Jane Fonda, R. 2. Ingrid

Bergmann, R. 1. Male model (PT) I. **148** Slimmer of the year, R. **149** Shrink-1, Florida (EAd) C.

21 What Clothes Say
151 Power dressing, R. **152** Jerry Hall and Ines de la Fressanges, R. **153** Man in golden suit, TW. **154** Woman on chair, TW. **155** Trying on hats (JRa) TIB. Cowboy (AA) MG. **156** Business men (SFe) I. Business man in school uniform (PFu) MG. **157** Business woman, TIB. **157** Woman smiling (DHl) TIB. **157** Pilot and little girl (JMcN) C. **158** Duchess of Windsor (CBn) R. **159** 1960s style, PFL. Woman holding hat, TW.

22 Bodytalk
160 Head in hands (BD) MG. Ballet class (MBl) I. **161** Crowd, R. **162** Celebrating Superbowl (AWe) MG. **163** Ascot races (BH) I.

23 Personal Style
164 Jackie Kennedy (x2), R. **165** Woman in red gloves, TW. **165** Woman outside tent, TW. **165** Men in suits (SFe) I. **166** Wedding (DB) C. **166** On holiday, TW. **167** Pierre Cardin, R. **167** Mariel Hemingway, R. **168** Diana Vreeland, R. **169** Madonna, R.

24 Looking Better with Age
170-171 Dancers, TIB. **171** Work out (ESa) FSP. **172** Sophia Loren (x2), R. **173** Lauren Bacall (x2), R. Jane Russell (x2), R. **174** Sean Connery (x2), KC. **175** Connery and Ford, KC.

25 Skincare
176 Couple on beach (SBo) I. **177** Sunbed (MY) C. Cucumber on eyes, TW. **178** Girl biting her nails, C. **179** Baby (AS) N. Kiss, R. **180** Salt water treatment, TIB. **181** Steaming face, TW. **182** Bathing with fishes, R. Fish eating dead skin, R. **183** Skin graft (CVd) FSP. **184** Three generations, TW. **185** Bathing in milk (JLa) B/C. **186** Sunbathing on roof (BL) N. **187** Sunblock on nose (SBo) I.

26 Putting Cosmetics to Work
188 Queen Elizabeth II (DL) C. **189** Putting on eye shadow, TW. American Indian (JRu) C. **190** Blend-in palette by kind permission of Rita Roberts. Matching make-up and skin colour by kind permission of Rita Roberts. **191** Undereye cover (BMa) TIB. **192** M Gorbachev, G/FSP. **192** President Gorbachev, F/L/FSP. **193** Applying blusher, R. Brushing forehead, TW. **194** Lipstick, TW. **194** Lipstick, TW. **195** Face, TW. Eye make-up, TW. **196** Simon Weston, R. **197** Girl with birthmark, R. Covering birthmark with make-up, R.

27 Being Made Over
198 Makeup store (BGl) MG. **199** Professional make-up (AlS) TIB. **200** Computer hairstyles, R. **201** Beauty salon (MMn) TIB.

28 Hairstyle and Haircare
202 1780s French fashion, ME. 1920s fashion, ME. **203** Girl holding up hair, TW. Tina Turner, R. **204** Sun roof, TW. **205** Infra-red hair styling, R. Punk hairstyle, R. **206** Mud hair treatment, TW. Strand of hair, TW. **207** Soldier and US flag (DL) WP/C. Long haired artist, (GCl) WP/C. **208** Cutting fringe,

TW. Girl with sunglasses, TSW. **209** Black hair, blue bow (BMa) TIB. French braid, TW. **212-213** Man (DS) MG. **213** Woman (EE) MG.

29 Beautiful Hands, Beautiful Feet
214 Moroccan wedding (DS) MG. **215** Woman, France (CMa) TIB. Sculptor's hands (NDMcK) H. Handshake, G/FSP. **216** County Jail, USA (SMcC) MG. **217** Dancer, Thailand, H. Manicure (MN) MG. **220-221** Ballet dancers (MMl) H. **221** Scene from "The Night Porter," KC. **222** Foot massage, TIB/G+J. **223** Pedicure and manicure at home (CMa) TIB. Reflexology (IB) MG.

30 Looking After Your Smile
224-225 Singapore girls, R. **226** Grace Jones and Rosanna Arquette, R. **227** False teeth, R. **228** Braces, SRG. **228-229** Lady smiling, TSW. **229** Teeth tattoos, R. Lips, TW.

31 Fragrance and Aromatherapy
230 Perfume and roses (PCp) V. Perfume factory (GBc) FSP. **231** Perfume bottle, ME. **232** Man splashing on perfume (ZG) TIB. **234** Back massage (LD) TIB. **235** Flower fields (GBc) FSP.

32 Professional Beauty Care
236 Facial consultation, Helena Rubinstein, New York City, TIB. **237** Facial (AlS) TIB. **238** Steam cabinet (FHr) C. Leg waxing by kind permission of Carlton Professional/Taylor Reeson Labs Ltd. **239** Electrolysis, TW. **240** "Myoskop Plus" (OA) L/FSP. Tattooing eyes (JMcH) C/V. **241** Slendertone treatment (AV) MG. Body vaccum suction by kind permission of Carlton Professional/Chichester College of Technology. **242** Plastic surgeon and computer graphics (BEd) G/FSP. **243** Plastic surgery (JGu) G/FSP.

33 Looking Good, Feeling Great
244 Hiking, TW. **245** Exercising, Ashram Hot Spa, California (MN) MG. Woman in cowboy clothes, Marseilles (A) MG. **246** At garden gate, EW. **247** Karen Finley with Harriet, New York City (AR) C/C.